*Protease Inhibitors as
Cancer Chemopreventive
Agents*

Protease Inhibitors as Cancer Chemopreventive Agents

Edited by

Walter Troll

New York University Medical Center
New York, New York

and

Ann R. Kennedy

University of Pennsylvania School of Medicine
Philadelphia, Pennsylvania

Springer Science+Business Media, LLC

Library of Congress Cataloging-in-Publication Data

Protease inhibitors as cancer chemopreventive agents / edited by
  Walter Troll, Ann R. Kennedy.
       p.   cm.
    Includes bibliographical references and index.
    ISBN 978-0-306-44390-9   ISBN 978-1-4615-2882-1 (eBook)
    DOI 10.1007/978-1-4615-2882-1
    1. Cancer--Chemoprevention. 2. Proteolytic enzyme inhibitors-
  -Therapeutic use.   I. Troll, Walter. II. Kennedy, Ann R.
    [DNLM: 1. Protease Inhibitors--therapeutic use. 2. Protease
  Inhibitors--metabolism. 3. Neoplasms--prevention & control.   QU
  136 P9665 1993]
  RC268.15.P77 1993
  616.99'405--dc20
  DNLM/DLC
  for Library of Congress   93-24959
                                                                   CIP

ISBN 978-0-306-44390-9

© 1993 Springer Science+Business Media New York
Originally published by Plenum Press New York in 1993

Contributors

Takaaki Aoyagi   Institute of Microbial Chemistry, Shinagawa-ku, Tokyo 141, Japan

Sila Banerjee   Department of Obstetrics and Gynecology, New York University Medical Center, New York, New York 10016

Anne H. Bates   Western Regional Research Center, Agricultural Research Service, U.S. Department of Agriculture, Albany, California 94710

Paul C. Billings   Department of Radiation Oncology, University of Pennsylvania School of Medicine, Philadelphia, Pennsylvania 19104

Yehudith Birk   Department of Biochemistry and Human Nutrition, Faculty of Agriculture, The Hebrew University of Jerusalem, Rehovot 76100, Israel

Donald E. Bowman   Departments of Biochemistry and Molecular Biology, School of Medicine, Indiana University, Indianapolis, Indiana 46202-5122

David L. Brandon   Western Regional Research Center, Agricultural Research Service, U.S. Department of Agriculture, Albany, California 94710

Ann F. Chambers   The London Regional Cancer Centre, University of Western Ontario, London, Ontario, Canada N6A 4L6

Janice D. Chang   Department of Biology, Massachusetts Institute of Technology, Cambridge, Massachusetts 02139

Rita Colella   Department of Biological Sciences, Rutgers University, Piscataway, New Jersey 08855. *Present address:* Department of Anatomical Sciences and Neurobiology, University of Louisville School of Medicine, Louisville, Kentucky 40292

Pelayo Correa   Department of Pathology, Louisiana State University Medical Center, New Orleans, Louisiana 70112

Lydia Cox   Department of Environmental Medicine, New York University Medical Center, New York, New York 10016

Diane C. Currie   Department of Environmental Medicine, New York University Medical Center, New York, New York 10016

David T. Denhardt   Department of Biological Sciences, Rutgers University, Piscataway, New Jersey 08855

Thomas H. Finlay   Department of Obstetrics and Gynecology, New York University Medical Center, New York, New York 10016

Peter Flecker   Institute for Physiological Chemistry, University of Mainz, W-6500 Mainz, Germany

Elizabeth Fontham   Department of Pathology, Louisiana State University Medical Center, New Orleans, Louisiana 70112

Krystyna Frenkel   Departments of Environmental Medicine and Pathology, New York University Medical Center, New York, New York 10016

Mendel Friedman   Western Regional Research Center, Agricultural Research Service, U.S. Department of Agriculture, Albany, California 94710

Seymour J. Garte   Department of Environmental Medicine, New York University Medical Center, New York, New York 10016

Susan S. Kadner   Department of Obstetrics and Gynecology, New York University Medical Center, New York, New York 10016

Joseph Katz   Department of Obstetrics and Gynecology, New York University Medical Center, New York, New York 10016

Ann R. Kennedy   Department of Radiation Oncology, School of Medicine, University of Pennsylvania, Philadelphia, Pennsylvania 19104

Mortimer Levitz   Department of Obstetrics and Gynecology, New York University Medical Center, New York, New York 10016

Daniel S. Longnecker   Department of Pathology, Dartmouth Medical School, Hanover, New Hampshire 03755

Joan Motz   Department of Environmental Medicine, New York University Medical Center, New York, New York 10016

Joseph Nickels, Jr.   Department of Microbiology and Molecular Genetics, Rutgers University, New Brunswick, New Jersey 08903

Uma Raju   Department of Obstetrics and Gynecology, New York University Medical Center, New York, New York 10016

George Ritchie   Department of Physics, Rider College, Lawrenceville, New Jersey 08648

B. D. Roebuck   Department of Pharmacology and Toxicology, Dartmouth Medical School, Hanover, New Hampshire 03755

Lorraine T. Schepis   Department of Molecular Biology, Princeton University, Princeton, New Jersey 08530

Tomio Takeuchi   Institute of Microbial Chemistry, Shinagawa-ku, Tokyo 141, Japan

Snait Tamir   Department of Obstetrics and Gynecology, New York University Medical Center, New York, New York 10016

Wataru Tanaka   Institute of Microbial Chemistry, Shinagawa-ku, Tokyo 141, Japan

Walter Troll   Department of Environmental Medicine, New York University Medical Center, New York, New York 10016

Kazuo Umezawa   Department of Applied Chemistry, Faculty of Science and Technology, Keio University, Kohoku-ku, Yokohama 223, Japan

Jonathan Yavelow   Department of Biology, Rider College, Lawrenceville, New Jersey 08648

Preface

Protease inhibitors (PIs) are widely distributed in plants and animals, and have a variety of functions, which include preventing digestion of seeds by insects and modifying blood clotting in animals. After it was noted that synthetic and natural inhibitors suppress two-stage carcinogenesis and breast cancer, extensive work investigating PIs as chemopreventive agents was started.

PIs are unique in that they interfere with cancer development in a variety of ways, including suppression of oxygen radicals, oncogenes, and metastases. Epidemiologic evidence supports their prevention of major human cancers in populations that consume foods containing them. Their supervised use in humans is on the threshold of development.

The epidemiologic discovery of the importance of lentils and other seeds rich in PIs in preventing many human cancers allowed us to look at the action of PIs as chemopreventive agents, as reviewed in Chapter 1 (Fontham and Correa). Chapter 2 (Kennedy) discusses the role of natural PIs (e.g., the Bowman–Birk inhibitor) as anticarcinogens and the possible limitations of their use. In Chapter 3 (Kennedy), the transformation of C3H/10T^{1}/$_{2}$ cells caused by carcinogens and promoters is shown to be suppressed by PIs. Bowman (Chapter 4) relates the discovery of inhibitors in soybeans that are distinct from the Kunitz inhibitor, and the occurrence of a similar inhibitor in peanuts and other legumes. Chapter 5 (Birk) is an overview of PIs of plant origin and their role in human nutrition. In Chapter 6, Brandon and colleagues report on the measurement of soybean trypsin inhibitors by monoclonal antibodies, their possible use for cellular delivery, and the effect of food processing on the survival of the inhibitors. Chapter 7 (Umezawa *et al.*) concerns low-molecular-weight inhibitors, isolated from streptomycetes, that have been shown to suppress cancer in animal and some human experiments and are also useful for *in vitro* and oncogene expression studies. PI synthesis by MCF-7 breast cancer cell lines is discussed in Chapter 8 (Finlay *et al.*). α_1-Trypsin and chymotrypsin inhibitors synthesized by breast cancers may inhibit metastasis. In Chapter 9, Flecker analyzes the structure–activity relationships of the Bowman–Birk inhibitor of serine proteinases, with a view toward the design of new cancer chemopreventive agents. Troll (Chapter 10) discusses the prevention of cancer by vitamin B_3 compounds, PIs that are available for human use. Billings (Chapter 11) details approaches to studying the target enzymes of anticarcinogenic PIs. In Chapter 12, Colella and colleagues document the anticarcinogenic activities of naturally occurring cysteine proteinase inhibitors. These PIs prevent metastasis of tumors and are distinct from serine PIs. Yavelow and colleagues (Chapter 13) identify a chymotrypsin cell membrane enzyme that acts as a possible receptor for chymotrypsin inhibitors. Frenkel (Chapter 14) describes the role of reactive oxygen species in biological damage and the effect of some chemopreventive agents. Chapters 15 (Garte *et al.*) and 16 (Chang and Kennedy) discuss PI suppression of the actions induced by the *ras* and c-*myc* oncogene, respectively. Chapter 17 (Levitz *et al.*) reviews the role of esterases in steroid hormone turnover. Esterases in breast cyst fluid hydrolyze steroid esters, modifying their action. The action of PIs in inducing pancreatic cancer in animal models is reviewed by Roebuck and Longnecker (Chapter 18).

Contents

Chapter 10

Chapter 11

Chapter 12

Chapter 18

Protease Inhibitors and Pancreatic Carcinogenesis

B. D. Roebuck and Daniel S. Longnecker

The Epidemiologic Approach to the Study of Protease Inhibitors

ELIZABETH FONTHAM and PELAYO CORREA

1. Introduction

Protease inhibitors differ from other cancer-related dietary items in that the weight of the evidence of their protective effects is based on experimental and *in vitro* models rather than on studies in humans. For that reason the present comments focus on how to approach the issue from an epidemiologic point of view, with the purpose of establishing whether or not there is a causal association between protease inhibitors and human cancer. The multifactorial etiology of human cancer is a generally accepted scientific proposition. Protease inhibitors, therefore, may be just one of the factors in a complex interplay of carcinogenic and anticarcinogenic influences.

2. Descriptive Epidemiology

The epidemiologic evidence for a cancer protective role of protease inhibitors comes primarily from correlation studies (Correa, 1981). These examine the frequency of cancer in different populations and relate it to other characteristics of such populations, in this case their diet. These types of studies are useful indicators for further research, but are insufficient for assessment of causality because of the so-called ecological fallacy which may lead investigators to assign

ELIZABETH FONTHAM and PELAYO CORREA • Department of Pathology, Louisiana State University Medical Center, New Orleans, Louisiana 70112.
Protease Inhibitors as Cancer Chemopreventive Agents, edited by Walter Troll and Ann R. Kennedy. Plenum Press, New York, 1993.

causal roles to characteristics of the populations which are unrelated to their cancer experience (confounders).

Cancer correlation studies have examined the association between inter-country cancer rates and dietary consumption of particular foods (e.g., milk, meat, eggs) or nutrients (e.g., fats, sugar, protein). Breast cancer, colon cancer, and pancreatic cancer rates have been positively correlated with per capita consumption of total fat and of nutrients derived from animal sources, in particular beef, pork, milk, and eggs (Wynder et al., 1970; Carroll et al., 1968; Gregor et al., 1969; Hems, 1970; Drasar and Irving, 1973; Armstrong and Doll, 1975; Segi et al., 1969). Cancers of the genital and reproductive organs including prostate, ovary, and endometrium have also been positively correlated with dietary intake of fats and animal protein (Lea, 1967). Similarly, strong negative correlations have been demonstrated with per capita consumption of grains and vegetable protein sources for many of these same cancers (Correa, 1981). Rice, maize, and beans are among those items negatively correlated with cancers of the breast, colon, and prostate. Whether this negative correlation reflects active protection from anticarcinogenic substances found in these foods or passive protection from the lack of concomitant consumption of foods which might increase risk of these cancers remains to be determined. Troll et al. (1984) have suggested that active protection may derive from protease inhibitors contained in cereals, beans, tubers, and seeds.

What makes causal hypothesis generation based on correlation more attractive in the case of protease inhibitors is the wealth of evidence from in vitro and animal studies. This adds biological plausibility to the hypothesis, an important ingredient in causality considerations. A wide range of protease inhibitors have been shown to reduce the occurrence of cancer in animal models. For example, inhibitors of trypsin and chymotrypsin have been shown to block tumor promotion in initiated mouse skin (Troll et al., 1970). Umezawa (1972) has demonstrated that leupeptin, a trypsin inhibitor, suppresses the induction of tumors of the skin in mice and of colon, esophagus, and mammary gland as well as leukemia in rats.

Protease inhibitors have also been used effectively to suppress carcinogenesis in vitro (Kennedy and Little, 1981; Yavelow et al., 1985). Schelp and Pongpaew (1988) have recently hypothesized that diets low in calories, fat, and animal protein and high in vegetables and fiber, which are sufficient to maintain nutritional health, stimulate production of endogenous protease inhibitors. These high levels of protease inhibitors, in particular α_2-macroglobulin, create an environment which protects against carcinogenesis.

3. Analytical Epidemiology

Correlation studies do not discriminate within a given population those persons who develop cancer from those who do not and therein resides their major weakness. Such discrimination is provided by analytic epidemiology studies which are of two main types: case–control and cohort studies. The former looks back at the life experience of cancer patients and of "controls" or "referent" persons who are supposedly free of the disease. Cohort or prospective studies register exposure data on subjects at a point in time and these persons are then followed throughout the years to discover if such exposures are linked to the development of cancer. These studies are of great value in the search for causality and could be applied to the study of protease inhibitors.

In spite of the absence of quantitative assessment of dietary protease inhibitor intake, the analytic epidemiologic approach has provided suggestive evidence in support of a chemopreventive role for protease inhibitors for certain cancers. Several studies of cancer in Seventh-Day Adventists have examined the role of diet in this population, about half of whom follow a lacto-ovo-vegetarian diet (Phillips, 1975). The relative risks of colon and breast cancer for reported dietary consumption of food items were estimated in a case–control study nested in a prospective study of Seventh-Day Adventists. A significant two- to threefold increased risk of colon cancer was associated with high intake of beef, lamb, fish, nonmilk dairy products, and other high-fat foods. A halving of risk (odds ratios 0.3–0.5) was found for high consumption of milk, vegetarian protein products, and green leafy vegetables. As noted, these foods are those which lacto-ovo-vegetarians are likely to consume to the exclusion of high-fat meat products. The vegeterian protein products are derived from soy or gluten protein. They contain no fiber, little or not fat, and are a dietary source of protease inhibitors. Green leafy vegetables are fat-free, high in fiber and other micronutrients with chemopreventive potential (β-carotene, ascorbic acid, indoles, phenols). Only consumption of fried potatoes was significantly associated with increased risk of breast cancer, odds ratio = 2.4. Other items, either fried or containing fat, were associated with increased risk but were not statistically significantly elevated and no other protective effects were reported. A more recent nested case–control analysis from this same cohort with a larger number of breast cancer cases has been reported (Mills *et al.*, 1988a). This study also failed to find an increased risk of breast cancer associated with consumption of foods of animal origin. In addition, the Adventist women who adhered to a vegetarian life-style (54%) were not at decreased risk of breast cancer death relative to Adventist women who consumed meat heavily or to comparable white women in the general U.S. population. However, the report did not specifically address consumption of dried beans, dried fruits, vegetarian protein and grains. Consumption of these items may vary even within the group adhering to a vegetarian life-style.

Dietary habits and pancreatic cancer risk were also examined in a prospective analysis of the Adventist Health Study (Mills *et al.*, 1988b). There was a suggestive increase in risk with increased consumption of meat, eggs, and coffee which was not statistically significant after controlling for cigarette smoking. A strong protective effect was found for consumption of vegetarian protein prod-

Table I. Relative Risk of Pancreatic Cancer Death
among Seventh-Day Adventists[a]

Foods	Intake[b]	Age–sex-adjusted relative risk	
Vegetarian protein products	Low	1.0	
(e.g., gluten, soy, or	Moderate	0.29	Trend
nuts)	High	0.40	$p = 0.02$
Beans, lentils, peas	Low	1.0	
	Moderate	0.47	Trend
	High	0.43	$p = 0.044$
Raisins, dates, other dried	Low	1.0	
fruit	Moderate	0.47	Trend
	High	0.35	$p = 0.009$

[a]From Mills *et al.* (1988b).
[b]Low, <1/week; moderate, 1–2/week; high, 3≥/week.

ucts, beans, lentils, peas, and dried fruit. This effect persisted after controlling for cigarette smoking, an established risk factor for pancreatic cancer (Table I). The protective association between consumption of nonmeat protein products was stronger than the increased risk from meat consumption. Although the food frequency questionnaire was limited to 35 foods and appropriately no nutrient or micronutrient intake indices were computed, the results are consistent with the hypothesis that foods containing protease inhibitors protect against cancers of the pancreas and colon.

4. Tools Needed for Epidemiologic Studies

Many of the tools needed for epidemiologic studies are in place except for two important ones: a valid measure of the protease inhibitor activity of foods as consumed by humans and/or a biologic marker in humans of consumption and bioavailability of protease inhibitors. Many studies of specific protease inhibitors obtained from specific food items are available, but a systematic account of their presence in the most common foods is lacking (Rackis *et al.*, 1986). Such information is available for many macro- and micronutrients believed to be associated with cancer risk. In the United States the Department of Agriculture publishes handbooks of the nutritive values of foods in raw, processed, and prepared forms. For example, Handbook Nos. 8 and 456 contain nutrient values for 2483 different food items with multiple entries for different ways the food might be consumed (raw, processed, cooked). For each item the following information is included: food energy (cal), protein (g), fat (g), carbohydrate (g), calcium (mg), phosphorus (mg), iron (mg), sodium (mg), potassium (mg), vitamin A (IU), thiamine (mg), riboflavin (mg), niacin (mg), and ascorbic acid (mg) (Watt and Merrill, 1975; Adams, 1975). These so-called food tables enable epidemiologists to calculate indices of consumption of a specific nutrient by summing the product of the frequency of intake of specific food items and the nutrient content of a specified portion of each relevant food item.

Such quantitative indices are possible only when measurements of a chemical compound are available for the most common food items. Further, for the quantitative estimates to have relevance to the human diet they must be based on foods as consumed. Food preparation, such as boiling, baking, frying, peeling, or chopping, must be taken into account. Protease inhibitors are affected by the processing of foods (Rackis *et al.*, 1986; Weder, 1986). Although detailed information on the influence of food processing on plant protease inhibitor activity is currently lacking, heating is known to inactivate inhibitors and the extent will vary by temperature, length of exposure, and pressure.

Since protease inhibitors are a class of compounds rather than one specific compound, the challenge in developing tools for epidemiologic use consists of providing measurements of the relevant compounds or developing a summary measure of protease inhibition potential which could result from more than one specific chemical compound. As an example, a number of trypsin inhibitors, chymotrypsin inhibitors, and elastase inhibitors are contained in soybeans and potatoes (Rackis *et al.*, 1986). Which of these, or combination of these, might be important in human carcinogenesis needs to be addressed prior to intervention.

A biologic marker of protease inhibitors would be a valuable addition to dietary intake data, but absorption information is also needed. Protease inhibitors from plants are proteins or polypeptides that are not absorbed by the gastrointestinal tract (Madar *et al.*, 1979; Troll and Yavelow, 1983). Hence, high dietary intake may result in high levels in the colon lumen and feces but may not result in a concomitant increase at internal organs, such as the breast.

In the past, certain dietary associations with cancer have been detected in epidemiologic studies without detailed information. A crude indicator of "low–medium–high" protease inhibitor activity could be used to analyze epidemiologic data, but not without pitfalls. Foods which have low, medium, or high protease inhibitor activity may also have a low, medium, or high content of other dietary constituents which confound the data. In addition, total protease inhibitor content may mask a specific effect from a particular type of protease inhibitor. Case–control studies of many thousands of cancer patients and their controls have collected detailed information on intake of specific foods. Similarly, several ongoing cohort studies have collected detailed dietary histories. If estimates of protease inhibitor activity were made available for such foods, analysis of existing data could be carried out addressing the issue of their association with cancer development.

5. Intervention Studies

The best available proof of causality is provided by intervention studies. These studies determine whether the introduction of a hypothetical protective factor is followed by a decrease in the frequency of the disease. If this were to be done with a specific protease inhibitor, sufficient amounts of an efficient, nontoxic compound would be needed and a target organ(s) chosen *a priori,* based on data from analytic and experimental studies. A less quantitative approach could be the introduction of protease inhibitor-rich food in the diet of a group of subjects whose cancer experience would then be compared with that of another group whose diet was not so modified. Adherence to the dietary regime, validation of intake, and unscheduled changes in the diet of the controls are important considerations in such studies.

A further difficulty in chemoprevention studies is the prolonged latency period in cancer development, usually measured in years or decades. Recently, greater use is being made of intermediate end-points as markers of progression in the neoplastic and the preneoplastic process. Adenomatous polyps might serve as a useful marker in a chemoprevention study of colon cancer and protease inhibitors. These techniques take advantage of the fact that most cancers are preceded by progressive phenotypic and genotypic changes in the tissues in which cancer eventually develops. Many such changes are specific for each type of tissue, especially those related to cytoplasmic protein synthesis or secretory products. Nuclear markers relate mostly to expansion of proliferative zones and oncogene expression. Opportunities for collaborative studies between population and laboratory researchers are provided by new techniques being developed in these areas.

6. Cancer Prevention

Considerable research is being carried out on the cancer preventive role of micronutrients, especially antioxidants. Similarities between such studies and those which could be done with protease inhibitors abound. The latter, however, may have an important advantage over the antioxidants in that *in vitro* studies suggest that the protective effect of protease inhibitors lasts much longer. Antioxidants as a rule cease to protect the subject or the cell when they are no longer present in abundant amounts.

7. Epilogue

Numerous epidemiologic studies have provided strong data linking dietary habits to cancer causation. Judgments about which component of the diet is implicated in the process have been made *a priori* and have influenced the design, conduct, analysis, and interpretations of the results of the studies. On the cancer initiation and promotion side, emphasis has been placed mostly on macronutrient consumption (especially fat), carcinogens present in food or produced by food processing, and contamination of food with carcinogens, either natural or synthetic (pesticides and the like). On the cancer inhibition side, most emphasis has been on fiber, antioxidant micronutrients, stimulators of immune defenses, and nonnutrient components of food. Protease inhibitors should be classified in the last category. It is entirely possible that the above dietary factors could interact in the enhancement or inhibition of carcinogenesis and that some factors will have agonistic or antagonistic relationships. The role of protease inhibitors has hardly been explored in human epidemiologic studies, mainly because of the lack of appropriate tools to measure their intake, absorption, and efficacy. If the basic scientists work in coordination with epidemiologists, it may be possible to develop and test such tools.

8. *References*

Adams, C. F., (ed.), *Nutritive Value of American Foods in Common Units*, Agriculture Handbook No. 456, U.S. Department of Agriculture, Washington, D.C.

Armstrong, B., and Doll, R., 1975, Environmental factors and cancer incidence in different countries with special reference to dietary practices, *Int. J. Cancer* **15**:617–631.

Carroll, K. K., Gammel, E. B., and Plunkett, E. R., 1968, Dietary fat and mammary cancer, *Can. Med. Assoc. J.* **23**:590–594.

Correa, P., 1981, Epidemiologic correlations between diet and cancer frequency, *Cancer Res.* **41**:3685–3690.

Drasar, G. S., and Irving, D., 1973, Environmental factors and cancer of the colon and breast, *Br. J. Cancer* **27**:167–172.

Gregor, O., Toman, R., and Frusona, F., 1969, Gastrointestinal cancer and nutrition, *Gut* **10**:1031–1034.

Hems, G., 1970, Epidemiologic characteristics of breast cancer in middle and late age, *Br. J. Cancer* **24**:226–234.

Kennedy, A. R., and Little, J. B., 1981, Effects of protease inhibitors on radiation transformation in vitro, *Cancer Res.* **41**:2103–2108.

Lea, A. J., 1967, Neoplasms and environmental factors, *Ann. R. Coll. Surg. Engl.* **41**:432–438.

Madar, Z., Gertter, A., and Birk, Y., 1979, The fate of Bowman–Birk trypsin inhibitor from soybeans in the digestive tract of chicks, *Comp. Biochem. Physiol. A* **62**:1057.

Mills, P. K., Annegers, J. F., and Phillips, R. L., 1988a, Animal product consumption and subsequent fatal breast cancer risk among Seventh Day Adventists, *Am. J. Epidemiol.* **127**(3):440–453.

Mills, P. K., Beeson, L., Abbey, D. E., Fraser, G. E., and Phillips, R. L., 1988b, Dietary habits and past medical history as related to fatal pancreas cancer risk among Adventists, *Cancer* **61**:2578–2585.

Phillips, R. L., 1975, Role of life-style and dietary habits in risk of cancer among Seventh-Day Adventists, *Cancer Res.* **35**:3513–3522.

Rackis, J. J., Wolf, W. J., and Baker, E. C., 1986, Protease inhibitors in plant foods: Content and inactivation, *Adv. Exp. Med. Biol.* **199**:299–347.

Schelp, F.-P., and Pongpaew, P., 1988, Protection against cancer through nutritionally-induced increase of endogenous proteinase inhibitors—A hypothesis, *J. Epidemiol.* **17**:287–292.

Segi, M., Kurihara, M., and Matsuyama, T., 1969, *Cancer Mortality of Selected Sites in 24 Countries*, No. 5 1964–65, Sendai: Japanese Department of Public Health, Tohoku University School of Medicine.

Troll, W., and Yavelow, J., 1983, Protease inhibitors as anticarcinogens, in: *Diet, Nutrition and Cancer: From Basic Research to Policy Implications* (D. A. Roe, ed.), Liss, New York.

Troll, W., Klassen, A., and Janoff, A., 1790, Tumorigenesis in mouse skin: Inhibition by synthetic inhibitors of proteases, *Science* **169**:1211–1213.

Troll, W., Frenkel, K., and Wiesner, R., 1984, Protease inhibitors as anticarcinogens, *J. Natl. Cancer Inst.* **73**:1245–1250.

Umezawa, K., 1972, *Enzyme Inhibitors of Microbial Origin*, University of Tokyo Press, Tokyo pp. 29–32.

Watt, B. K., and Merrill, A. L., (eds.), 1975, *Composition of Foods: Raw, Processed Prepared*, Agriculture Handbook No. 8., U.S. Department of Agriculture, Washington, D.C.

Weder, J. K. P., 1986, Inhibition of human proteinases by grain legumes, *Adv. Exp. Med. Biol.* **199**:239–279.

Wynder, E. L., Kajitani, T., Dodo, H., and Takano, A., 1970, Environmental factors of cancer of the colon and rectum. II. Japanese epidemiologic data, *Cancer (Philadelphia)* **23**:1210–1220.

Yavelow, J., Collins, M., Birch, Y., Troll, W., and Kennedy, A. R., 1985, Nanomolar concentrations of Bowman-Birk soybean protease inhibitor suppress x-ray induced transformation in vitro, *Proc. Natl. Acad. Sci. USA* **82**:5395–5399.

2

Anticarcinogenic Activity of Protease Inhibitors
Overview

ANN R. KENNEDY

1. Review of Data Showing Anticarcinogenic Activity of Protease Inhibitors

Cancer is one of the leading causes of death in the United States. There is known to be a great variation in cancer incidence with diet, as has been recently reviewed (Grobstein *et al.*, 1982). Epidemiological data suggest that environmental, specifically nutritional, factors play a major role in the etiology of cancer at many different sites (Grobstein *et al.*, 1982; Doll and Peto, 1981; Correa, 1981; Phillips, 1975). There are now many different epidemiological studies which suggest that components of vegetables, particularly legumes (Correa, 1981), might play a beneficial role in lowering the incidence of cancer (some examples of such studies are given in the references cited above). Legumes are known to contain high levels of protease inhibitors (Birk, 1974). Rice, maize, and beans, all of which are known to contain high levels of protease inhibitors (Birk, 1974, 1975), in the diet are associated with a reduced incidence of colon, breast, and prostate cancers (Correa, 1981). The intake of breads and cereals, food sources which are also known to contain high levels of protease inhibitors, has been associated with a lowered incidence of oral and pharyngeal cancers (Winn *et al.*, 1984). Other studies with high levels of protease inhibitors in the

ANN R. KENNEDY • Department of Radiation Oncology, School of Medicine, University of Pennsylvania, Philadelphia, Pennsylvania 19104.

Protease Inhibitors as Cancer Chemopreventive Agents, edited by Walter Troll and Ann R. Kennedy. Plenum Press, New York, 1993.

diet have also suggested a reduced risk of developing colorectal and breast cancers (Blondell, 1988). The role of vegetable-derived protease inhibitors as active cancer chemopreventive agents is discussed in several other chapters in this volume (e.g., Chapter 1).

A large body of experimental data suggest that protease inhibitors from various sources have strong anticarcinogenic activity *in vivo* (Troll, 1976; Troll *et al.*, 1970, 1979a,b, 1980; Becker, 1981; Corasanti *et al.*, 1982; Fukui *et al.*, 1975; Yamamoto *et al.*, 1974; Yamamura *et al.*, 1978; Nomura *et al.*, 1980; Berenblum *et al.*, 1974; Kennedy and Billings, 1987; Umezawa, 1972; Rossman and Troll, 1980; Hozumi *et al.*, 1972; Verloes and Kanarek, 1976; Weed *et al.*, 1985; Messadi *et al.*, 1986; Witschi and Kennedy, 1989; St. Clair *et al.*, 1990; Billings *et al.*, 1990b); these *in vivo* data are summarized in Table I.

Protease inhibitors are widely distributed in both the plant and animal kingdoms. They are found in many common foods, including legumes, cereals, oilseeds, nuts, fruits, vegetables, eggs, potatoes, and other dairy and animal products. Many vegetables contain protease inhibitors which could be useful as cancer chemopreventive agents, as has been reviewed (Birk, 1975; Liener and Kakade, 1980; Rackis *et al.*, 1986). Soybeans are unusually rich in protease inhibitor activity; protease inhibitors comprise as much as 6% of the total soybean protein. Several protease inhibitors are present in soybeans. The best characterized of these inhibitors are soybean trypsin inhibitor (SBTI) (Kunitz, 1947) and the Bowman–Birk inhibitor (BBI) (Birk, 1975). SBTI has a molecular weight of about 21,000 and has primarily trypsin inhibitory activity; BBI has a molecular weight of about 8000 and inhibits chymotrypsin and trypsin (Birk, 1975). The other soybean protease inhibitors have not been as fully characterized as BBI and SBTI, but are known to inhibit trypsin (Hwang *et al.*, 1977). The chick pea inhibitor (CPI) is part of the Bowman–Birk family of protease inhibitors (which are naturally present in all legumes) which inhibits both trypsin and chymotrypsin; CPI is effective in suppressing transformation *in vitro* at the lowest concentration of any legume-derived protease inhibitor which has been studied (see Chapter 3). The Bowman–Birk family of protease inhibitors presumably inhibit carcinogenesis because of their ability to inhibit chymotrypsin (Yavelow *et al.*, 1985; Kennedy, 1985). Certain other protease inhibitors have the ability to inhibit chymotrypsin. For example, the chymotrypsin inhibitor from potatoes inhibits chymotrypsin (Birk, 1975; Smirnoff *et al.*, 1979; Ryan and Kassell, 1970); unlike the Bowman–Birk type of protease inhibitors, this protease inhibitor does not have a distinct trypsin inhibitory region. Fruits are also known to contain protease inhibitors that inhibit chymotrypsin; for example, bananas have a particularly high chymotrypsin inhibitor content (Rackis *et al.*, 1986).

As our *in vitro* studies indicated that protease inhibitors were highly effective as anticarcinogenic agents (see Chapter 3), we began to plan studies to evaluate this class of compounds as human cancer chemopreventive agents. Several previous studies suggested that protease inhibitors could be useful as

Table I. Protease Inhibitor Suppression of Carcinogenesis in Vivo

Carcinogen	Protease inhibitor	Animal model system	Reference
7,12-dimethylbenz(a)anthracene (DMBA) (promoter = croton oil or phorbol ester)	TLCK[a] TPCK[b] TAME[c]	Mouse skin tumorigenesis	Troll et al. (1970)
DMBA (promoter = croton oil)	Leupeptin	Mouse skin tumorigenesis	Hozumi et al. (1972)
Azoxymethane	Leupeptin	Rat colon carcinogenesis	Yamamoto et al. (1974)
Radiation	α_2-macroglobulin	Mouse lymphatic leukemia	Berenblum et al. (1974)
DMBA	Leupeptin	Rat mammary tumorigenesis	Fukui et al. (1975)
Chemical carcinogenesis	Leupeptin	Rat colon, esophagus, and mammary gland carcinogenesis; mouse leukemia, skin carcinogenesis	Matsushima et al. (1976)
DMBA	N,N-dimethylamino (p-p'-guanidinobenzoyloxy) benzilcarbonyloxyglycolate	Rat mammary tumorigenesis	Yamamura et al. (1978)
4-Nitroquinoline oxide and PMA	Soybean diet	Mouse skin tumorigenesis	Troll et al. (1979a)
Urethane	Antipain	Mouse lung tumorigenesis	Nomura et al. (1980)
X-irradiation	Soybean diet	Rat mammary carcinogenesis	Troll et al. (1980)
DMBA	TPCK	Mouse skin tumorigenesis	Slaga et al. (1980)
Spontaneous	Edi Pro A (isolated soy protein)	Mouse liver tumorigenesis	Becker (1981)
Dimethylhydrazine	ε-Aminocaproic acid	Mouse colon tumorigenesis	Corasanti et al. (1982)
3-Methylcholanthrene	N,N-dimethyl carbamoyl-methyl 4-(4-guanidinobenzoyloxy) phenylacetate methanesulfate (FOY-305)	Mouse skin carcinogenesis	Ohkoshi and Fujii (1983)

(continued)

Table I. (Continued)

Carcinogen	Protease inhibitor	Animal model system	Reference
Dimethylhydrazine	Bowman–Birk	Mouse colon tumorigenesis	Weed et al. (1985), St. Clair et al. (1990), Billings et al. (1990b)
DMBA	Bowman–Birk	Hamster oral carcinogenesis	Messadi et al. (1986)
	FOY-305	Rat liver carcinogenesis	Yamauchi et al. (1987)
3-Methylcholanthrene	Bowman–Birk	Mouse lung tumorigenesis	Witschi and Kennedy (1989)
Dimethylhydrazine	Bowman–Birk	Mouse liver tumorigenesis	St. Clair et al. (1990)

[a]TLCK, tosyl lysine chloromethyl ketone.
[b]TPCK, tosyl phenylalanine chloromethyl ketone.
[c]TAME, tosyl arginine methyl ester.

human cancer chemopreventive agents. While some synthetic protease inhibitors, such as TLCK, TPCK, and TAME, are effective antitumorigenic agents in the mouse skin system (Troll et al., 1970; Rossman and Troll, 1980), these agents are extremely toxic. This toxicity severely limits their potential use as dietary additives. Relatively nontoxic protease inhibitors, such as antipain, leupeptin, chymostatin, and others from actinomycetes, have also been shown to suppress carcinogenesis in vivo and in vitro. These inhibitors are small, oligopeptide-like compounds which can effectively inhibit protease activity in the micromolar range. We have observed that the most effective of these protease inhibitors for the suppression of malignant transformation in vitro is chymostatin, an inhibitor of chymotrypsin (Kennedy, 1985). The problem with use of the inhibitors from actinomycetes as dietary supplements is that they are extremely expensive when bought from commercial sources, and large-scale trials would be prohibitive in cost. A further problem with many of these inhibitors (such as antipain) is that they have the undesirable side effect of inhibiting blood clotting, and thus may not be the best possible cancer chemopreventive protease inhibitors.

Three studies in particular served as models to us as we planned our own in vivo studies. Troll et al. (1980) showed that a diet containing raw soybeans (and a high level of protease inhibitor activity) could suppress radiation-induced mammary carcinogenesis in rats. Corasanti et al. (1982) reported a suppression of colon carcinogenesis by ε-aminocaproic acid, and Becker (1981) observed a suppression of liver carcinogenesis in mice by Edi Pro A, a soy-protein extract made by the Ralston Purina Company. While the protease inhibitor animal studies of Becker (1981), Troll et al. (1980), and Corasanti et al. (1982) suggested that a protease inhibitor could suppress carcinogenesis, they did not provide all of the information which is needed before protease inhibitors can be considered for human cancer chemoprevention trials. The limitations of these previous studies, in terms of designing a cancer chemopreventive agent, are as follows: (1) The major problem with the data presented by Troll et al. (1980) is that the rats given the soybean diet weighted significantly less than the untreated rats. Because caloric restriction alone can suppress carcinogenesis (Grobstein et al., 1982), it cannot be concluded that there was a direct effect of the protease inhibitors on the suppression of carcinogenesis. (2) The data reported by Corasanti et al. (1982) showed that even a very weak protease inhibitor, such as ε-aminocaproic acid, can produce a significant suppressive effect on colon carcinogenesis. The major problem with the study by Corasanti et al. (1982) is that ε-aminocaproic acid is too toxic to be considered reasonable for use as a human cancer chemopreventive agent. (3) Becker (1981) showed that Edi Pro A could suppress liver carcinogenesis arising in a strain of mice in which 85% of the animals spontaneously develop liver cancer. While these data suggest that there is an edible soybean protease inhibitor which can inhibit carcinogenesis, the model chosen for use may not be applicable to most human cancer as the mice used in those experiments are a "genetically susceptible" population. Given the data reported by Becker (1981), however, Edi Pro A might have been a reasonable substance to use in cancer chemoprevention protocols. We chose not to use it in our studies because Edi Pro A contains mainly SBTI; as discussed above, we believe that it is the ability to inhibit chymotrypsin (i.e., not trypsin) which is important for anticarcinogenic activity. Furthermore, Edi Pro A is no longer available. The Ralston Purina Company fears that our studies, and those of other investigators, could damage the reputation of their final product. [When Edi Pro A is sold commercially, the protease inhibitor activity is destroyed by heat to result in a fully nutritious product, as officials at Ralston Purina believe that high levels of trypsin inhibitory activity can result in decreased protein utilization (see below for a discussion of this phenomenon).]

As there appeared to be no protease inhibitor preparation commercially available which would be suitable for large-scale cancer chemoprevention protocols, we have attempted to produce a protease inhibitor-containing extract of soybeans which could serve as a human cancer chemopreventive agent. Our studies utilizing this BBI-containing extract (and pure BBI) are summarized below.

To be practical as a human cancer chemopreventive agent, it is believed that the active ingredient in soybeans must be at least partially purified to reduce the volume of material necessary to obtain anticarcinogenic activity (as well as to remove any agents which may enhance carcinogenesis or mask the activity of anticarcinogenic agents; see Section 3.1). The protease inhibitor content of various soybean preparations is known and it is conceivable that sufficient anticarcinogenic activity can be obtained from normal dietary sources. Our previous studies have suggested that, at 0.1% of the diet, either pure BBI or an extract of soybeans containing BBI (and other soybean protease inhibitors), carcinogenesis can be suppressed in animals (St. Clair et al., 1990; Billings et al., 1990b). For an adult, a normal dietary intake is 1600 g/day (Snyder et al., 1974). If we assume that our studies in animals are appropriate for extrapolation to human populations, 1600 mg/day (0.1% of 1600 g/day) of protease inhibitors would be needed for anticarcinogenic activity. This amount of protease inhibitor activity could be consumed in a normal diet. In the normal Western diet, approximately 330 mg/day is consumed (Doell et al., 1981; Billings et al., 1990a). The remaining protease inhibitor activity could be obtained from soybean products high in protease inhibitor activity. For example, commercially available "soya bean drink" contains approximately 600 mg protease inhibitor/quart and tofu contains approximately 150 mg/cup (Dr. Paul Billings, personal communication). Other estimates of protease inhibitor activity in soy products can be found in the literature (Doell et al., 1981; Rackis et al., 1986).

It is conceivable that lower amounts of soybean-containing products may be necessary to reduce the risk of cancer if other soybean-derived anticarcinogenic agents are present. Other compounds in soybeans which may have anticarcinogenic activity include isoflavones (dietary estrogens), phytic acid, phytosterols, and saponins; the different types of anticarcinogenic activities in soybeans have recently been reviewed (Messina and Barnes, 1991b). We are enthusiastic about the use of dietary protease inhibitors to prevent or reduce the incidence of cancer in the human population.

As discussed below, our studies have shown that soybean protease inhibitors can suppress carcinogenesis *in vivo* at many different sites. We believe that a suitable level of anticarcinogenic protease inhibitors in the diet can be found which will not lead to any problems because: (1) there are normal human populations with high levels of protease inhibitors in the diet which show no adverse effects (i.e., the Japanese and Seventh-Day Adventists) (Armstrong and Doll, 1975) and (2) we have observed no undesirable side effects, including pancreatic changes, decreased growth rate, or decline in general health, in animals maintained at high levels of anticarcinogenic dietary protease inhibitor activity for their entire life span (Weed *et al.*, 1985; Kennedy, unpublished data).

2. Potential Adverse Effects of Anticarcinogenic Protease Inhibitors

2.1. Effects of Protease Inhibitors on Growth

Protease inhibitors in vegetables have been regarded as antinutritional substances, primarily because growth-inhibiting effects have been attributed to them. Questions about the role of protease inhibitors in nutrition began with the findings of Osborne and Mendel (1917) that soybeans would not support the growth of young rats unless the soybeans were heat-treated. As it was thought that protease inhibitors were largely inactivated by heat treatment, it was assumed that it was inactivation of the protease inhibitors by the heat treatment that led to soybean products that did not suppress growth. In fact, the Bowman–Birk type of protease inhibitors are quite resistant to heat treatment, and are found in an active form in many processed foods such as canned chick peas, kidney beans, and so forth (Yavelow *et al.*, 1982). The evidence suggesting that protease inhibitors are antinutritional has been largely circumstantial, based on studies which have not utilized purified compounds for study. When purified protease inhibitors have been studied for their effects on growth, the studies have shown that protease inhibitors do not have the deleterious effects on growth that have been widely attributed to them, as discussed in Chapter 5.

While the protease inhibitors in soybeans do not appear to have the primary suppressive effects on animal growth, it is clear that some components of soybeans do have growth-suppressing effects. There are many antinutritional and toxic factors in legumes, as has been reviewed by Liener (1989). For example, soybeans contain high levels of polyphenolic substances known as tannins. Tannins inhibit all of the digestive enzymes in a nonspecific manner (Gallaher and

Schneeman, 1986). Tannins are responsible for poor digestibility of proteins and growth inhibition when fed to animals; the antinutritional characteristics of tannins have been discussed in detail elsewhere (Liener, 1989; Rackis *et al.*, 1986). Other antinutritional substances found in soybeans (and other legumes) include: hemagglutinins (lectins), goitrogens, cyanogens, lathyrogens, phytate (phytic acid), flatulence producers, and gossypol (Liener, 1989). While any or all of these substances could contribute to the growth-suppressing effects of raw soybeans, it is likely that the soybean protein itself is the major factor producing growth suppression (Gallaher and Schneeman, 1986). When trypsin inhibitors were removed from raw soybean meal by affinity chromatography and the raw meal lacking protease inhibitors was fed to rats, the degree of growth depression was only a bit less than with the raw meal containing the trypsin inhibitors (Kakade *et al.*, 1973). This experiment suggested that much of the growth-suppressing effect was due to the protein itself. In their native state, plant proteins are refractory to proteolytic attack, which results in poor amino acid availability (Grau and Carroll, 1958; Bozzini and Silano, 1978). As heat treatment of soybean meal is known to increase the digestibility of soybean protein, heat treatment would thus bring about an alleviation of growth depression produced by soybean protein in its native state (Gallaher and Schneeman, 1986). While the precise contribution of protease inhibitors to the growth-suppressing effects of raw soybean is controversial, it is clear that heat treatment of soybeans results in products which support the normal growth of animals.

2.2. Effects of Protease Inhibitors on the Pancreas

2.2.1. Regulation of Pancreatic Secretions/Effects of Soybean Protease Inhibitors on Pancreatic Secretions

For the rat, a negative feedback mechanism exists for pancreatic enzyme secretion and cholecystokinin (CCK) is known to be a major regulatory hormone (Green and Lyman, 1972). CCK is secreted by cells of the proximal small intestine as a response to an increase in the level of trypsin activity in the intestinal lumen (Green and Lyman, 1972). CCK–pancreozymin is the humoral agent released from the intestine; it has the ability to stimulate pancreatic secretion and cause both pancreatic hypertrophy and hyperplasia (Rothman and Wells, 1967; Mainz *et al.*, 1973; Yanatori and Fujita, 1976). The exact details of the feedback response are still controversial. Evidence has been presented that a "monitor peptide" is secreted with the pancreatic juice and signals CCK secretion by the intestinal mucosa (Fushiki and Iwai, 1989; Miyasaka *et al.*, 1989). If the intestinal mucosa is low in trypsin inhibitor activity, these peptides are destroyed by proteolytic activity and CCK secretion is reduced. CCK secretion is increased when trypsin inhibitors are present in the diet; it is assumed that trypsin inhibition protects the CCK-releasing peptides from being destroyed. It is thought that CCK induces hyperplasia and hypertrophy of the acinar tissue (as well as having some effect on the ductal elements) of the pancreas as a response to greater needs for pancreatic functions (Morgan, 1987).

CCK is thought to be an essential promoter involved in pancreatic carcinogenesis in the rat (for review see Chapter 18).

Whether a feedback system involving CCK exists in humans or, in fact, in any species other than rats is unknown, as discussed in Chapter 18. It is known that the administration of camostate, which induces CCK in rats (see Chapter 18), does not induce an increase in plasma levels of CCK in humans (Watanabe *et al.*, 1986; Adler *et al.*, 1986, 1988). Although controversial, there is some evidence that humans do have feedback control of pancreatic enzyme secretions (as discussed by Toskes, 1986, and Liener *et al.*, 1988). If such a system does exist for the human pancreas, this does not mean that the human pancreas will respond to soy trypsin inhibitors (STI) with enlargement. A negative feedback mechanism for pancreatic enzyme secretion (similar to that of rats) exists in hamsters (Andrén-Sandberg and Ihse, 1983), pigs, and calves, but these species do not develop pancreatic cancer (or even enlargement in the case of pigs and calves) in response to trypsin inhibitors (reviewed by Gallaher and Schneeman, 1986). The existence of feedback control of the pancreas appears to be absent in some species, such as the dog (Sale *et al.*, 1977; Diaz *et al.*, 1982).

The effect of protease inhibitors on the negative feedback control system is not specific; protease inhibitors affect the system in the same manner as do other proteins, but are a somewhat more potent stimulus (Green and Lyman, 1972; Green *et al.*, 1973). It is of interest that proteins have the same "deleterious" effects on the rat pancreas attributed to protease inhibitors. Raw soybean protein fractions lacking trypsin inhibitor activity cause pancreatic enlargement in rats as do the protease inhibitor-containing fractions (Naim *et al.*, 1982).

It is specifically trypsin inhibition, and not chymotrypsin inhibition, involved in triggering the feedback response, and ultimately the production of pancreatic enlargement in rats, as reviewed in Chapter 5. As it is chymotrypsin inhibition which is involved in anticarcinogenic activity (Kennedy, 1985; Yavelow *et al.*, 1985), the anticarcinogenic activity can be separated from the trypsin inhibitory activity which has the potential to produce deleterious side effects on the pancreas in some species.

2.2.2. Histopathological Changes in the Pancreas Associated with Soybean Products

High levels of unheated soybean products in the diet of rats have been associated with pancreatic hyperplasia and hypertrophy; in a few rats fed in this manner for very long periods of time, pancreatic cancer developed (Naim *et al.*, 1982; McGuiness *et al.*, 1980; Gumbmann *et al.*, 1985; Crass and Morgan, 1982; as reviewed by McGuiness *et al.*, 1984, and Morgan, 1987). The carcinogenic effect of soybeans has been widely attributed to the protease inhibitors in soybeans (Liener and Kakade, 1980; Rackis *et al.*, 1986; Flavin, 1982), although the evidence is circumstantial and, perhaps, not correct.

There appears to be no doubt that the soybean protease inhibitors are involved in the stimulation of growth in the rat pancreas, causing primarily hypertrophy and some hyperplasia (Melmed *et al.*, 1976; Crass and Morgan, 1982; Kakade *et al.*, 1967), but whether these lesions are related to the development of pancreatic cancer is controversial (see Chapter 5). As there are species, such as the mouse, which respond to soybean protease inhibitors by developing pancreatic hyperplasia and hypertrophy, but do not develop cancer and there are other species, such as the hamster, which respond to soybean protease inhibitors with pancreatic enlargement and a reduced pancreatic cancer risk (Liener and Hasdai, 1986), these phenomena may not be related. Even in rats fed soybean protease inhibitors, the occurrence of hyperplasia/hypertrophy and cancer in the pancreas are separable phenomena (Richter and Schneeman, 1987). Other components of soybeans could be responsible for the carcinogenic effect, as discussed below.

Enlargement of the pancreas associated with soybean protease inhibitors is a readily reversible process (McGuiness *et al.*, 1984), as expected for the effects of a promoting agent (reviewed by Weinstein, 1978). (The evidence for considering soybean products as "promoters" of rat pancreatic carcinogenesis is discussed in Section 2.2.4.) Even when rats are fed on raw soya flour diets for as long as 6 months, and then receive non-soya-containing diets, the pancreatic weights, protein contents, and morphological appearances of the pancreata revert to normal swiftly (McGuiness *et al.*, 1984).

The pancreata of most species do not respond, as does the pancreas of the rat, to high levels of soybeans in the diet (Birk, 1975, 1985, and this volume; Folsch *et al.*, 1974); examples of species which do not respond in this fashion are: dogs (Wolf and Cowan, 1975; Patten *et al.*, 1971a,b), the adult guinea pig (Patten *et al.*, 1973), calves (Kakade *et al.*, 1976; Gorrill and Thomas, 1967), pigs (Struthers *et al.*, 1983; Hooks *et al.*, 1965; Yen *et al.*, 1977), cebus monkeys (Ausman *et al.*, 1985; Struthers *et al.*, 1983), and chacma baboons (Robbins *et al.*, 1988).

There are a few species whose pancreata respond with enlargement, as do the pancreata of rats, to high levels of soybeans in the diet, notably chickens (Chernick *et al.*, 1948; Nitsan and Alumot, 1964; Gertler and Nitsan, 1970; Nitsan and Nir, 1977), young (but not adult) guinea pigs (Patten *et al.*, 1973), quails (Birk, 1985; Madar *et al.*, 1974), mice (Schingoethe *et al.*, 1970), and hamsters (Hasdai and Liener, 1983). From the data concerning the species variation in response, it has been suggested (by Kakade *et al.*, 1976; Liener, 1979a,b; Liener and Kakade, 1980) that animals whose pancreata are 0.3% of body weight or more (such as the mouse, chick, rat, and young guinea pig) show pancreatic enlargement with feeding of STI, while those animals whose pancreata are less than 0.3% of body weight (the adult guinea pig, pig, dog, and calf) do not exhibit pancreatic enlargement. With this relationship, the human pancreas is not expected to enlarge because of trypsin inhibitors, as it weighs about 0.09% to 0.12% of body weight.

Thus, the available evidence suggests that soybean protease inhibitors will not bring about pancreatic enlargement. Even if they do, however, this does not mean that these protease inhibitors will produce pancreatic cancer. As noted above, pancreatic enlargement produced by soybean protease inhibitors does not lead to pancreatic cancer in mice and, in hamsters, the soybean protease inhibitors suppress pancreatic cancer development even though they cause pancreatic enlargement (Liener and Hasdai, 1986).

2.2.3. Is Soybean-Product-Associated Pancreatic Cancer in Rats the Result of Protease Inhibitors?

As discussed in Chapter 18, when rats are fed a diet containing raw, full-fat soybean flour, pancreatic cancer can occur, and carcinogen-induced pancreatic carcinogenesis can be enhanced, but whether the effect is caused by protease inhibitors is not clear. Several studies have suggested that protease inhibitors may be only partially responsible for the deleterious effects of soybeans on the pancreas; for example, Kakade et al. (1973) and Liener (1979a) present data showing that trypsin inhibitors are responsible for only approximately 40% of the stimulatory effects of raw soy flour on the pancreas. The actual effect may be even less than that estimate. It is known that there is a high content of unsaturated fat in soybeans [raw soy flour contains approximately 20% fat (Richter and Schneeman, 1987)]; the unsaturated fat from soybeans is known to enhance pancreatic carcinogenesis in rats (Roebuck et al., 1987). When soybeans are defatted, the hyperplastic, hypertrophic, and carcinogenic effects of the soybean products (containing high levels of the soybean protease inhibitors) in the pancreas of rats are not observed (for review, see Richter and Schneeman, 1987). Further evidence that the soybean protease inhibitors may not be responsible for the deleterious effects of raw soybeans on the pancreas is that protein fractions lacking trypsin inhibitory activity cause pancreatic enlargement in rats (Naim et al., 1982).

The fact that the hypertrophic, hyperplastic, and carcinogenic effects of raw soybean products on the pancreas can be abolished by heat treatment of the soybean flour (McGuiness et al., 1980; Folsch et al., 1974; Roebuck et al., 1987) suggests that BBI (and the other BBI-type protease inhibitors in soybeans) is not responsible for these effects, as this protease inhibitor is highly resistant to degradation by normal levels of heat treatment* (Bowman, 1946; Birk, 1961).

*Whereas the proteolytic activity of BBI is relatively unaffected by heat treatment, such treatment does destroy most of the protease inhibitor activity in soybeans. Heat treatment not only inactivates most of the trypsin inhibitors, but also destroys some of the amino acids and generally reduces amino acid availability. As the amount of heat necessary to destroy all of the trypsin-inhibitor

2.2.4. Relationship of Experiments on Azaserine-Induced Pancreatic Cancer to Soybean-Associated Pancreatic Pathology in Rats

In the experiments which have been performed to determine the effects of constituents of soybeans on the pancreas, pure compounds have not been used, so that observed effects can often be attributed to other components of the soybeans or the diet utilized. In several experiments performed on azaserine-induced rat pancreatic carcinogenesis, a synthetic protease inhibitor, called FOY-305 (or camostate), has been used, as discussed in Chapter 18. These studies suggest that this protease inhibitor might have two opposing effects on pancreatic carcinogenesis, a promoting effect on early preneoplastic lesions, caused by its ability to enhance CCK secretion, but then a direct suppressive effect on pancreatic carcinogenesis after its absorption from the intestine and transport to the pancreas. It has been shown that growth of basophilic putative neoplastic foci in the pancreas is inhibited by camostate (and stimulated by CCK) (Douglas et al., 1989). As suggested in Chapter 18, these studies on the pancreas suggest that the overall effect of protease inhibitors absorbed from the gastrointestinal tract may be to suppress pancreatic carcinogenesis, even in the rat model system. In azaserine-induced pancreatic carcinogenesis in rats, protease inhibitors appear to act as promoters only during the early postinitiation phase (i.e., the first 2 months and not the last 2 months of the postinitiation phase) of carcinogenesis (Roebuck et al., 1987). In these studies, both a protease inhibitor-containing protein fraction and a fraction containing unsaturated fat from soybeans increased the size of azaserine-induced preneoplastic foci in the pancreas but did not increase the number of foci occurring in the "initiated" pancreas (Roebuck et al., 1987). These studies suggest that the soybean protease inhibitor-containing fraction (as well as the fraction containing unsaturated fat) can act as a growth promoter for carcinogen-induced pancreatic carcinogenesis in rats, but the protease inhibitor-containing fraction had no ability to induce cancer by itself or act as a cocarcinogen with azaserine to enhance pancreatic carcinogenesis. [A purified trypsin inhibitor has also been shown to act as a promoter for azaserine-induced pancreatic carcinogenesis (Douglas et al., 1989).] Similar conclusions have been reached in experiments involving spontaneous pancreatic carcinogenesis; the evidence suggests that soybean products do not cause cancer by themselves but instead can serve as a promoter for multistage carcinogenesis in the pancreas (McGuiness et al., 1984).

In the studies which have shown pancreatic cancer development in rats maintained on high levels of soybeans in the diet, "spontaneous" carcinogenesis could be induced by a variety of carcinogens in the environment of the animals.

---

activity would damage the nutritive value of proteins, most commercially available soy products are heat-treated to an extent that results in 5–20% of the original trypsin-inhibitor activity remaining intact (Rackis et al., 1986).

For example, *N*-nitrosamines, known to cause pancreatic cancer in animals (McGuiness *et al.*, 1984), have been found in animal food and bedding material (Silverman and Adams, 1983).

2.2.5. Apparent Thresholds for Pancreatic Effects in Rats

There appears to be a threshold in rats both for stimulation of CCK and for bringing about pancreatic enlargement. The threshold for negative feedback regulation by luminal proteases occurs when luminal protease activity is reduced by 90% in the rat; at this point, increased pancreatic secretion occurs (Miyasaka and Green, 1984). It is widely believed that there is a threshold for pancreatic pathology (hypertrophy) in rats (Rackis *et al.*, 1975; Churella *et al.*, 1976; McGuiness *et al.*, 1984; Liener, 1989). This threshold for pancreatic enlargement in rats occurs when the animals are fed raw soyflour in an amount which represents 5% of the total protein in the diet (McGuiness *et al.*, 1984).

2.2.6. Pancreatic Cancer in Humans: Relationship of Soybean Products to Pancreatic Cancer

The cause of human pancreatic cancer is unknown. There is a strong association with cigarette smoking (Mack, 1982) as well as an association with high levels of dietary fat (Norell *et al.*, 1986; Durbec *et al.*, 1983; Carroll and Khor, 1975; Wynder, 1975; Gold *et al.*, 1985). Experimental pancreatic carcinogenesis in rats has also shown a strong association with high levels of dietary fat, as discussed above.

There are several reasons for believing that soybean-derived protease inhibitors and other soybean constituents will not have a carcinogenic effect on the human pancreas as they may have on the rat pancreas:

1. Human trypsin is more resistant to inhibition by the soybean-derived protease inhibitors than is the trypsin of other mammals, suggesting that dietary soybean-derived trypsin inhibitors will not have a sufficiently strong effect to bring about pancreatic pathology (reviewed by Flavin, 1982).

2. The size (percentage of body weight) of the human pancreas is such that it falls into a classification of species which do not respond to soybean trypsin inhibitors (products) by pancreatic enlargement (or cancer development), as discussed in detail above.

3. Rats have different essential amino acid requirements than do humans; of particular importance is that their requirements for sulfur-containing amino acids, such as methionine, are not like those of humans (Bodwell and Hopkins, 1985; Bodwell *et al.*, 1981). The metabolic pathway by which rats (chicks and presumably other species responding to soybean-

derived trypsin inhibitors with pancreatic enlargement) metabolize soybean products is unusual and clearly different from those operating in
humans (e.g., see Young et al., 1984; Scrimshaw et al., 1983). As
soybean protein is known for its deficiency in sulfur-containing amino
acids (Liener and Kakade, 1980), rats respond to this food source in a
manner unlike that of many species, including humans. Rats are considered a poor model for humans in the determination of the soybean
protein efficiency ratio (PER), an assay utilized to assess the nutritional
qualities of human food proteins; alternatives to the rat model system are
discussed in detail elsewhere (e.g., see Bodwell and Hopkins, 1985;
Torun et al., 1982; Pineda et al., 1982; Soy Protein Council, 1987).
Thus, rats are considered an unsuitable species by which to judge the
likely effects of soybean protease inhibitors on any organ system, including the pancreas, and the results of studies on soybean products in rats
cannot be assumed to represent the likely response of humans to those
products.

Although the effect of soybean-derived protease inhibitors on human pancreatic carcinogenesis is unknown, the evidence suggests that they will inhibit
the development of pancreatic cancer. The Seventh-Day Adventists are known to
have high levels of soybeans (and other legumes such as peas and lentils) in their
diet and reduced rates of pancreatic cancer (Mills et al., 1988). There is no
evidence to suggest that soybean-derived protease inhibitors increase the risk of
pancreatic cancer. Other populations with high levels of soybean products in the
diet, such as the Japanese, show no increased risk of pancreatic cancer (Armstrong and Doll, 1975).

2.3. Potential Effects of Protease Inhibitors on the Immune System

Another potential toxicity problem involves the possible effect of protease
inhibitors on the immune system. This is considered a potential toxicity problem
based on the report by Goldstein et al. (1979) which showed that protease
inhibitors can prevent the induction of O_2^- and H_2O_2 in polymorphonuclear
leukocytes by tumor-promoting agents. Even though this effect of protease inhibitors is specifically in response to an undesirable cellular effect brought about by
tumor-promoting agents, the results discussed above have suggested to some that
protease inhibitors might interfere with the normal functioning of the immune
system.

In addition, the possible role of proteases in the normal functioning of the
immune system (in particular, neutrophils and macrophages) has also raised the
question of whether or not protease inhibitors might in some way compromise
the normal functioning of the immune system. For several reasons, an effect of
dietary protease inhibitors on the immune system is unlikely. There are currently

two major hypotheses on the mechanism of target-cell killing by macrophages: (1) cytolysis dependent on reactive oxygen intermediates and (2) cytolysis dependent on lysosomal enzymes (Leb et al., 1985). α-Tocopherol was found to be highly effective at inhibiting both antibody-dependent monocyte cytotoxicity (ADCC) and phorbol myristate acetate (PMA)-induced monocyte cytotoxicity (Corwin and Gordon, 1982). It is generally thought that this indicates that the production of H_2O_2 and oxygen free radicals are of primary importance for macrophage function. In spite of this, α-tocopherol is commonly used as a dietary supplement with no apparent ill effects. In fact, a slight stimulatory effect of α-tocopherol on the immune system (i.e., the opposite effect of that observed in vitro) has been observed in vivo (Corwin and Gordon, 1982; Lim et al., 1981). Two protease inhibitors, an ovomucoid trypsin inhibitor and SBTI, have been studied in separate investigations for their effects on macrophage function; in the first, the ovomucoid trypsin inhibitor had a slight inhibitory effect on cell killing (Leb et al., 1985); in the second, SBTI was tested for inhibition of elastolytic activity and found to be negative (Chapman and Stone, 1984). With respect to neutrophils, proteolytic activity is thought to play a major role in unwanted tissue destruction, such as emphysema. There has consequently been much medical research to find a protease inhibitor which might antagonize this protease-associated pathological condition. While SBTI was found to be more effective at inhibiting the elastolytic activity of neutrophils than macrophages in vitro, it is not expected to be effective in vivo (Harlan et al., 1981). The close association between effector cells and target cells makes access of protease inhibitors to proteases involved in tissue destruction or cell killing difficult (this would be true for neutrophils as well as for macrophages). Thus, we feel it is highly unlikely that there will be deleterious effects of protease inhibitors on the normal functioning of the immune system. Thus far, studies performed to determine whether BBI has an effect on cells of the immune system have shown no effect (Goldfarb et al., 1989).

3. The Soybean-Derived BBI as an Anticarcinogenic Agent

3.1. Review of Data on the Anticarcinogenic Activity of BBI

Our early studies showed BBI to be so effective in its ability to suppress malignant transformation in vitro that we decided to determine its ability to suppress carcinogenesis in animal model systems. As a crude extract of the inhibitor would potentially be of greater applicability in our future animal and human cancer chemopreventive studies (than pure BBI—due to the cost of its isolation and purification, etc.), we began to evaluate various extracts of soybeans containing BBI as potential anticarcinogenic preparations. Unfortunately, finding an effective extract proved to be a difficult task, for unknown reasons.

Many of the extracts we produced were not effective as anticarcinogenic agents in *in vitro* transformation assays and some even enhanced transformation (e.g., soybean flour, as discussed in Yavelow *et al.*, 1985). There are, in fact, some compounds in soybeans, such as the soybean lectin, which might be expected to work like a promoting agent for carcinogenesis. We believe that there are compounds in soybeans which are capable of masking the ability of BBI to serve as an anticarcinogenic agent and which are removed by various purification procedures, such as those described by Birk (Kassell, 1970) and Hwang *et al.* (1977). Pure BBI is an effective anticarcinogenic agent when produced by either the Birk (Kassell, 1970) or the Hwang *et al.* (1977) procedures; however, none of the "intermediate" extracts produced by either of those published procedures have anticarcinogenic activity [as measured by the ability to suppress radiation-induced transformation *in vitro* (Kennedy, unpublished data)]. We did manage to produce an anticarcinogenic extract of soybeans by acetone pretreatment of the starting material followed by the Birk purification procedure, as described in detail elsewhere (Yavelow *et al.*, 1985). The anticarcinogenic extract we produced has the same ability as pure BBI to suppress malignant transformation *in vitro;* the anticarcinogenic activity of the extract is thought to be the result solely of the presence of BBI (Yavelow *et al.*, 1985). The extract produced by our procedure contains five separate soybean protease inhibitors (including BBI, but not including SBTI), all of which are similar to BBI in molecular weight and trypsin inhibitory activity; these other trypsin inhibitors have been only partially characterized (Hwang *et al.*, 1977). We have observed that our extract, at a low concentration (0.01 µg/ml) in the medium, has essentially the same ability as pure BBI to suppress malignant transformation *in vitro* induced by radiation in C3H10T1/2 cells (Yavelow *et al.*, 1985) and induced by radiation, benzo(*a*)pyrene, and β-propiolactone (carcinogen treatments being given both with and without the cocarcinogen, pyrene) in 3T3 cells (Baturay and Kennedy, 1986). The BBI-containing extract has also been shown to reduce the levels of spontaneously occurring chromosome abnormalities in cells of patients with Bloom's syndrome; for this *in vitro* effect, the crude extract works approximately as well as does pure BBI (Kennedy *et al.*, 1984).

At this point, we have studied both pure BBI and the BBI-containing extract extensively in *in vitro* and *in vivo* experimentation. As discussed above, we have shown that BBI prevents or suppresses radiation- and chemical carcinogen-induced malignant transformation *in vitro* (Yavelow *et al.*, 1983, 1985; Kennedy, 1985; Baturay and Kennedy, 1986) and carcinogenesis in animals in several different model systems. In our studies on BBI, we have shown that BBI and/or the BBI-containing extract suppresses carcinogenesis: (1) in three different species (mice, rats, hamsters); (2) in several different organ systems/tissue types [colon, lung, liver, esophagus, and cheek pouch (oral epithelium)]; (3) in different cell types [epithelial cells (in the colon, liver, lung, esophagus, and cheek pouch) as well as connective tissue cells (fibroblasts—*in vitro* and those in the liver which give rise to angiosarcomas)]; (4) when given to animals by several different routes of administration [including injection (i.p. or i.v.), direct application, and through the diet]; and (5) leading to different types of cancers [e.g., squamous cell carcinomas (oral epithelium), adenocarcinomas (colon), angiosarcomas (liver)]. The specific animal model carcinogenesis systems in which BBI and/or the BBI-containing extract have been shown to have a suppressive effect on carcinogenesis include: (1) dimethylhydrazine (DMH)-induced colon (Weed *et al.*, 1985; St. Clair *et al.*, 1990; Billings *et al.*, 1990b) and liver (St. Clair *et al.*, 1990) carcinogenesis in mice, (2) 7,12-dimethylbenz(*a*)anthracene-induced oral carcinogenesis in hamsters (Messadi *et al.*, 1986; Kennedy *et al.*, 1993), and (3) 3-methylcholanthrene-induced lung carcinogenesis in mice (Witschi and Kennedy, 1989), and methylbenzylnitrosamine-induced esophageal carcinogenesis in rats (von Hofe *et al.*, 1991). Several of these *in vivo* studies have been reviewed elsewhere (Kennedy and Billings, 1987) and are summarized here.

In the colon, BBI completely prevented carcinogenesis induced by a low carcinogen dose (Figs. 1 and 2) (Weed *et al.*, 1985; St. Clair *et al.*, 1990) and suppressed carcinogenesis induced by a high carcinogen dose (Fig. 3) (Billings *et*

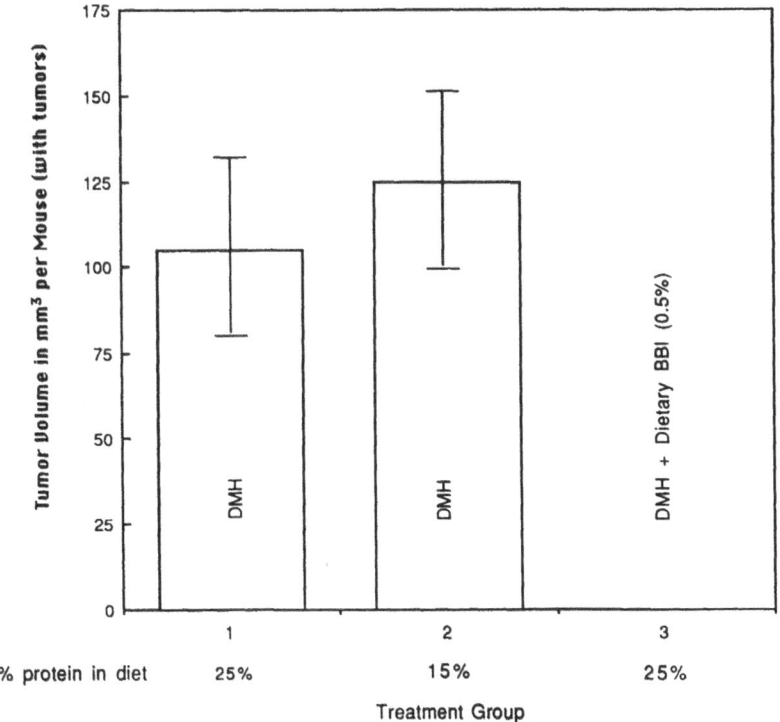

Figure 1. Results of our initial study performed to determine the effect of the Bowman–Birk inhibitor (BBI), given in the diet, on dimethylhydrazine (DMH)-induced adenomatous tumors of the colon and rectum. Details of this study are given in Weed *et al.* (1985).

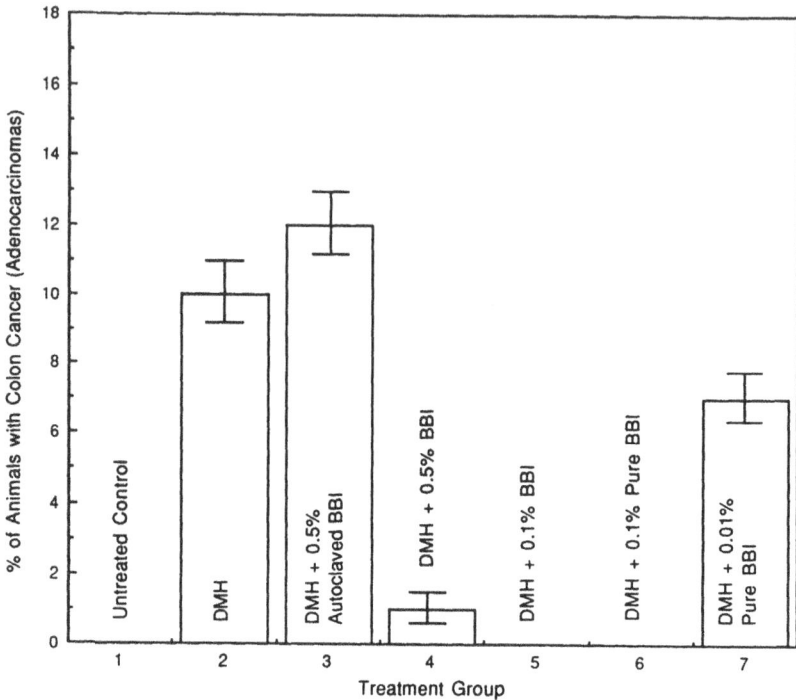

Figure 2. Effects of the BBI extract and pure BBI on DMH-induced adenocarcinomas of the gastrointestinal tract. BBI extract (0.1–0.5%) and 0.1% pure BBI suppress colon carcinogenesis, while 0.01% pure BBI did not have a significant suppressive effect on colon carcinogenesis in this study. It can be observed that BBI can completely prevent/suppress colon carcinogenesis induced by a low dose of DMH. Details of this study are given in St. Clair *et al.* (1990).

al., 1990b). BBI affected adenomatous tumors of the mouse colon which are histopathologically similar to those which occur in the most common form of human colon cancer. The types of gastrointestinal tract tumors studied are illustrated in Figs. 4–7. In the liver, BBI prevented the DMH-induced elevation in the incidence of angiosarcomas (St. Clair *et al.*, 1990), as shown in Fig. 8, as well as premalignant lesions (e.g., hyperplasia, as shown in Fig. 9). Oncogenic lesions of the liver are shown in Figs. 10–15. In both the colon and liver carcinogenesis studies, BBI was given in the diet.

In the oral carcinogenesis studies performed, BBI was topically applied to the hamster check pouch. In the initial study, we observed that the BBI extract (at 1.0% in a distilled water solution) suppressed oral carcinogenesis in a statistically significant fashion, as shown in Fig. 16. In other studies, pure BBI has been shown to suppress DMBA-induced oral carcinogenesis, and lower concentrations of the BBI extract (than previously studied) have been shown to have an

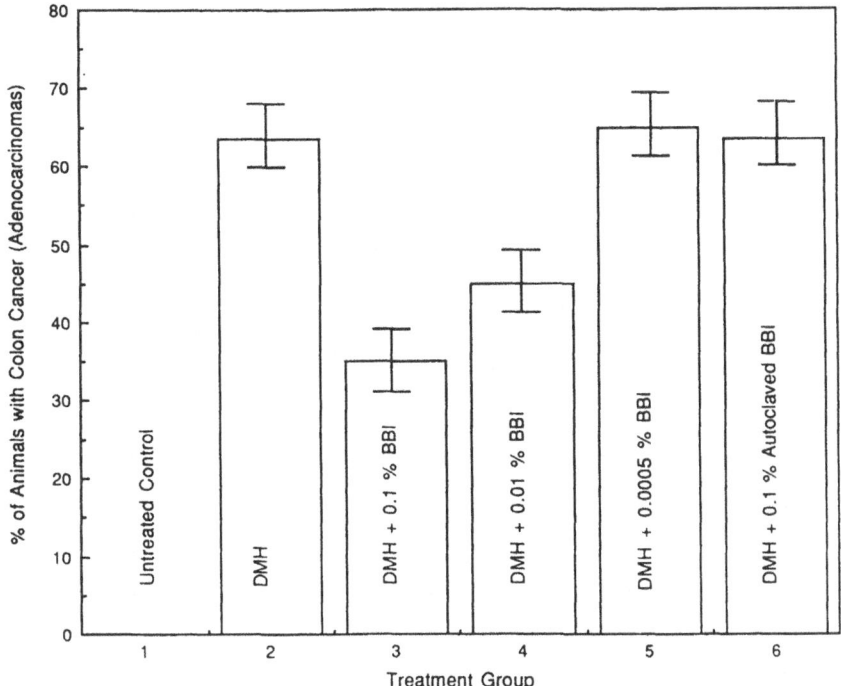

Figure 3. Suppressive effects of the BBI extract on DMH-induced adenocarcinomas. BBI 0.1% had a significant suppressive effect on colon carcinogenesis while the suppressive effect of 0.01% BBI was not statistically significant in this study. Details of this study are given in Billings *et al.* (1990b). BBI 0.1% suppressed the incidence of cancer by approximately one-half in this study in which a high carcinogen dose was utilized; with a lower carcinogen dose, BBI can totally prevent colon carcinogenesis, as shown in Figs. 1 and 2.

irreversible suppressive effect on carcinogenesis, even when given at a long time period after exposure to the carcinogenic agent. These data are shown in histogram form in Fig. 17 (from Kennedy *et al.*, 1993).

In our lung carcinogenesis studies, BBI has been given primarily as i.p. injections. BBI has been shown to reduce the percentage of animals bearing lung tumors, as well as the number of lung tumors per animal, as shown in Fig. 23. In one experiment, the suppression of tumorigenesis was compared when BBI was given i.p. versus p.o. The results suggested that the same amount of BBI given p.o. was about one-half as effective as observed for the i.p. route of administration; these results are shown in Fig. 24. A typical rodent lung tumor of the sort studied in our lung tumorigenesis experiments is shown in Fig. 25.

Before beginning our tumor induction experiments in the esophagus, we considered various ways of increasing the uptake of BBI into esophageal epithelial cells. We believed that we achieved optimal delivery of the BBI into the

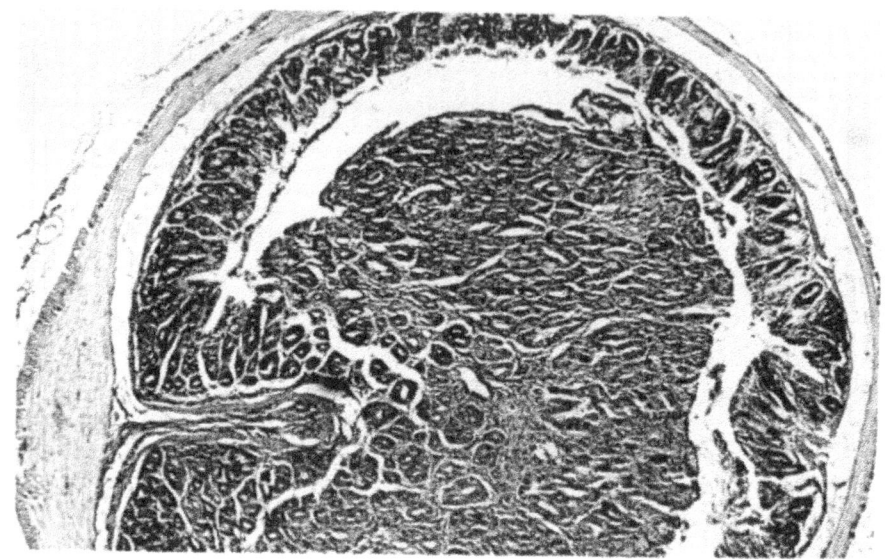

Figure 4. Adenomatous tumor of the colon in CD-1 male mouse treated with DMH. (×45)

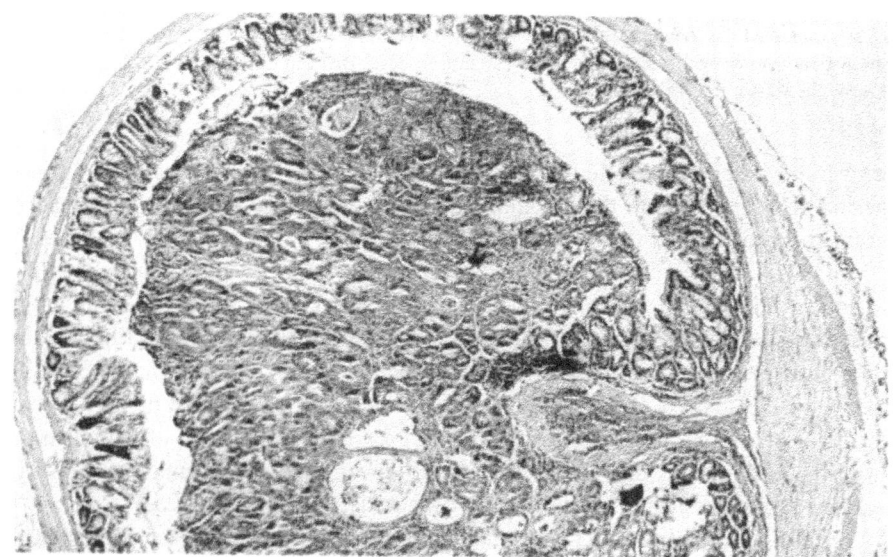

Figure 5. Adenomatous tumor of the colon in CD-1 male mouse treated with DMH. (×45)

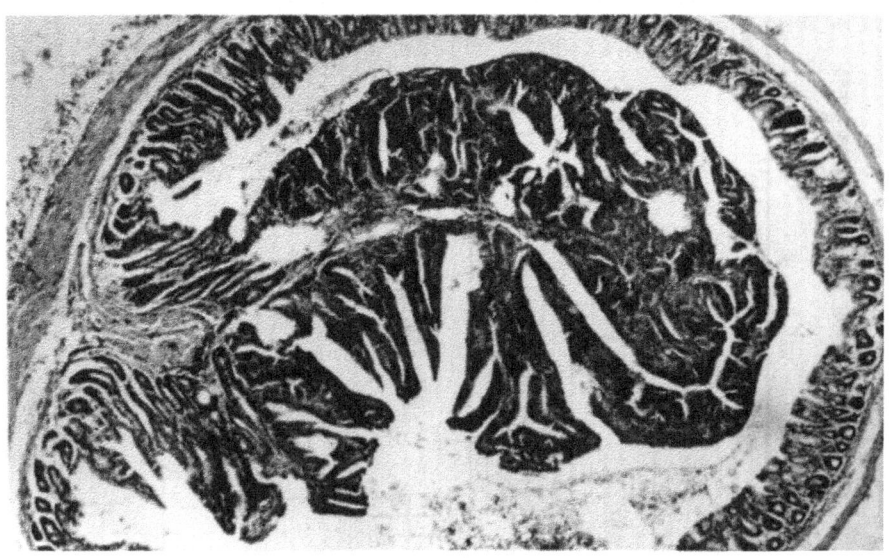

Figure 6. Adenomatous tumor of the colon in CD-1 male mouse treated with DMH. (×30)

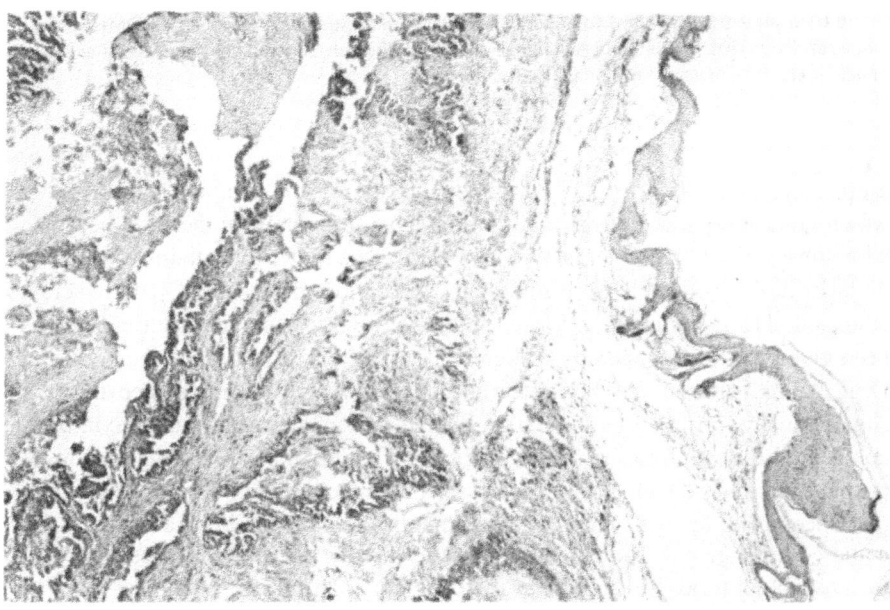

Figure 7. Anal gland squamous carcinoma (with invasive characteristics) in CD-1 male mouse treated with DMH. (×45)

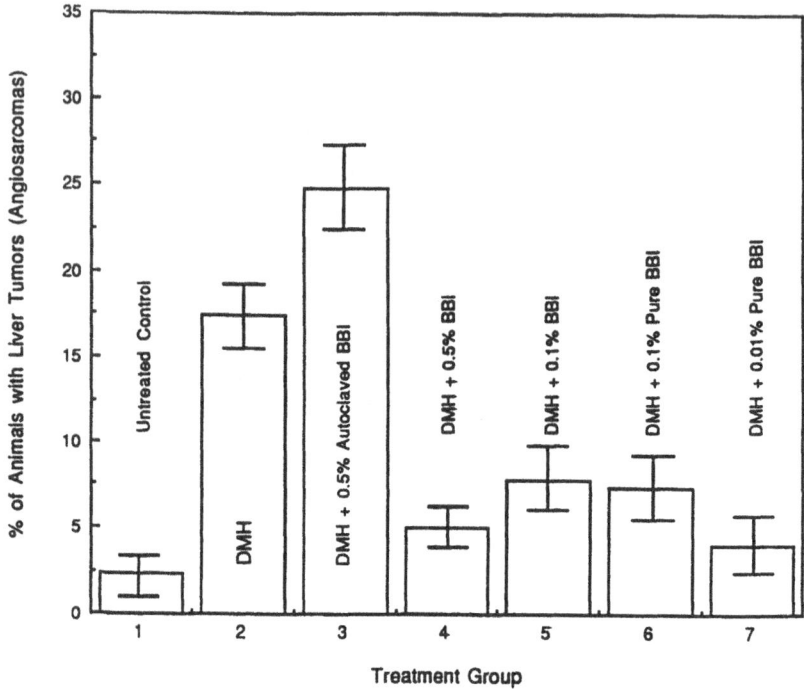

Figure 8. Suppression of DMH-induced angiosarcomas of the liver by 0.1–0.5% BBI extract and 0.1–0.01% pure BBI. While 0.01% pure BBI did not have a significant effect on DMH-induced colon carcinogenesis in this study (see Fig. 2), it did significantly suppress the incidence of angiosarcomas in the liver. Details are given in St. Clair *et al.* (1990).

esophageal epithelial cells of rats by incorporating the inhibitor into a tablet which rats ate separately from their normal laboratory chow in these studies. The base substance of the tablet is Witepsol H15. This material contains mono- and diglycerides of vegetable fatty acids and triglycerides of C_{12} and C_{18} fatty acids. Witepsol H15 is commercially used in the formulation of suppositories and has been given a GRAS (generally recognized as safe) classification by the Food and Drug Administration. As this material melts at 37°C, it was deemed the best suited for providing a coating action over the esophagus and thus maximizing contact of the inhibitor with the esophageal epithelium. A small amount of peanut butter was also included in the tablet to make it more palatable to the rats. (The peanut butter was shown not to contain protease inhibitor activity which could complicate our studies.) Animals received one tablet three times a week in the absence of food (i.e., food was removed at 9:00 a.m., the tablet was given at 10:00 a.m., and the normal chow was returned at 4:00 p.m., after the tablet had been eaten). The specific formulation of the tablet is given in Table II. In our first experiment, the amount of BBI in each tablet was calculated to be such that the

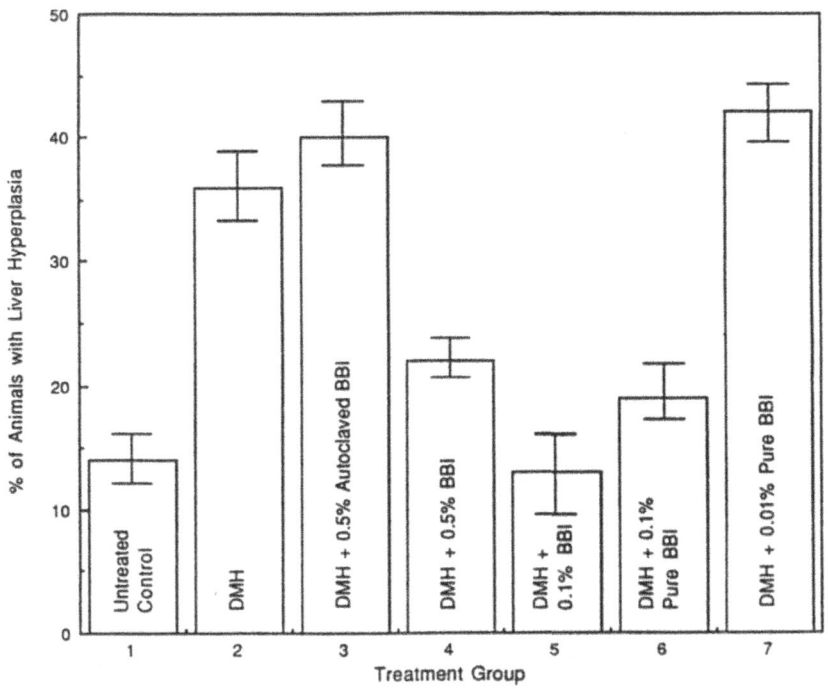

Figure 9. Suppressive effects of 0.1–0.5% BBI extract and 0.1% pure BBI on hyperplasia in the liver induced by DMH. As can be observed, BBI is capable of suppressing the incidence of lesions considered "premalignant." Details are given in St. Clair *et al.* (1990).

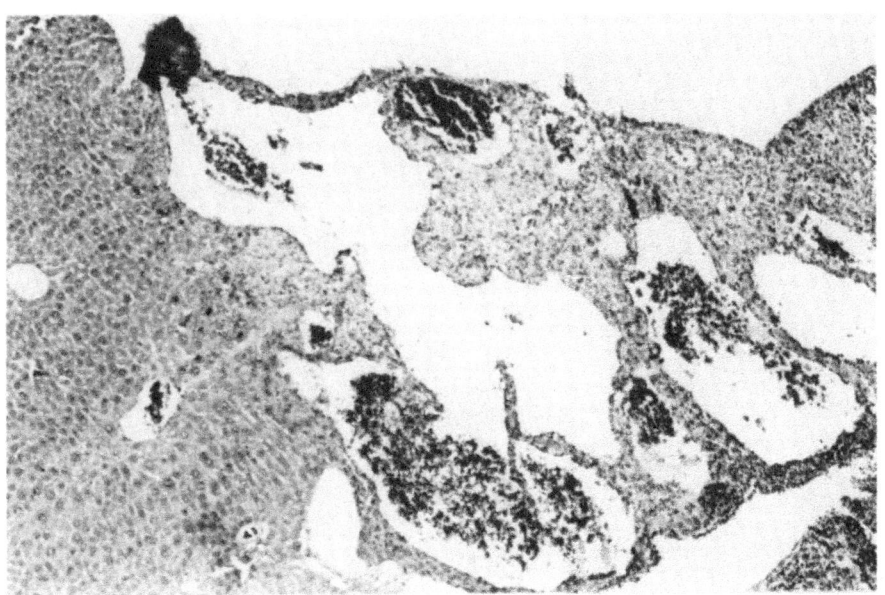

Figure 10. Angiosarcoma of the liver in a DMH-treated mouse. (×45)

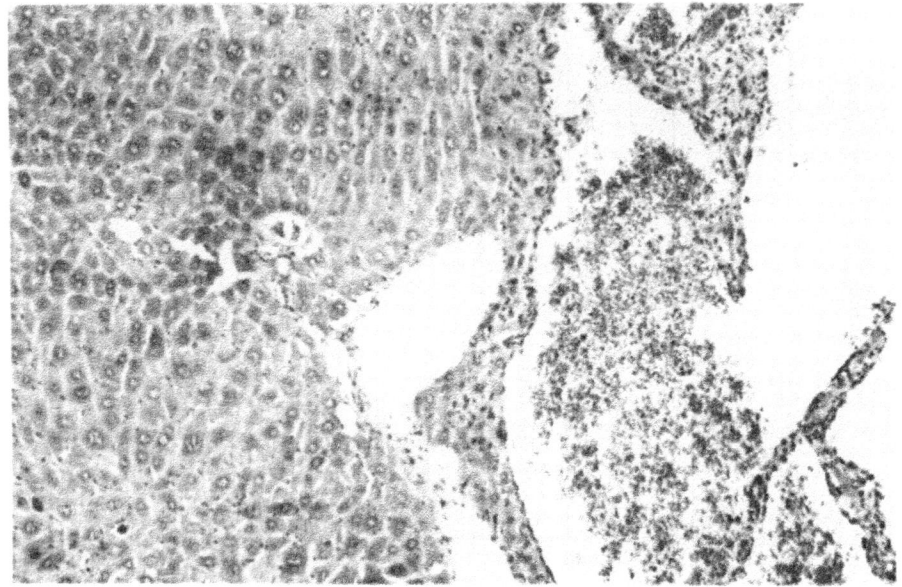

Figure 11. Higher-power view of angiosarcoma shown in Fig. 10. (×90)

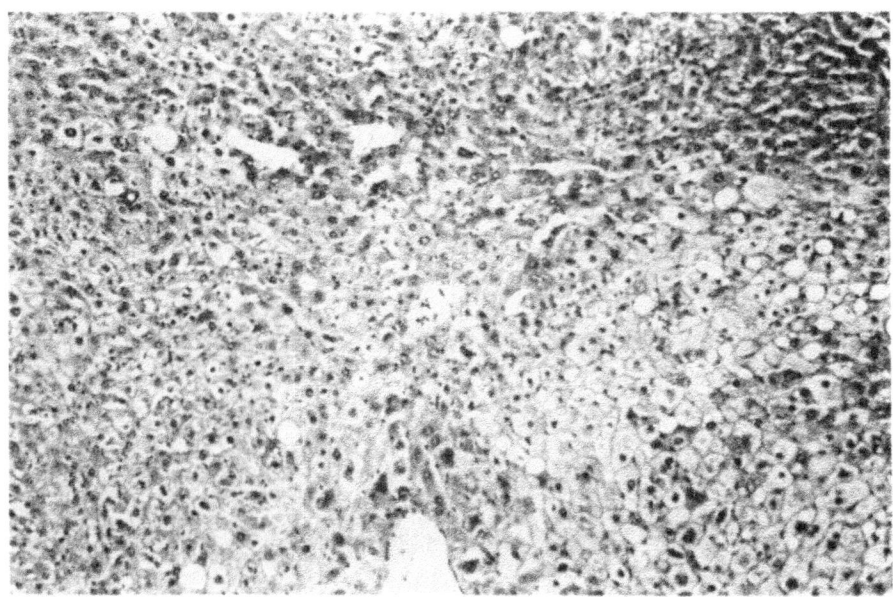

Figure 12. Angiosarcoma and nodular hyperplasia in the liver of a DMH-treated mouse. (×90)

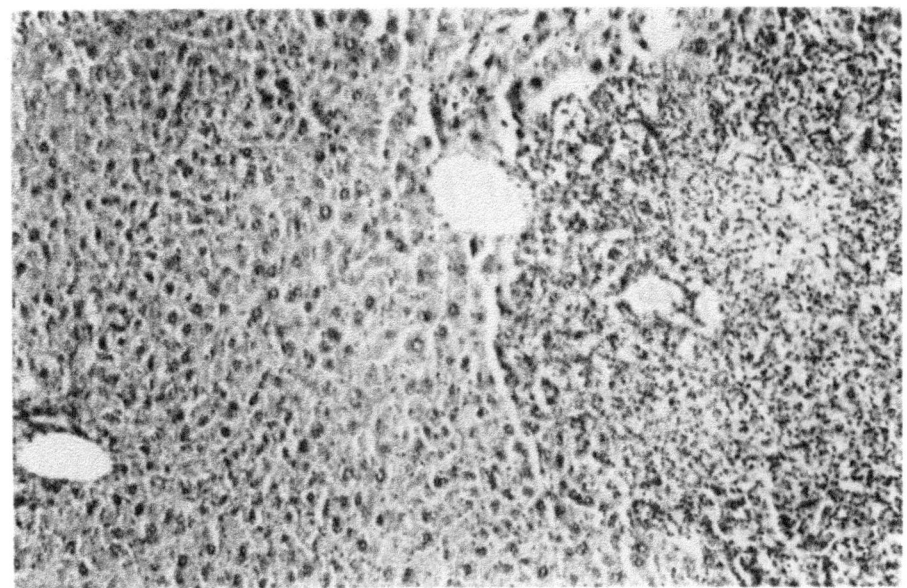

Figure 13. Nodular hyperplasia in the liver of a DMH-treated mouse. (×45)

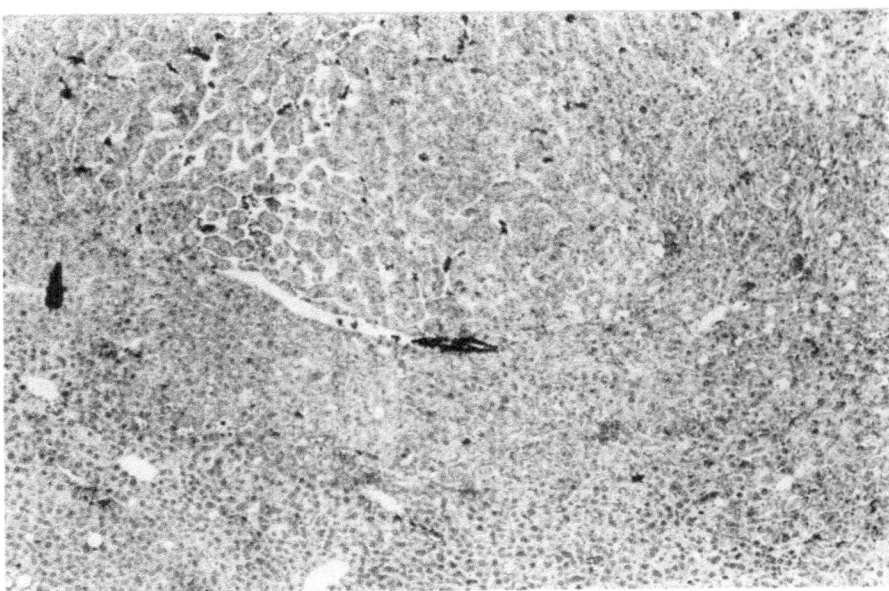

Figure 14. Hepatocellular carcinoma in the liver of a DMH-treated mouse. (×90)

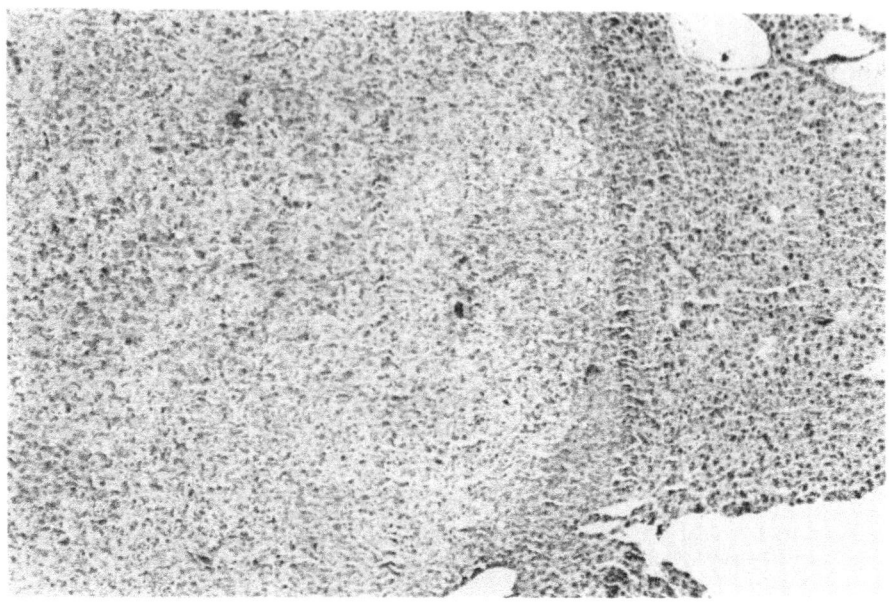

Figure 15. Hepatocellular carcinoma in a DMH-treated mouse. (×90)

rats received a comparable dose of BBI (over the period of the experiment) to that which they would receive from BBI when administered as 0.5% of their diet.

Since Witepsol has already been approved for human use (and has, in fact, already been in use for a relatively long time), it seemed to be a particularly useful substance for our studies designed to develop a way to deliver protease inhibitors to the cells at risk for the development of esophageal cancer.

The results of our studies on esophageal carcinogenesis are given in Table III and Fig. 26; esophageal cancers are shown in Figs. 27–29. In our experiments, we observed a suppressive effect of BBI on both premalignant lesions and tumors of the esophagus in MBNA-treated rats. It is of interest that we observed less "lymphocytic infiltrate" in the BBI-treated animals (Table III and Fig. 26). These results are consistent with results noted earlier in our colon carcinogenesis studies described in St. Clair *et al.* (1990); the protease inhibitor-treated animals had fewer "extensive lymphoid aggregates" than observed in control animals exposed to DMH alone. These results from our colon carcinogenesis studies are shown in Table IV.

These results of ours suggest that pure BBI and the BBI extract may be anti-inflammatory.* It has been shown previously that certain protease inhibitors have

---

*These preparations may not be anti-inflammatory, however. There may be less "lymphocytic infiltrate" etc. in the animals of the carcinogen/BBI treatment groups (compared with carcinogen-only treatment groups) simply because there are fewer tumors in these groups and the tumors are capable of eliciting an immune response.

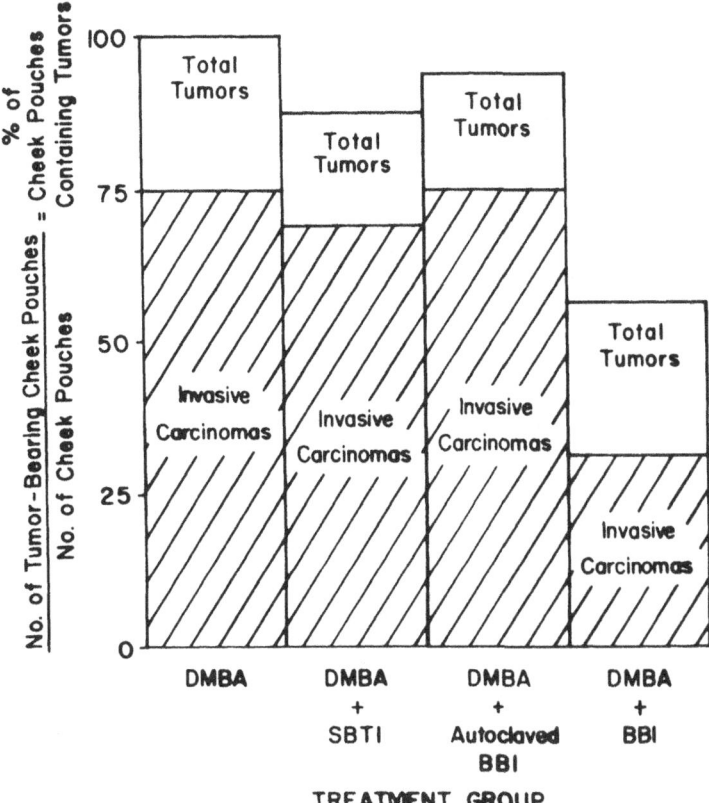

Figure 16. Suppressive effect of BBI on oral carcinogenesis induced in hamsters by dimethyl-benz(*a*)anthracene (DMBA). SBTI, soybean trypsin inhibitor; BBI, Bowman–Birk inhibitor; auto-claved BBI, Bowman–Birk inhibitor preparation in which protease inhibitor activity has been de-stroyed by heat. Note lack of effect of SBTI and autoclaved BBI on oral carcinogenesis. Details of these studies are given in Messadi *et al.* (1986).

anti-inflammatory properties (Goldstein *et al.*, 1979; Witz *et al.*, 1980; Troll *et al.*, 1982). This effect on the immune system from the BBI extract does not affect the survival level of animals; animals maintained on the BBI extract for essen-tially their entire life span had the same survival level as observed for animals maintained on the same diet lacking the BBI addition (Weed *et al.*, 1985; Ken-nedy, unpublished data).

In all of our studies with BBI, the possible anti-inflammatory property is the only potential side effect which we have observed. This potential side effect may be viewed as a positive one. The anticarcinogenic protease inhibitors have been shown to inhibit inflammation specifically associated with tumor promotion (Goldstein *et al.*, 1979; Witz *et al.*, 1980; Troll *et al.*, 1982), which is a stage of carcinogenesis subject to inhibition; thus, the inhibition of promotion by protease inhibitors may be viewed as a beneficial effect. Thus far, no investigators have

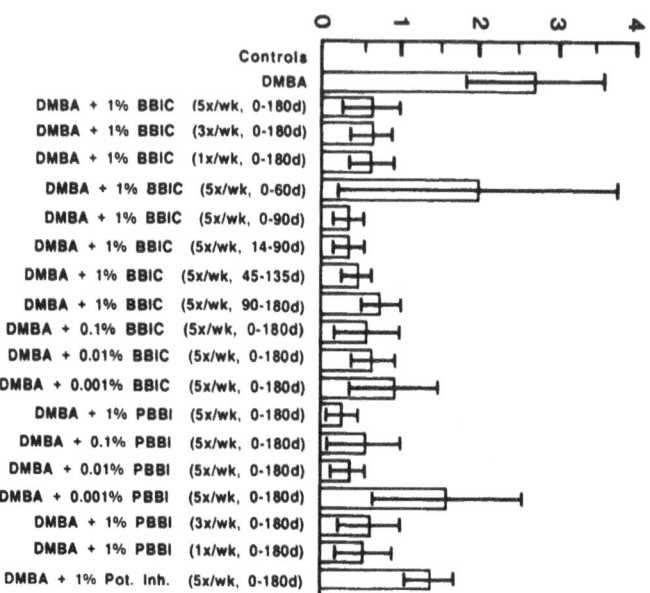

Figure 17. Results of study performed to determine further information about the suppressive effects of the purified BBI (PBBI) and the BBI-containing extract (BBIC) on DMBA-induced oral carcinogenesis in hamsters. In this study, it was observed that BBIC and PBBI were capable of suppressing carcinogenesis at concentrations ranging from 1 to 0.01% and were equally effective when given as a 1% solution 5 times per week, 3 times per week, or once per week. Given as a 1% solution, BBIC was effective at suppressing oral carcinogenesis when given at the following times during the assay period: 0–180, 0–90, 14–90, and 45–135 days. Thus, BBI treatment can be given long after carcinogen exposure and still have an irreversible suppressive effect on the carcinogenic process. Details of these experiments are given in Kennedy *et al.* (1993).

shown effects of BBI on the normal function of cells of the immune system (Goldfarb *et al.*, 1989). Other potential side effects which have been of concern to us have been adverse effects on animal growth and on the pancreas: concerns about these side effects were discussed in Section 2.

Our experiments, as well as those of other investigators (Becker, 1981; Corasanti *et al.*, 1982), have not shown weight loss at anticarcinogenic levels of soybean protease inhibitors in the diet. Given the potential problems with trypsin inhibition, however, we have carefully evaluated body weight and the pancreas/body weight ratio in all of our studies involving animals treated with BBI (and other protease inhibitors), and have found that protease inhibitor treatment has not altered these parameters in our studies while serving as an anticarcino-

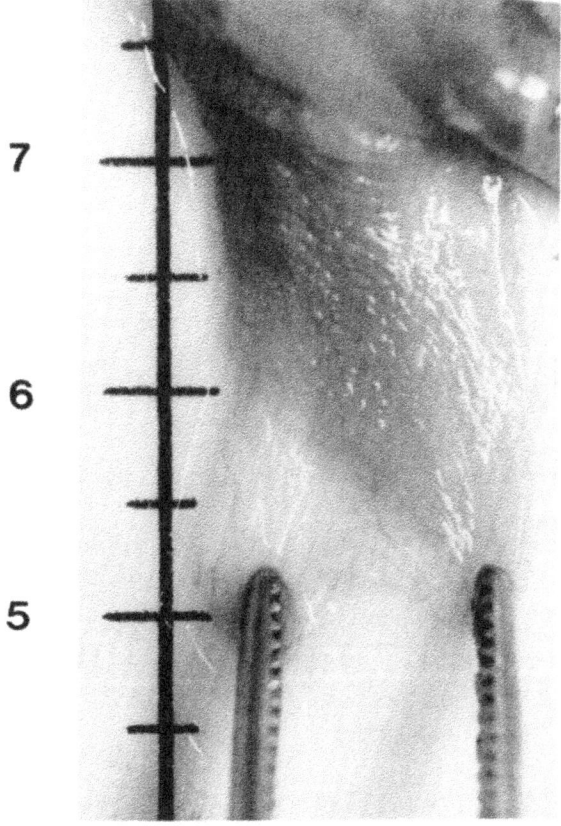

Figure 18. Normal (untreated) hamster cheek pouch.

genic agent. Growth charts for some of the animals in our carcinogenesis studies are shown in Figs. 30–32. Pancreas/body weight ratios are given in several of our publications on animal carcinogenesis; an example of data on pancreas/body weight ratios is shown in Fig. 33. Histopathological analysis of the pancreata of the animals has shown no effects due to protease inhibitor treatment in any of our long-term experiments.

In summary, our work has shown that pure BBI and the extract of soybeans containing BBI have anticarcinogenic activity at nontoxic levels. BBI has also been shown to have anticarcinogenic activity *in vitro* at nontoxic levels (Yavelow *et al.*, 1983, 1985; Kennedy, 1985; Baturay and Kennedy, 1986; Kennedy *et al.*, 1984). None of our *in vitro* studies have shown toxicity of pure BBI or the BBI extract at any level studied (Yavelow *et al.*, 1983, 1985; Kennedy, 1985; Baturay and Kennedy, 1986; Kennedy *et al.*, 1984). The only toxicity attributable to BBI

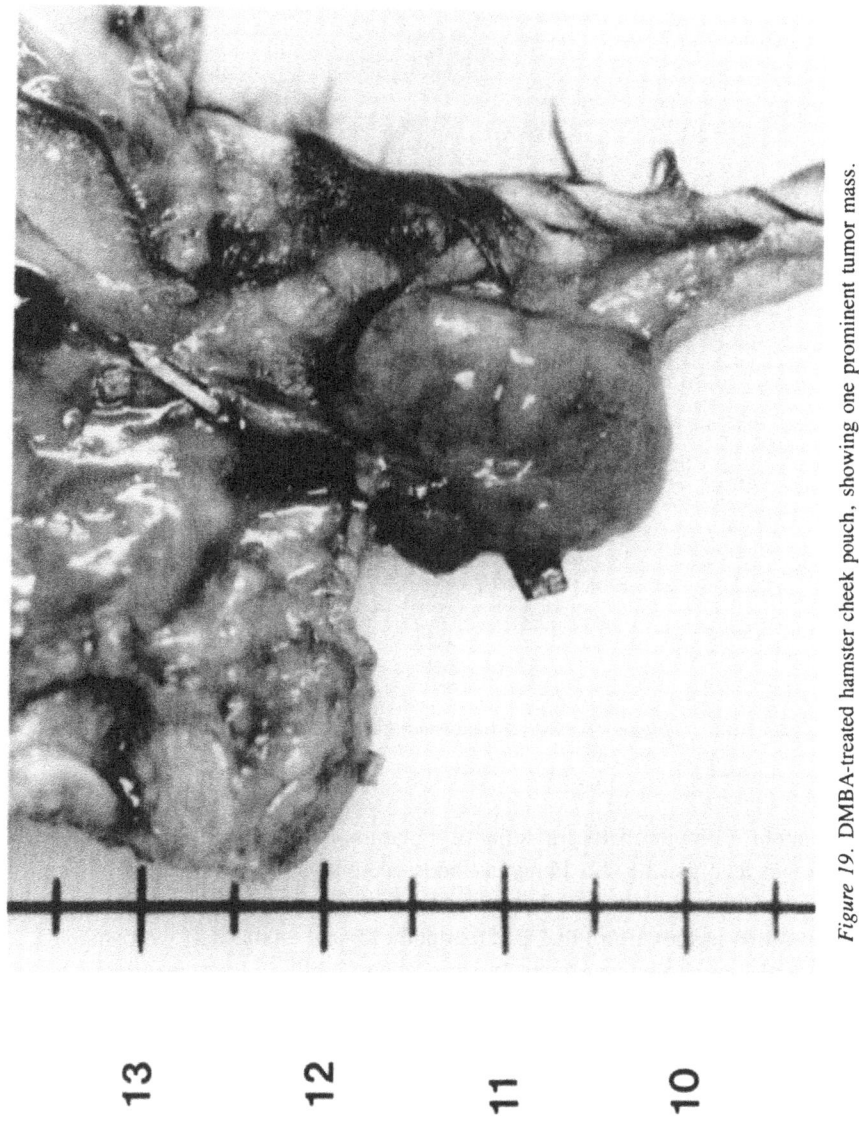

Figure 19. DMBA-treated hamster cheek pouch, showing one prominent tumor mass.

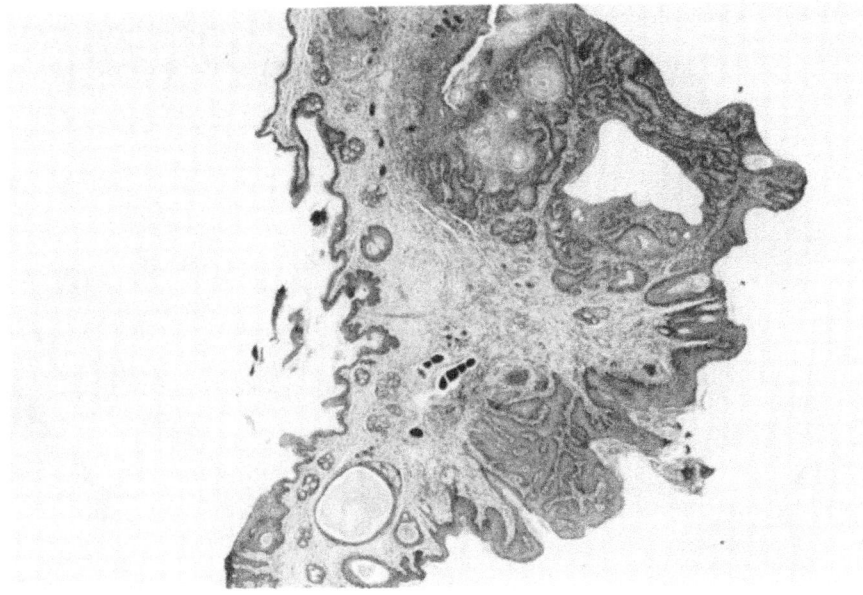

Figure 20. Invasive squamous cell carcinoma in cheek pouch of hamster treated with DMBA. (×25)

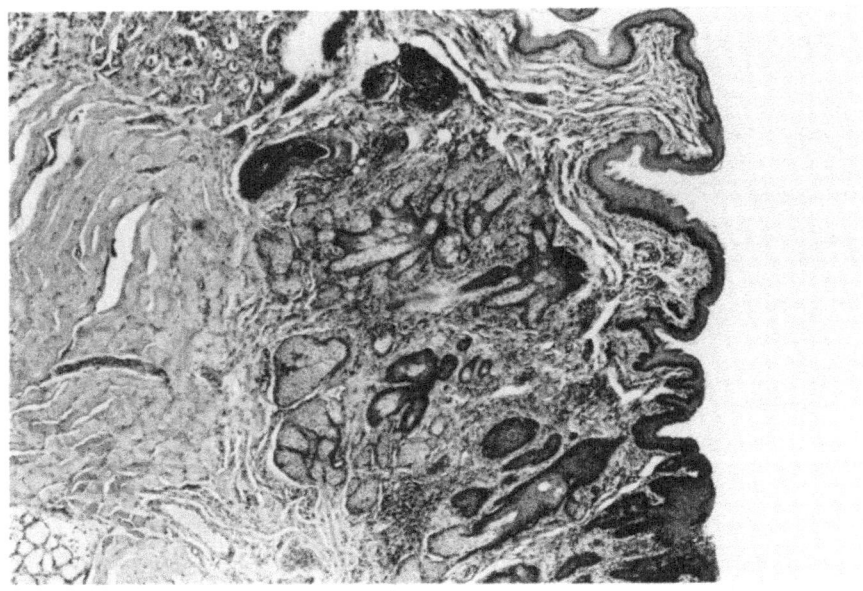

Figure 21. Invasive squamous cell carcinoma in cheek pouch of hamster treated with DMBA. (×25)

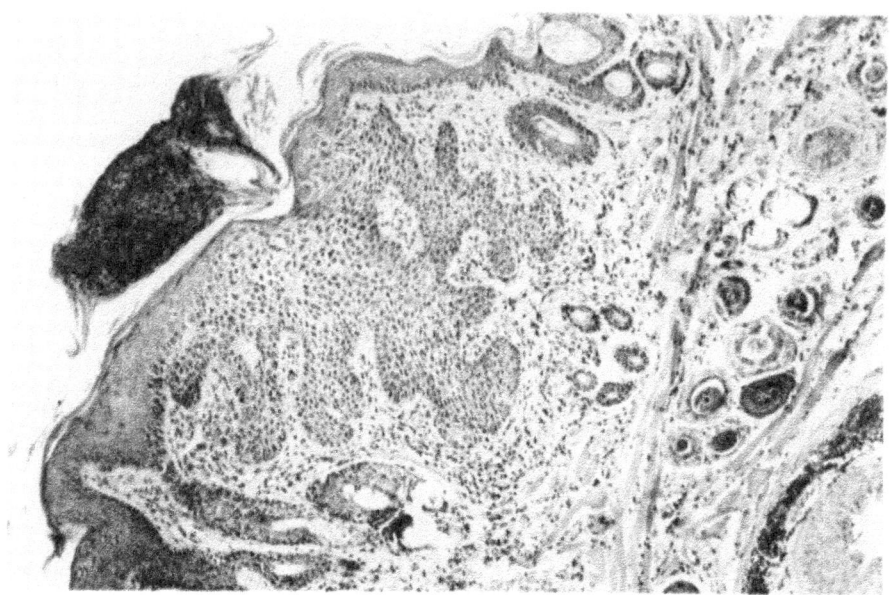

Figure 22. Cheek pouch hyperplasia in DMBA-treated hamster. (×90)

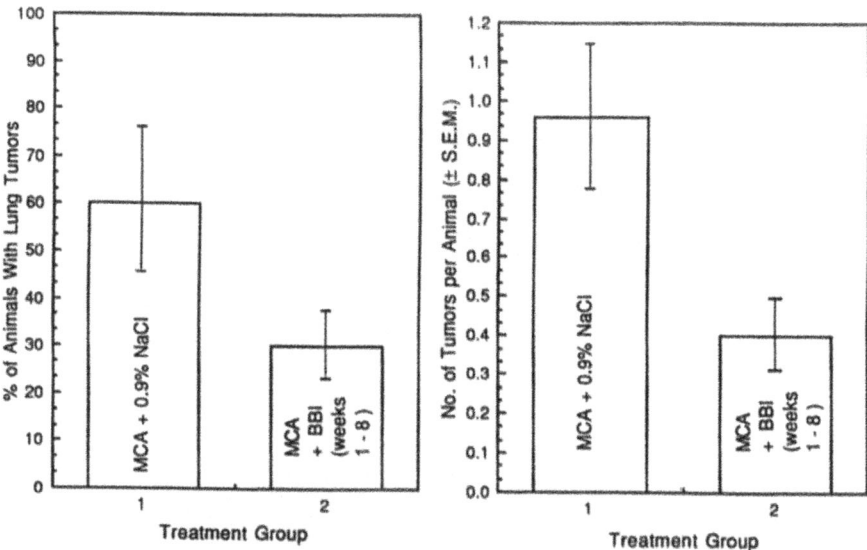

Figure 23. BBI suppression of lung tumorigenesis induced by 3-methylcholanthrene (MCA) in strain A mice. BBI was capable of suppressing both the percentage of animals bearing lung tumors and the number of lung tumors per animal. Details of this study are given in Witschi and Kennedy (1989).

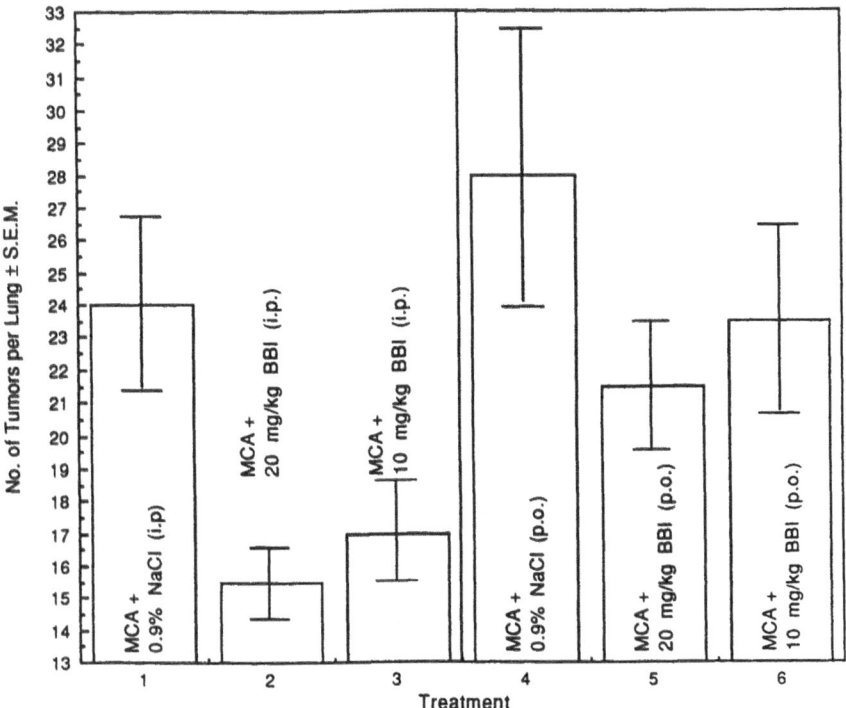

Figure 24. Results of lung tumorigenesis study in which BBI was given as i.p. injections or p.o. From these results, it is believed that a dose of 20 mg/kg BBI p.o. is comparable to a dose of 10 mg/kg BBI i.p., in terms of effectiveness as an anticarcinogenic agent in the lung. Details are given in Witschi and Kennedy (1989).

which has been observed in any of our BBI studies was in our teratogenesis studies. In these studies, a high level of BBI was shown to be toxic to the developing fetus while having no apparent effect on the pregnant mice; in these same studies, nontoxic levels of protease inhibitors (BBI and antipain) were shown to prevent some birth abnormalities and have no effect on the incidence of other birth defects (von Hofe *et al.*, 1990). In these studies of ours on the antiteratogenic effects of BBI (von Hofe *et al.*, 1990) and in several of our previous studies on the suppression of lung tumorigenesis by BBI (Witschi and Kennedy, 1989), BBI was injected into animals (i.p.) with no apparent problems. [In our lung carcinogenesis studies, many i.p. injections of BBI were given over periods of several weeks, and no toxicity was apparent (Witschi and Kennedy, 1989).] Thus, the only BBI toxicity that has been observed involves a toxic effect on the fetus during the early part of pregnancy (following i.p. injection into pregnant mice).

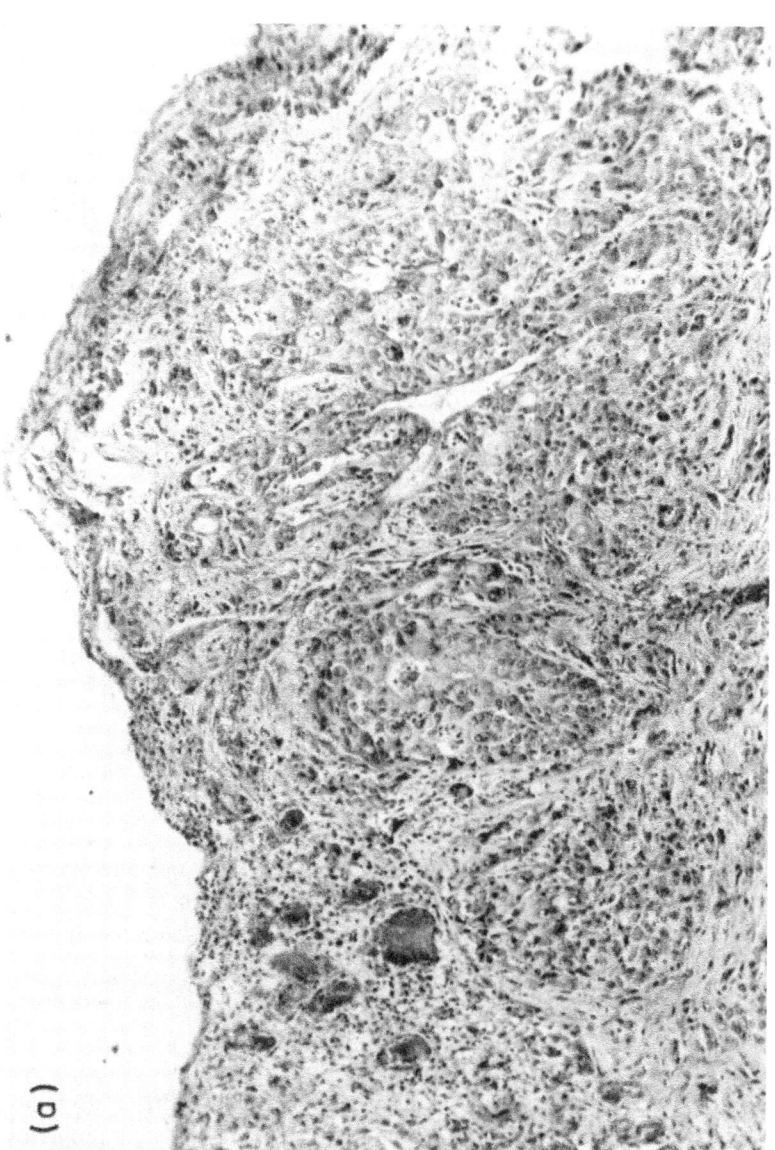

(a)

Figure 25. Peripheral rodent lung tumor of the sort studied by Witschi and Kennedy (1989). In the portion of the tumor shown in panel (a), there is acinar formation and some mucus production. In another part of the tumor, shown in panel (b), the pattern is predominantly epidermoid, with keratin pearls.

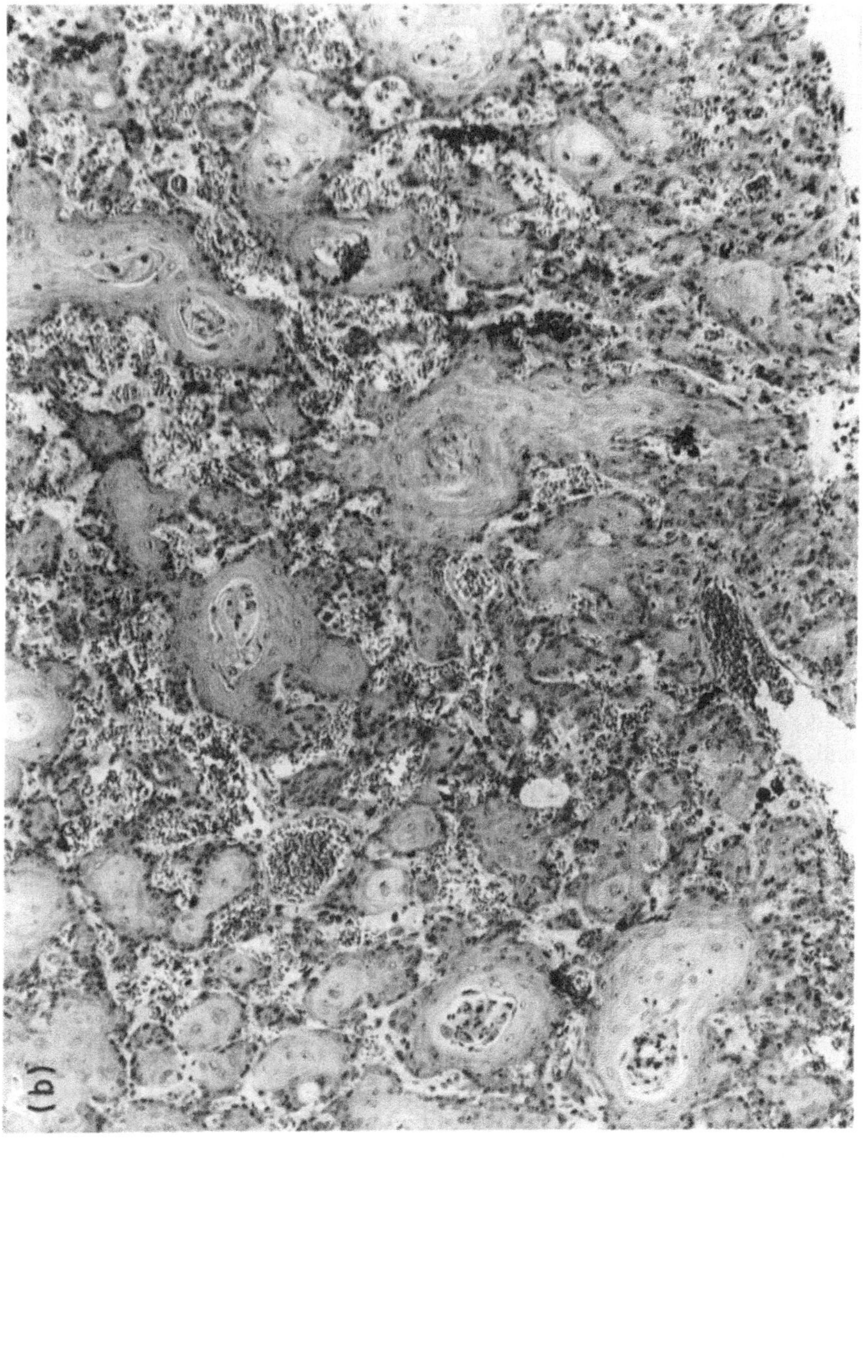

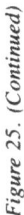

(b)

Figure 25. (Continued)

Table II. Tablets Utilized in the Study
of MBNA-Induced Rat Esophageal Carcinogenesis

	Ingredients	mg/tablet
Bowman–Birk inhibitor (inactivated)	Bowman–Birk inhibitor (inactivated)	180
	Peanut butter	100
	Witepsol H15	720
		1000 mg
Bowman–Birk inhibitor	Bowman–Birk inhibitor	180
	Peanut butter	100
	Witepsol H15	720
		1000 mg

3.2. Limitations of BBI as a Human Cancer Chemopreventive Agent

We have previously shown that BBI, when ingested in the diet, reaches the colon in an active form, but that very little is taken up into the bloodstream and delivered to other organ systems (Yavelow *et al.*, 1983). Thus, we believe that BBI (or our extract containing BBI) could be used effectively as a dietary additive to inhibit carcinogenesis in the gastrointestinal (GI) tract at the present time, but that there may not be sufficient amounts of BBI getting to organs outside of the GI tract via this route of administration. To increase the amount of anticarcinogenic protease inhibitor reaching other organs, we are performing research based on the following approaches: (1) modify BBI such that more of the compound is taken up by the GI epithelium and (2) design a smaller (i.e., lower molecular weight) protease inhibitor which will be taken up more readily into the bloodstream. We now have data which suggest that a modified version of BBI is potentially useful in our future studies. BBI covalently attached to polylysine (which is known to increase the uptake of high-molecular-weight compounds into cells) works as effectively at inhibiting *in vitro* transformation as does native BBI (Persiani *et al.*, 1991). In our distribution studies, we have observed that considerably more BBI–polylysine is present in the lungs than native BBI (Persiani *et al.*, 1991); studies to determine whether BBI–polylysine is an improved anticarcinogenic agent for the lungs are in progress.

In addition, there is evidence that smaller versions of BBI will be effective as a chemopreventive agent. There is a published procedure by which the halves of BBI can be obtained using a chemical procedure (Birk, 1975; Ikenaka *et al.*, 1974; Odani and Ikenaka, 1973). The two separate halves of BBI have been obtained by us from Dr. Yehudith Birk (Hebrew University, Israel) and we have observed that the BBI half containing the chymotrypsin inhibitory site has retained all of the activity of whole BBI to inhibit radiation transformation, while

Table III. Effect of BBI on MBNA-Induced Esophageal Carcinogenesis in Rats

Treatment group	Lesions and S.E.	Esophageal lesions[a]								
		Hyperker.	Paraker.	Sim. Hyp.	Pap. Hyp.	Dysplasia	Lym. Inf.	Papillomas (A)	Carcinomas (B)	A + B
1. MBNA (34 rats)	Total No. of lesions	93	41	110	67	60	90	54	11	65
	Average No. of lesions/rat	2.76	1.21	3.24	1.97	1.76	2.65	1.59	0.32	1.91
	S.E.	0.21	0.17	0.22	0.21	0.24	0.22	0.19	0.10	0.24
2. MBNA + BBI (34 rats)	Total No. of lesions	58	34	63	46	38	56	30	6	36
	Average No. of lesions/rat	1.71[b]	1.00[c]	1.85[d]	1.35[c]	1.12[e]	1.65[f]	0.88[g]	0.18[c]	1.06[h]
	S.E.	0.15	0.15	0.15	0.15	0.13	0.15	0.16	0.07	0.18

[a] Abbreviations: Hyperker., hyperkeratosis; Paraker., parakeratosis; Sim. Hyp., simple hyperplasia; Pap. Hyp., papillary hyperplasia; Lym. Inf., Lymphocytic infiltrate.
[b] $p < 0.0005$ (t-test for two independent samples).
[c] $p > 0.05$.
[d] $p < 0.000005$.
[e] $p < 0.05$.
[f] $p < 0.0005$.
[g] $p < 0.005$.
[h] $p < 0.01$.

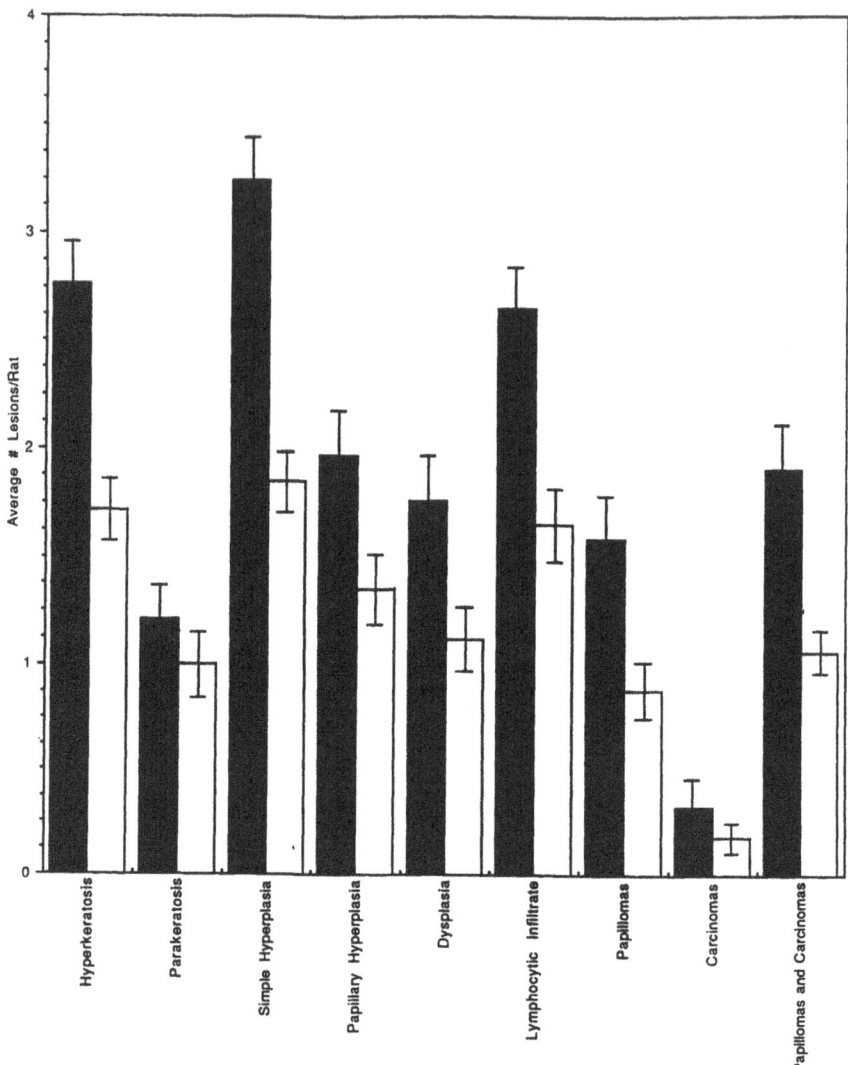

Figure 26. BBI extract suppression of esophageal carcinogenesis. BBI was observed to inhibit both premalignant lesions and tumors in the esophagus. Details are given in Table III (■, MBNA, mean ± standard error; □, MBNA + BBI, mean ± standard error) (von Hofe, Newberne, and Kennedy, 1991).

the trypsin inhibitor half of BBI does not have the ability to affect transformation. Even "half" of BBI is still quite large, however; we believe that a considerably smaller protease inhibitor will be necessary to serve as an ideal cancer chemopreventive agent. The design of smaller protease inhibitors is theoretically feasible, as we have shown that low-molecular-weight compounds (tripeptide analogues;

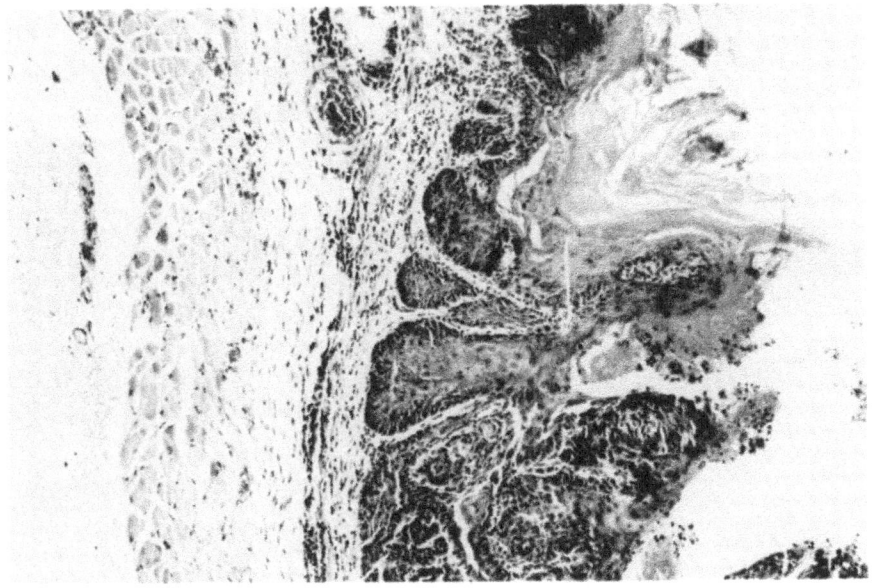

Figures 27–29. Invasive cancers of the esophagus in MBNA-treated rats. (×90)

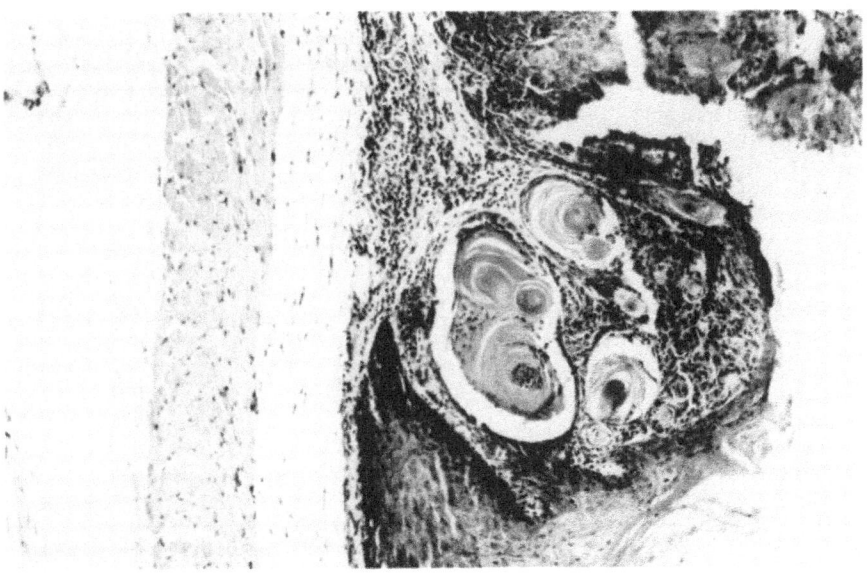

Figure 28

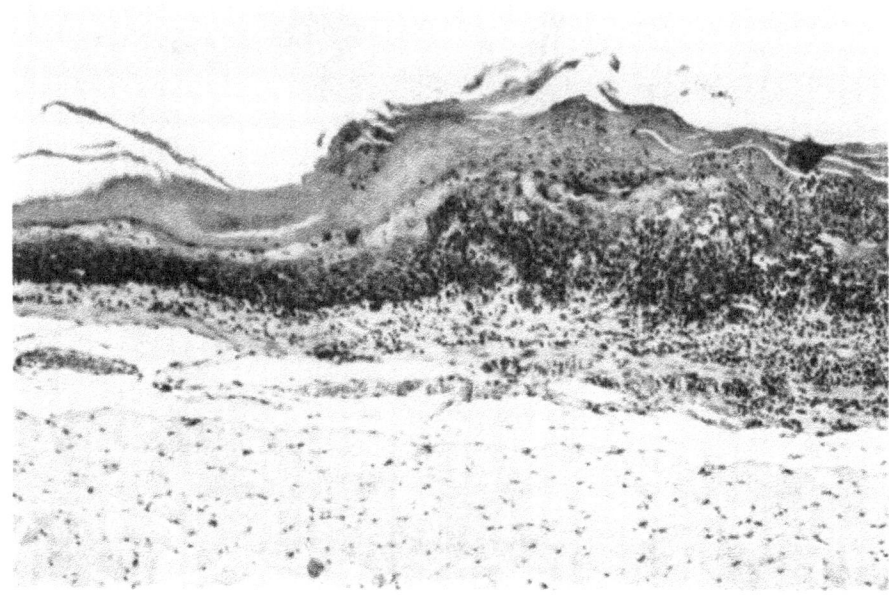

Figure 29

Table IV. BBI Suppression of Extensive Lymphoid Aggregates
and Colon Carcinogenesis Induced by Dimethylhydrazine[a]

Treatment	Yield of malignant tumors (adenocarcinomas)[b]	Colon extensive lymphoid aggregates[c]
1. Control (no treatment)	0/38	1/38 = 0.03
2. 0.1% PBBI	0/10	0/10
3. 0.5% BBI	0/54	2/54 = 0.04
4. 0.1% BBI	0/5	0/5
DMH groups		
5. DMH	6/62 = 0.10	5/62 = 0.08
6. DMH + BBI (auto-claved)	2/25 = 0.08	1/25 = 0.04
7. DMH + 0.5% BBI	1/92 = 0.01	3/92 = 0.03
8. DMH + 0.1% BBI	0/24	0/24
9. DMH + SBBI (suc-cinylated)	2/28 = 0.07	0/28
10. DMH + 0.1% PBBI	0/27	0/27
11. DMH + 0.01% PBBI	3/27 = 0.11	1/27 = 0.04

[a]Total number of lesions/total number of animals in group or total number of animals with lesions/total number of animals in group.
[b]Statistical analysis (χ^2): Groups 5 versus 7, 5 versus 8, and 5 versus 10, $p < 0.05$.
[c]Statistical analysis (χ^2): Groups 5 versus 7, 8, and 10, $p < 0.05$.

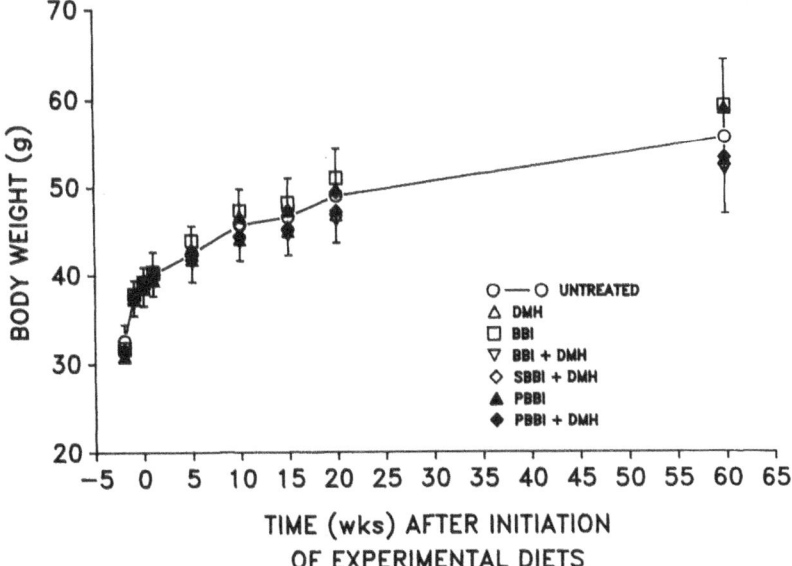

Figure 30. Growth charts for the animals on cancer chemopreventive diets containing protease inhibitors; none of the diets had an effect on animal body weight, while carcinogenesis was being suppressed in the colon (Fig. 2) and liver (Fig. 8). Details are given in St. Clair *et al.* (1990).

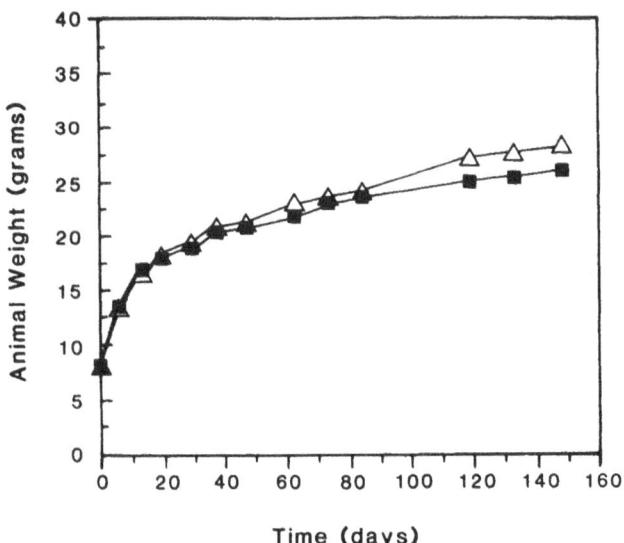

Figure 31. Results of a study performed to determine the effect of BBI on growth of irradiated animals (C57BL mice). Each point represents the average weight of 50 animals in each experimental group. □, x-ray treatment; △, x-ray treatment + 0.5% BBI extract. In this study, it is of interest that the average weights of the protease inhibitor-treated animals were actually somewhat higher than the non-protease inhibitor-treated animals.

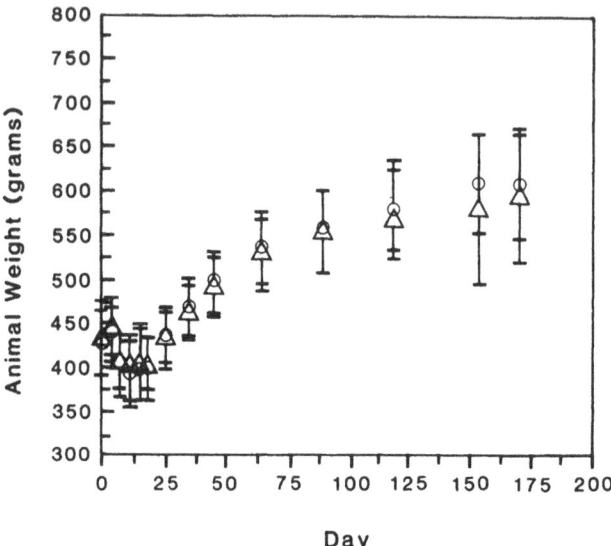

Figure 32. Growth charts of rats in experiments to determine whether BBI affected MBNA-induced esophageal carcinogenesis in rats. Rats received approximately 0.5% BBI (or autoclaved BBI in which all protease inhibitor activity was removed by autoclaving) in the diets. O, NMBzA + BBI; △, NMBzA + ABBI.

examples include chymostatin and antipain) can inhibit malignant transformation. It is worth pointing out that presently no protease inhibitor is commercially available which has "ideal" characteristics as a chemopreventive agent.

We believe that the important properties of our ideal protease inhibitor to be used as a cancer chemopreventive agent include the ability to inhibit transformation *in vitro,* chemical stability, water solubility, low molecular weight, the abilities to inhibit the enzyme chymotrypsin and to be internalized by cells (for a discussion of this, see Billings *et al.,* 1989), and the inability to inhibit the blood clotting process. BBI has all of these "ideal" properties except for its relatively high molecular weight.

4. Mechanism of Action of the Anticarcinogenic Protease Inhibitors

Many hypotheses have been proposed to explain the anticarcinogenic actions of protease inhibitors. As discussed in Chapter 3, we will not be able to determine the actual mechanism by which any cancer chemopreventive agent has its effect until the mechanism of carcinogenesis is determined with certainty. Our own hypotheses for the protease inhibitor suppressive effects on carcinogenesis include effects on specific oncogenes and specific proteases thought to be in-

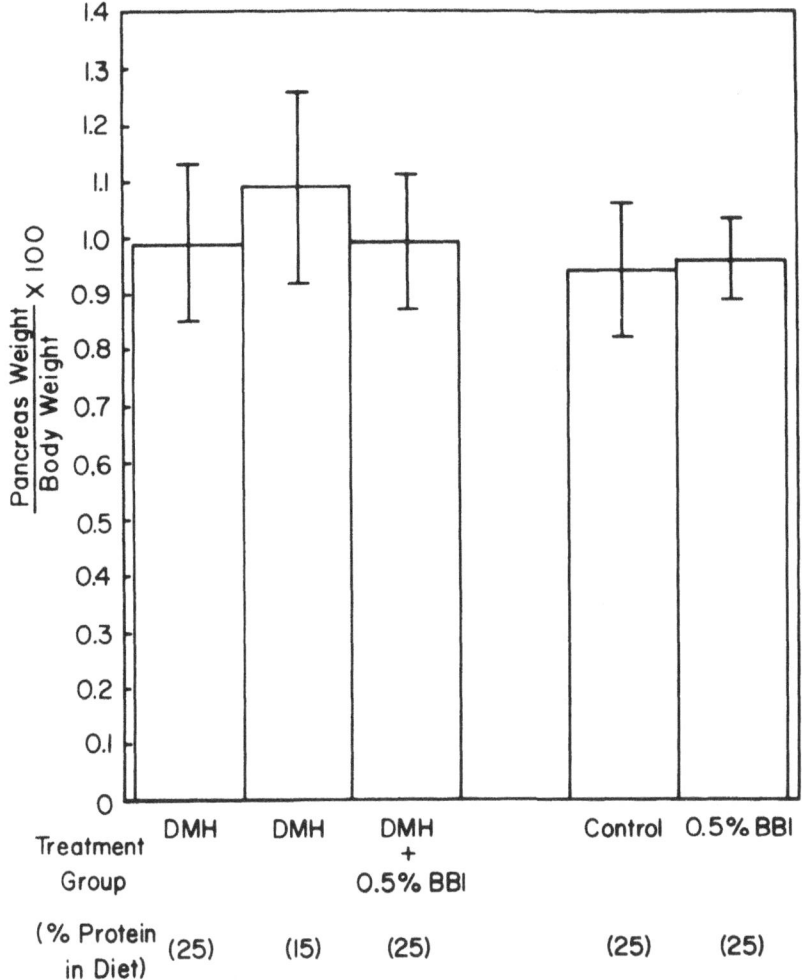

Figure 33. Lack of effect of anticarcinogenic BBI-containing diet on the pancreas/body weight ratio of animals in the study. Results of study by Weed *et al.* (1985).

volved in the conversion of a cell to malignancy, as discussed in Chapter 3. Our current thoughts on other proposed mechanisms of action of the anticarcinogenic protease inhibitors are presented briefly here.

Schelp and Pongpaew (1988) have proposed that elevated levels of endogenous protease inhibitors, in particular α_2-macroglobulin, serve to protect against carcinogenesis in those with diets low in calories, fat, and animal protein but high in vegetable content; it is thought that high levels of α_2-macroglobulin in such populations produce low cancer incidence rates for the colon, rectum, breast, and prostate. Data have been presented which indicate that α_2-macroglobulin levels do increase in response to diets which do not totally fulfill normal energy and protein requirements, as reviewed by Schelp and Pongpaew (1988). While this mechanism may operate for people in underdeveloped countries, as suggested by Schelp and Pongpaew, it does not explain the suppression of tumorigenesis in animal experiments in which the basal diets have fulfilled normal energy and protein requirements [as, e.g., in the studies by Becker (1981), Corasanti *et al.* (1982), Weed *et al.* (1985), Messadi *et al.* (1986), St. Clair *et al.* (1990), Witschi and Kennedy (1989), and Billings *et al.* (1990b)]. Thus, we believe that other mechanisms are responsible for the suppression of carcinogenesis by protease inhibitors in the animal experiments in which the animals have been maintained on diets sufficient for their energy and protein needs.

It has been proposed that protease inhibitors suppress carcinogenesis by their ability to prevent free radical-induced changes in cells as they have been shown to block free radical production in sea urchin eggs (Coburn *et al.*, 1981) and mammalian cells. It has been shown that certain protease inhibitors prevent the influx of polymorphonuclear leukocytes (PMN) as well as the release of free radicals by PMN in response to TPA (Goldstein *et al.*, 1979; Witz *et al.*, 1980; Troll *et al.*, 1982). The antipromotional characteristics of protease inhibitors have been specifically attributed to this effect. There is also some evidence that protease inhibitors can serve as antioxidants, through direct interactions with free radicals (Shasby, 1985). While there is much evidence to suggest that TPA may bring about its effects through the induction of free radicals (e.g., see Kennedy, 1986; Kennedy and Symons, 1987), it is difficult to explain the reversibility of promotion if free radical-produced effects are involved, since free radical effects are generally thought to be irreversible in nature. For example, free radicals are known to produce DNA damage, which can lead to mutations. [Radiation biology involves the study of effects attributed to free radical damage. The DNA-damaging and mutation-inducing characteristics of ionizing radiation are discussed in detail elsewhere; for example, see the BEIR V Report (1990).] Mutations are irreversible events which do not disappear when the inducing agent is removed. Promoting agents such as TPA have many reversible effects in cells that are thought to be involved in promotion, since promotion is known to be a reversible process (at least at early stages) (reviewed by Weinstein, 1978). (For a further discussion of the reversibility of promotion, see Kennedy, 1984). Thus, the early phase of promotion (or the second stage of "two-stage" carcinogenesis) is likely to be reversible in nature. While it is generally thought that the first stage of carcinogenesis is irreversible in nature (reviewed by Weinstein, 1978; Ryser, 1971), our own work suggests that the initiation phase of carcinogenesis is also reversible in nature, since it can be reversed by protease inhibitor treatment (see Chapter 3).

While the role of free radical-produced effects in carcinogenesis is still unclear, it is clear that certain anticarcinogenic protease inhibitors can prevent the release of O_2^- and H_2O_2 from PMN. The ability of a particular protease inhibitor to prevent the PMN respiratory burst is correlated with the ability of the protease inhibitor to prevent malignant transformation, with the ability to inhibit chymotrypsin being of some importance in both of these phenomena (e.g., see Kennedy, 1985; Frenkel et al., 1987). The connection between the ability of protease inhibitors to prevent malignant transformation and the respiratory burst in PMN is unknown.

It is possible that protease inhibitors could owe their anticarcinogenic activity to a selective toxicity for tumor cells. Noonan and Noonan (1977) reported that one protease inhibitor (TLCK) did show a selective toxicity for transformed cells. While selective toxicity could easily explain the anticarcinogenic activity of protease inhibitors, such selective toxicity for transformed cells by protease inhibitors has not been observed in our studies (e.g., see Kennedy and Little, 1981) or those of Kuroki and Drevon (1979).

Some protease inhibitors offer protection against radiation-induced lethality in vivo, as measured by survival levels in chickens and mice. The spectrum of protease inhibitors offering protection against radiation-induced mortality has suggested that a kallikrein-like enzyme (playing a role in vascular permeability) is likely to be involved in this effect (reviewed by Palladino et al., 1982). The spectrum of protease inhibitors serving as anticarcinogenic agents for radiation-induced transformation in vitro is quite different (see Chapter 3), suggesting that different processes are involved in these phenomena. The anticarcinogenic protease inhibitors do not affect the survival levels of cells irradiated in vitro in our studies (e.g., see Kennedy and Little, 1981).

It is widely assumed that cancer cells are capable of invading normal tissue through the action of proteases; thus, proteases and protease inhibitors have been studied extensively in cancer research, as reviewed by Quigley (1979). In general, malignant cells exhibit elevated proteolytic activity relative to normal cells (Quigley, 1979) and the sera of cancer patients exhibit abnormal levels of certain protease inhibitors (e.g., see Bernacka et al., 1988; Chawla et al., 1984; Nash et al., 1980). A natural assumption would be that certain protease inhibitors owe their anticarcinogenic activity to their ability to inhibit the proteases produced by malignant cells. While some protease inhibitors may have the ability to affect the proteases in malignant cells [e.g., see the inhibition of such proteases by diisopropyl phosphorofluoridate (Kaneko et al., 1986) and Chapter 12], the anticarcinogenic protease inhibitors discussed as cancer chemopreventive agents (i.e., those which suppress the process involved in the development of malignancy) do not affect the proteases most studied for their ability to invade normal tissue. For example, collagenases have long been associated with malignant cells and tumors (e.g., see Taylor et al., 1970; Dresden et al., 1972; Bauer et al., 1979). Type IV collagen-specific collagenase is thought to play an important role in invasion and metastasis (Sheela and Barrett, 1982; Liotta et al., 1980), as this collagenase is specific for the type IV collagen which occurs in basement membranes. It has been observed that anticarcinogenic protease inhibitors such as antipain and BBI do not affect type IV collagenase (Kennedy, unpublished data). The proteases affected by the anticarcinogenic protease inhibitors are ones which are presumably involved in the conversion of a cell to the malignant state, as discussed elsewhere in this volume (Chapters 3, 11, and 13). It is not surprising that the anticarcinogenic protease inhibitors do not affect specific proteases produced by malignant cells, as they have no effect on transformed cells in our *in vitro* studies (e.g., see Kennedy and Little, 1981).

There are many other possible mechanisms for the observed protease inhibitor anticarcinogenic activity. For example, it is reasonable to expect that the anticarcinogenic protease inhibitors affect protein kinase C (PKC). PKC is an enzyme involved in signal transduction and tumorigenesis, as it serves as the primary receptor for TPA (for reviews, see Ashendel, 1984; Nishizuka, 1984). The binding of TPA to PKC at the diacylglycerol binding site results in activation of the enzyme (for review, see Nishizuka, 1984). It is known that limited proteolysis of PKC with calpain converts the enzyme into a permanently active form of the enzyme, called protein kinase M (Inoue *et al.*, 1977; Takai *et al.*, 1977). The activity of calpain can be inhibited by high concentrations of several different thiol protease inhibitors (Ishiura, 1981; Solomon *et al.*, 1985; Sugita *et al.*, 1980; Takai *et al.*, 1979). A correlation does not exist, however, between anticarcinogenic activity and the ability of a protease inhibitor to inhibit the activity of calpain. For example, some protease inhibitors lacking anticarcinogenic activity, such as TLCK, inhibit calpain, while other protease inhibitors which do have anticarcinogenic activity, such as antipain and BBI, do not affect calpain even when evaluated at very high concentrations (Solomon *et al.*, 1985). Our own studies suggest that protease inhibitors do not suppress promotion *in vitro* through effects on PKC (Su *et al.*, 1991).

There are many hypotheses to explain the anticarcinogenic activity of other chemopreventive agents as well. It is possible that several of them may work through the induction of a protease inhibitor. For example, retinoic acid induces a novel protease inhibitor (in which the active site is the same as that of antithrombin III) (Wang and Gudas, 1990) and a glucocorticord hormone (dexamethasone) acts like a protease inhibitor in that it has been shown to inhibit the basal and induced transcription of a protease (collagenase) (Jonat *et al.*, 1990).

5. Summary

Protease inhibitors are highly promising as human cancer chemopreventive agents. For all cancer chemopreventive agents, potential toxicity problems need to be addressed. As discussed in detail above, certain adverse health effects have been attributed, perhaps incorrectly, to protease inhibitors. It is perceived that some problems could result from the chemoprevention of cancer with dietary protease inhibitors; these are: (1) pathologic alterations could develop in the pancreas while cancer is being inhibited in other organs and (2) there may be decreased protein utilization, resulting in weight loss. We believe that a suitable level of protease inhibitors in the diet can be found which will not lead to the problems cited above because: (1) there are normal human populations with high levels of protease inhibitors in the diet which show no increased risk of pancreatic cancer [i.e., the Japanese and Seventh-Day Adventists (Armstrong and Doll, 1975; Doell *et al.*, 1981; Phillips, 1975; Phillips *et al.*, 1980); in fact, the Seventh-Day Adventists have a decreased risk of developing pancreatic cancer (Mills *et al.*, 1988)] and (2) we have observed no undesirable side effects, including pancreatic changes, decreased growth rate, or decline in general health, in animals maintained on high levels of anticarcinogenic dietary protease inhibitor activity for as long as their entire life span, as discussed in detail above. Thus, it is highly likely that protease inhibitor supplementation to the diet will prevent the development of cancer without adverse health effects in human populations.

ACKNOWLEDGMENTS. Research in the Kennedy laboratory discussed in this report is supported by NIH Grants CA22704, CA46496, and CA34680.

6. References

Adler, G., Mullenhoff, A., Bozkurt, T., Koop, I., Goke, B., Beglinger, C., and Arnold, R., 1986, Pancreatic function and plasma CCK in humans after ingestion of a proteinase inhibitor (FOY-305), *Dig. Dis. Sci.* **31**:1123.

Adler, G., Mullenhoff, A., Bozkurt, T., Goke, B., Koop, I., and Arnold, R., 1988, Comparison of the effect of single and repeated administrations of a protease inhibitor (camostate) on pancreatic secretion in man, *Scand. J. Gastroenterol.* **23**:158–162.

Andrén-Sandberg, A., and Ihse, I., 1983, Regulatory effects on the pancreas of intraduodenal pancreatic juice and trypsin in the Syrian golden hamster, *Scand. J. Gastroenterol.* **18**:697–706.

Armstrong, B., and Doll, R., 1975, Environmental factors and cancer incidence and mortality in different countries, with special reference to dietary factors, *Int. J. Cancer* **15**:617–631.

Ashendel, C. L., 1985, The phorbol ester receptor: A phospholipid-regulated protein kinase, *Biochim. Biophys. Acta* **822**:219–242.

Ausman, L. M., Harwood, J. P., King, N. W., Sehgal, P. K., Nicolosi, R. J., Hegsted, M. D., Liener, I. E., Donatucci, D., and Tarcza, J., 1985, The effects of long-term soy protein and milk protein feeding on the pancreas of Cebus albifrons monkeys, *J. Nutr.* **115**:1691–1701.

Baturay, N. Z., and Kennedy, A. R., 1986, Pyrene acts as a cocarcinogen with the carcinogens, benzo(a)pyrene, β-propiolactone and radiation in the induction of malignant transformation of cultured mouse fibroblasts; soybean extract containing the Bowman–Birk inhibitor acts as an anticarcinogen, *Cell Biol. Toxicol.* **2**:21–32.

Bauer, E. A., Uitto, J., Walters, R. C., and Eisen, A. Z., 1979, Enhanced collagenase production by fibroblasts derived from human basal cell carcinomas, *Cancer Res.* **39**:4594–4599.

Becker, F. F., 1981, Inhibition of spontaneous hepatocarcinogenesis in C3H/Hen mice by Edi Pro A, an isolated soy protein, *Carcinogenesis* **2**:1213–1214.

BEIR V Report, 1990, Health effects of exposure to low levels of ionizing radiation: BEIR V, A. C.

Upton (Chairman) *et al.*, Committee on the Biological Effects of Ionizing Radiations; Board of Radiation Effects Research Commission on Life Sciences, National Research Council, National Academy Press, Washington, D.C., pp. 1–400.

Berenblum, I., Burger, M., and Knyszynski, A., 1974, Inhibition of radiation-induced lymphatic leukemia in C57BL mice by 195 alpha-2-globulin (α2-MG) from human blood serum, *Radiat. Res.* **60:**501–505.

Bernacka, K., Kuryliszyn-Moskal, A., and Sierakowski, S., 1988, The levels of alpha-antitrypsin and alpha-antichymotrypsin in the sera of patients with gastrointestinal cancers during diagnosis, *Cancer* **62:**1188–1193.

Billings, P. C., Morrow, A. R., Ryan, C. A., and Kennedy, A. R., 1989, Inhibition of radiation-induced transformation of C3H/10T1/2 cells by carboxypeptidase inhibitor I and inhibitor II from potatoes, *Carcinogenesis* **10:**687–691.

Billings, P. C., Longnecker, M. P., Keary, M., and Taylor, P. R., 1990a, Protease inhibitor content of human dietary samples, *Nutr. Cancer* **14:**81–93.

Billings, P. C., Newberne, P., and Kennedy, A. R., 1990b, Protease inhibitor suppression of colon and anal gland carcinogenesis induced by dimethylhydrazine, *Carcinogenesis* **11:**1083–1086.

Birk, Y., 1961, Purification and some properties of a highly active inhibitor of trypsin and α-chymotrypsin from soybeans, *Biochim. Biophys. Acta* **54:**378–381.

Birk, Y., 1974, Structure–activity relationship of several trypsin and chymotrypsin inhibitors from legume seeds, in: *Proteinase Inhibitors* (N. Fritz, H. Tschesche, L. J. Green, and E. Truscheit, eds.), Springer-Verlag, Berlin, pp. 355–361.

Birk, Y., 1975, Proteinase inhibitors from plant sources, *Methods Enzymol.* **45:**695–751.

Birk, Y., 1985, The Bowman–Birk inhibitor, *Int. J. Peptide Protein Res.* **25:**113–131.

Blondell, J. M., 1988, Urban–rural factors affecting cancer mortality in Kentucky, 1950–1969, *Cancer Detect. and Prevent.* **11:**209–223.

Bodwell, C. E., and Hopkins, D. T., 1985, Nutritional characteristics of oilseed proteins, in: *New Protein Foods*, Volume 5 (A. A. Altschul and H. L. Wilcke, eds.), Academic Press, New York, pp. 221–257.

Bodwell, C. E., Adkins, J. S., and Hopkins, D. T. 1981, *Protein Quality in Humans: Assessment and in Vitro Estimation*, AVI Publishing, Westport, Conn., pp. 278–301.

Bowman, D. E., 1946, Differentiation of soybean antitryptic factors, *Proc. Soc. Exp. Biol. Med.* **63:**547–550.

Bozzini, A., and Silano, V., 1978, Control through breeding methods of factors affecting nutritional quality of cereals and grain legumes, in: *Nutritional Improvement of Food and Feed Proteins* (M. Freidman, ed.), Plenum Press, New York, pp. 249–274.

Carroll, K. K., and Khor, H. T., 1975, Dietary fat in relation to tumorigenesis, *Prog. Biochem. Pharmacol.* **10:**308–353.

Chapman, H. A., Jr., and Stone, O. L., 1984, Comparison of live human neutrophil and alveolar macrophage elastolytic activity *in vitro:* Relative resistance of macrophage elastolytic activity to serum and alveolar proteinase inhibitors, *J. Clin. Invest.* **74:**1693–1700.

Chawla, R. K., Rausch, D. J., Miller, F. W., Vogler, W. R., and Lawson, D. H., 1984, Abnormal profile of serum proteinase inhibitors in cancer patients, *Cancer Res.* **44:**2718–2723.

Chernick, S. S., Lepkovsky, S., and Chaikoff, I. L., 1948, A dietary factor regulating the enzyme content of the pancreas; changes induced in size and proteolytic activity of the chick pancreas by the ingestion of raw soybean meal, *Am. J. Physiol.* **155:**33–41.

Churella, H. R., Yao, B. C., and Thompson, W. A. B., 1976, Soybean trypsin inhibitor activity of soy infant formulas and its nutritional significance for the rat, *J. Agric. Food Chem.* **24:**393–397.

Coburn, M., Schuel, H., and Troll, W., 1981, A hydrogen peroxide block to polyspermy in the sea urchin, Arbacia punctulata, *Dev. Biol.* **84:**235–238.

Corasanti, J. G., Hobika, G. H., and Markus, G., 1982, Interference with dimethylhydrazine induction of colon tumors in mice by ε-aminocaproic acid, *Science* **216:**1020–1021.

Correa, P., 1981, Epidemiologic correlations between diet and cancer frequency, *Cancer Res.* **41**:3685–3690.

Corwin, L. M., and Gordon, R. K., 1982, Vitamin E and immune regulation, in: *Vitamin E: Biochemical, Hematological, and Clinical Aspects* (B. Lubin and L. J. Machlin, eds.), N.Y. Acad. Sci., New York, pp. 437–451.

Crass, R. A., and Morgan, R. G. H., 1982, The effect of long-term feeding of soya bean flour diets on pancreatic growth in the rat, *Br. J. Nutr.* **47**:119–129.

Diaz, G. R., Devaux, M. A., Johnson, C. D., Adrich, Z., and Sarles, H., 1982, Physiological conditions for the study of basal and meal-stimulated exocrine pancreatic secretion in the dog. Absence of feedback inhibition of basal secretion, *Can. J. Physiol. Pharmacol.* **60**:1287–1295.

Doell, B. H., Ebden, C. J., and Smith, C. A., 1981, Trypsin inhibitor activity of conventional foods which are part of the British diet and some soya products, *Qual. Plant. Plant Foods Hum. Nutr.* **31**:139–150.

Doll, R., and Peto, R., 1981, The causes of cancer: Quantitative estimates of avoidable risks of cancer in the United States today, *J. Natl. Cancer Inst.* **66**:1193–1308.

Douglas, B. R., Woutersen, R. A., Jansen, J. B. M. J., de Jong, A. J. L., Rovati, L. C., and Lamers, C. B. H. W., 1989, Modulation by CR-1409 (lorglumide), a cholecystokinin receptor antagonist, of trypsin inhibitor-enhanced growth of azaserine-induced putative preneoplastic lesions in rat pancreas, *Cancer Res.* **49**:2438–2441.

Dresden, M. H., Heilman, S. A., and Schmidt, J. D., 1972, Collagenolytic enzymes in human neoplasms, *Cancer Res.* **32**:993–996.

Durbec, J. P., Chevilotte, G., Bidart, J. M., Berthezene, P., and Sarles, H., 1983, Diet, alcohol, tobacco and risk of cancer of the pancreas—A case control study, *Br. J. Cancer* **47**:463–470.

Flavin, D. F., 1982, The effect of soybean trypsin inhibitors on the pancreas of animals and man, *Vet. Hum. Toxicol.* **24**:25–28.

Folsch, U. R., Winckler, K., and Wormsley, K. G., 1974, Effect of a soybean diet on enzyme content and ultrastructure of the rat exocrine pancreas, *Digestion* **11**:161–171.

Frenkel, K., Chrzan, K., Ryan, C., Wiesner, R., and Troll, W., 1987, Chymotrypsin-specific protease inhibitors decrease H_2O_2 formation by activated human polymorphonuclear leukocytes, *Carcinogenesis* **8**:1207–1212.

Fukui, Y., Takamura, C., Yamamura, M., and Yamamoto, M., 1975, Effect of leupeptin on carcinogenesis of rat mammary tumor induced by 7,12-dimethylbenz(a)-anthracene, Proc. Japan Cancer Assoc., 34th Annual Meeting, p. 20.

Fushiki, T., and Iwai, K., 1989, Two hypotheses on the feedback regulation of pancreatic enzyme secretion, *FASEB J.* **3**:121–126.

Gallaher, D., and Schneeman, B. O., 1986, Nutritional and metabolic response to plant inhibitors of digestive enzymes, *Adv. Exp. Med. Biol.* **199**:167–184.

Gertler, A., and Nitsan, Z., 1970, The effect of trypsin inhibitors on pancreotopeptidase E, trypsin, chymotrypsin, and amylase in the pancreas and intestinal tract of chicks receiving raw and heated soya bean diets, *Br. J. Nutr.* **24**:803–804.

Gold, E. B., Gordis, L., Diener, M. D., Seltser, R., Boitnott, J. K., Bynum, T. E., and Hutcheon, D. F., 1985, Diet and other risk factors for cancer of the pancreas, *Cancer* **55**:460–467.

Goldfarb, R. H., Kitson, R. P., Giffen, C. Z., and Yavelow, J., 1989, Anticarcinogenic and antiproteolytic Bowman–Birk inhibitor (BBI): Failure to inhibit both LAK cell proteases and LAK cell-mediated killing of tumor cells, Proc. Am. Assoc. Cancer Res. (March, 1989), Volume 30, Abstract No. 711, p. 179.

Goldstein, B. D., Witz, G., Amoruso, M., and Troll, W., 1979, Protease inhibitors antagonize the activation of polymorphonuclear leukocyte oxygen consumption, *Biochem. Biophys. Res. Commun.* **88**:854–860.

Gorrill, A. D. L., and Thomas, J. W., 1967, Body weight changes, pancreas size and enzyme activity, and proteolytic enzyme activity and protein digestion in intestinal contents from calves fed soybean and milk protein diets, *J. Nutr.* **92**:215–223.

Grau, C. R., and Carroll, R. W., 1958, Evaluation of protein quality, in: *Processed Plant Protein Foodstuffs* (A. M. Altschul, ed.), Academic Press, New York, pp. 153–189.

Green, G. M., and Lyman, R. L., 1972, Feedback regulation of pancreatic enzyme secretion as a mechanism for trypsin inhibitor induced hypersecretion in rats, *Proc. Soc. Exp. Biol. Med.* **140**:6–12.

Green, G. M., Olds, B. O., Matthews, G., and Lyman, R. L., 1973, Protein as a regulator of pancreatic enzyme secretion in the rat, *Proc. Soc. Exp. Biol. Med.* **142**:1162–1167.

Grobstein, C., Cairns, J., Berliner, R. *et al.*, 1982, Diet, Nutrition and Cancer, Committee on Diet, Nutrition and Cancer, Assembly of Life Sciences, National Research Council, National Academy of Sciences, Washington, D.C.

Gumbmann, M. R., Spangler, W. L., Dugan, G. M., Rackis, J. J., and Liener, I. E., 1985, The USDA trypsin inhibitor study, IV: The chronic effects of soyflour and soy protein isolate in rats after two years, *Qual. Plant. Plant Foods Hum. Nutr.* **35**:275–314.

Harlan, J. M., Killen, P. D., Harker, L. A., Striker, G. E., and Wright, D. G., 1981, Neutrophil-mediated endothelial injury *in vitro:* Mechanisms of cell detachment, *J. Clin. Invest.* **68**:1394–1403.

Hasdai, A., and Liener, I. E., 1983, Growth, digestibility, and enzymatic activities in the pancreas and intestines of hamsters fed raw and heated soy flour, *J. Nutr.* **113**:662–668.

Hooks, R. D., Hays, V. W., Speer, V. C., and McCall, J. T., 1965, Effects of raw soybeans on pancreatic enzyme concentrations and performance of pigs, *Fed. Proc. Fed. Am. Soc. Exp. Biol.* **24**:894.

Hozumi, M., Ogawa, M., Sugimura, T., Takeuchi, T., and Umezawa, H., 1972, Inhibition of tumorigenesis in mouse skin by leupeptin, a protease inhibitor from actinomycetes, *Cancer Res.* **32**:1725–1728.

Hwang, D. L. R., Davis-Lin, K. T., Yang, W. K., and Foard, D. T., 1977, Purification, partial characterization and immunological relationships of multiple low molecular weight proteinase inhibitors of soybean, *Biochim. Biophys. Acta* **495**:369–382.

Ikenaka, T., Odani, S., and Koide, T., 1974, Proteinase inhibitors, *Proc. 2nd Int. Res. Conf.* (Baker Symp. V), Grosse Leder, 1973, Springer-Verlag, Berlin, p. 325.

Inoue, M., Kishimoto, A., Takai, Y., and Nishizuka, Y., 1977, Studies on a cyclic nucleotide-independent protein kinase and its proenzyme in mammalian tissues, *J. Biol. Chem.* **252**:7610–7616.

Ishiura, S., 1981, Calcium-dependent neutral protease from chicken skeletal muscle. I. Purification and characterization, *J. Biochem.* **84**:225–230.

Jonat, C., Rahmsdorf, H. J., Park, K.-K., Cato, A. C. B., Gebel, S., Ponta, H., and Herrlich, P., 1990, Antitumor promotion and antiinflammation: Down-modulation of AP-1 (Fos/Jun) activity by glucocorticoid hormone, *Cell* **62**:1189–1204.

Kakade, M. L., Barton, T. L., Schaible, P. J., and Evan, R. J., 1967, Biochemical changes in the pancreas of chicks fed raw soybeans and soybean meal, *Poult. Sci.* **46**:1578–1585.

Kakade, M. L., Hoffa, D. E., and Liener, I. E., 1973, Contribution of trypsin inhibitors to the deleterious effects of unheated soybeans fed to rats, *J. Nutr.* **103**:1772–1778.

Kakade, M. L., Thompson, R. D., Englestad, W. W., Behrens, G. C., Yoder, R. D., and Crave, F. M., 1976, Failure of soybean trypsin inhibitors to exert deleterious effects in calves, *J. Dairy Sci.* **59**:1484–1489.

Kaneko, A., Enomoto, K., Oyamada, M., Sawada, N., Dempo, K., and Mori, M., 1986, Induction of a novel Ca^{2+}-dependent chymotrypsin-like serine protease by tumor promoters in rat livers, *J. Natl. Cancer Inst.* **77**:121–125.

Kassell, B., 1970, Trypsin and chymotrypsin inhibitors from soybeans, *Methods Enzymol.* **19**:853–862.

Kennedy, A. R., 1984, Discussion (pp. 127–136) of "Analysis of phorbol ester receptors: A biochemical approach to understanding the mechanism of action of tumor promoters," by P. M.

Blumberg, B. Konig, N. A. Sharkey, S. Jaken, K. L. Leach, and A. G. Jeng, in: *Molecular and Cellular Approaches to Understanding Mechanisms of Toxicity,* pp. 108–127, Proceedings of a conference held in Boston on September 1–2, 1983 (A. H. Tashjian, Jr., ed.), published by the President and Fellows of Harvard College.

Kennedy, A. R., 1985, The conditions for the modification of radiation transformation *in vitro* by a tumor promoter and protease inhibitors, *Carcinogenesis* **6:**1441–1446.

Kennedy, A. R., 1986, Role of free radicals in the initiation and promotion of radiation-induced and chemical carcinogen induced cell transformation, in: *Oxygen and Sulfur Radicals in Chemistry and Medicine* (A. Breccia, M.A. J. Rodgers, and G. Semerano, eds.), Edizioni Scientifiche, "Lo Scarabeo," Bologna, Italy, pp. 201–209.

Kennedy, A. R., and Billings, P. C., 1987, Anticarcinogenic actions of protease inhibitors, in: *Anticarcinogenesis and Radiation Protection* (P. A. Cerutti, O. F. Nygaard, and M. G. Simic, eds.), Plenum Press, New York, pp. 285–295.

Kennedy, A. R., and Little, J. B., 1981, Effects of protease inhibitors on radiation transformation *in vitro, Cancer Res.* **41:**2103–2108.

Kennedy, A. R., and Symons, M. C. R., 1987, "Water structure" vs "radical scavenger" theories as explanations for the suppressive effects of DMSO and related compounds on radiation induced transformation *in vitro. Carcinogenesis* **8:**683–688.

Kennedy, A. R., Radner, B., and Nagasawa, H., 1984, Protease inhibitors reduce the frequency of spontaneous chromosome abnormalities in cells from patients with Bloom syndrome, *Proc. Natl. Acad. Sci. USA* **81:**1827–1830.

Kennedy, A. R., Billings, P. C., Maki, P. A., and Newberne, P., 1993, Effects of various protease inhibitor preparations on oral carcinogenesis in hamsters induced by 7,12-dimethylbenz(a) anthracene, *Nutrition and Cancer* **19:**191–200.

Kunitz, M., 1947, Crystalline soybean trypsin inhibitor, *J. Gen. Physiol.* **30:**291–310.

Kuroki, T., and Drevon, C., 1979, Inhibition of chemical transformation in C3H/10T1/2 cells by protease inhibitors, *Cancer Res.* **39:**2755–2761.

Leb, L., Beatson, P., Fortier, N., Newburger, P. E., and Snyder, L. M., 1985, Modulation of mononuclear phagocyte cytotoxicity by alpha-tocopherol (vitamin E), *J. Leuk. Biol.* **37:**449–459.

Liener, I. E., 1979a, Significance for humans of biologically active factors in soybeans and other food legumes, *J. Am. Oil Chem. Soc.* **56:**121–129.

Liener, I. E., 1979b, Protease inhibitors and lectins, in: *International Review of Biochemistry* (A. Veuberger and T. H. Jakes, eds.), University Park Press, Baltimore, pp. 97–122.

Liener, I. E., 1989, Control of anti-nutritional and toxic factors in oilseeds and legumes, in: *Food Uses of Whole Oil and Protein Seeds* (E. W. Lusas, D. R. Erikson, and W.-K. Nip, eds.), American Oil Chemists Society, Champaign, Ill., pp. 344–371.

Liener, I. E., and Hasdai, A., 1986, The effect of long-term feeding of raw soy flour on the pancreas of mouse and hamster, *Adv. Exp. Med. Biol.* **199:**189–197.

Liener, I. E., and Kakade, M. L., 1980, Protease inhibitors, in: *Toxic Constituents of Plant Foodstuffs* (I. E. Liener, ed.), Academic Press, New York, pp. 7–71.

Liener, I. E., Goodale, R. L., Deshmukh, A., Satterberg, T. L., Ward, G., DiPietro, C. M., Bankey, P. E., and Borner, J. W., 1988, Effect of a trypsin inhibitor from soybeans (Bowman–Birk) on the secretory activity of the human pancreas, *Gastroenterology* **94:**419–427.

Lim, T. S., Putt, N., Safranski, D., Chung, C., and Watson, R. R., 1981, Effect of vitamin E on cell-mediated immune responses and serum corticosterone in young and maturing mice, *Immunology* **44:**289–295.

Liotta, L. A., Tryggvason, K., Garbisa, S., Hart, I., Foltz, C. M., and Shafie, S., 1980, Metastatic potential correlates with enzymatic degradation of basement membrane collagen, *Nature* **284:**67–68.

McGuiness, E. E., Morgan, R. G. H., Levison, D. A., Frape, D. L., Hopwood, D., and Wormsley,

K. G., 1980, The effect of long-term feeding of soya flour on the rat pancreas, *Scand. J. Gastroenterol.* **15**:497–502.

McGuiness, E. E., Morgan, R. G. H., and Wormsley, K. G., 1984, Effects of soybean flour on the pancreas of rats, *Environ. Health Perspect.* **56**:205–212.

Mack, T. M., 1982, Pancreas, in: *Cancer Epidemiology and Prevention* (D. Schottenfeld and J. Fraumeni, eds.), Saunders, Philadelphia, pp. 638–667.

Madar, Z., Birk, Y., and Gertler, A., 1974, Native and modified Bowman–Birk trypsin inhibitor— Comparative effect on pancreatic enzymes upon ingestion by quails, *Comp. Biochem. Physiol.* **48B**:251–256.

Mainz, D. L., Black, O., and Webster, P. D., 1973, Hormonal control of pancreatic growth, *J. Clin. Invest.* **52**:2300–2304.

Matsushima, T., Kakizoe, T., Kawachi, T., Hara, K., Sugimura, T., Takeuchi, T., and Umezawa, H., 1976, Effects of protease inhibitors of microbial origin on experimental carcinogenesis, in: *Fundamentals in Cancer Prevention* (P. N. Magee *et al.*, eds.), University of Tokyo Press, Tokyo, University Park Press, Baltimore, pp. 57–69.

Melmed, R. N., El-Aaser, A. A. A., and Holt, S. J., 1976, Hypertrophy and hyperplasia of the neonatal rat exocrine pancreas induced by orally administered soybean trypsin inhibitor, *Biochim. Biophys. Acta* **421**:280–282.

Messadi, D. V., Billings, P., Shklar, G., and Kennedy, A. R., 1986, Inhibition of oral carcinogenesis by a protease inhibitor, *J. Natl. Cancer Inst.* **76**:447–452.

Messina, M. J., and Barnes, S., 1991, Workshop report from the Division of Cancer Prevention and Control: The role of soy products in reducing the risk of cancer, *J. Natl. Cancer Inst.* **83**:541–546.

Mills, P. K., Beeson, W. L., Abbey, D. E., Fraser, G. E., and Phillips, R. L., 1988, Dietary habits and past medical history as related to fatal pancreas cancer risk among Adventists, *Cancer (Philadelphia)* **61**:2578–2585.

Miyasaka, K., and Green, G. M., 1984, Effect of partial exclusion of pancreatic juice on rat basal pancreatic secretion, *Gastroenterology* **86**:114–119.

Miyasaka, K., Nakamura, R., Funakoshi, A., and Kitani, K., 1989, Stimulatory effect of monitor peptide and human pancreatic secretory trypsin inhibitor on pancreatic secretion and cholecystokinin release in conscious rats, *Pancreas* **4**:139–144.

Morgan, R. G. H., 1987, Raw soy flour and pancreatic cancer in experimental animals, in: *Experimental Pancreatic Carcinogenesis* (D. G. Scarpelli, J. K. Reddy, and D. S. Longnecker, eds.), CRC Press, Boca Raton, Fla., pp. 159–174.

Naim, M., Gertler, A., and Birk, Y., 1982, The effect of dietary raw and autoclaved soya-bean protein fractions on growth, pancreatic enlargement and pancreatic enzymes in rats, *Br. J. Nutr.* **47**:281–288.

Nash, D. R., McLarty, J. W., and Fortson, N. G., 1980, Pretreatment, prediagnosis immunoglobulin, and alpha$_1$-antitrypsin levels in patients with bronchial carcinoma, *J. Natl. Cancer Inst.* **64**:721–724.

Nishizuka, Y., 1984, The role of protein kinase C in cell surface signal transduction and tumor promotion, *Nature* **308**:693–698.

Nitsan, Z., and Alumot, E., 1964, Overcoming the inhibition of intestinal proteolytic activity caused by raw soybean in chicks of different ages, *J. Nutr.* **84**:179–184.

Nitsan, Z., and Nir, I., 1977, A comparative study of the nutritional and physiological significance of raw and heated soybeans in chicks and goslings, *Br. J. Nutr.* **37**:81–91.

Nomura, T., Hata, S., Enomoto, T., Tanaka, H., and Shibata, K., 1980, Inhibiting effects of antipain on urethane induced lung neoplasia in mice, *Br. J. Cancer* **42**:624–626.

Noonan, N. E., and Noonan, K. D., 1977, The effect of TLCK on transcription and its role in modifying cell growth, *J. Cell. Physiol.* **92**:137–144.

Norell, S. E., Ahlbom, A., Erwald, R., Jacobson, G., Lindberg-Navier, I., Olin, R., Tornberg, B., and Wiechel, K. L., 1986, Diet and pancreatic cancer: A case–control study, *Am. J. Epidemiol.* **124**:894–902.

Odani, S., and Ikenaka, T. J., 1973, Scission of soybean Bowman–Birk proteinase inhibitor into two small fragments having either trypsin or chymotrypsin inhibitor activity, *J. Biochem.* **74**:857–860.

Ohkoshi, M., and Fujii, S., 1983, Effect of the synthetic protease inhibitor N,N-dimethylcarbamoyl-methyl 4-(4-guanidinobenzoyloxy) phenylacetate methanesulfate on carcinogenesis by 3-methylcholanthrene in mouse skin, *J. Natl. Cancer Inst.* **71**:1053–1057.

Osborne, T. B., and Mendel, L. B., 1917, The use of soybean as food, *J. Biol. Chem.* **32**:369–387.

Palladino, M. A., Galton, J. E., Troll, W., and Thorbecke, G. J., 1982, γ-Irradiation-induced mortality: Protective effect of protease inhibitors in chickens and mice, *Int. J. Radiat. Biol.* **41**:183–191.

Patten, J. R., Richards, E. A., and Wheeler, J., 1971a, The effect of raw soybean on the pancreas of adult dogs, *Proc. Soc. Exp. Biol. Med.* **137**:58.

Patten, J. R., Richards, E. A., and Wheeler, J., 1971b, The effect of dietary soybean trypsin inhibitor on the histology of dog pancreas, *Life Sci.* **10**(2):145–150.

Patten, J. R., Patten, J. A,. and Pope, H., 1973, II. Sensitivity of the guinea pig to raw soya bean in the diet, *Food Cosmet. Toxicol.* **11**:577–583.

Persiani, S., Yeung, A., Shen, W. C., and Kennedy, A. R., 1992, Polylysine conjugates of Bowman–Birk protease inhibitor as targeted anticarcinogenic agents, *Carcinogenesis* **12**:1149–1152.

Phillips, R. L., 1975, Role of lifestyle and dietary habits in risk of cancer among Seventh Day Adventists, *Cancer Res.* **35**:3515–3522.

Phillips, R. L., Garfinkel, L., Kuzma, J. W., Beeson, W. L., Lotz, T., and Brin, B., 1980, Mortality among California Seventh-Day Adventists for selected cancer sites, *J. Natl. Cancer Inst.* **65**:1097–1107.

Pineda, O., Torun, B., Viteri, F. E., and Arroyave, G., 1982, Protein quality in relation to estimates of essential amino acid requirements, in: *Protein Quality in Humans: Assessment and In Vitro Estimation* (C. E. Bodwell, J. S. Adkins, and D. T. Hopkins, eds.), AVI Publishing, Westport, Conn., pp. 29–42.

Quigley, J. P., 1979, Proteolytic enzymes of normal and malignant cells, in: *Surfaces of Normal and Malignant Cells* (R. O. Hynes, ed.), Wiley, New York, pp. 247–255.

Rackis, J. J., McGhee, J. E., and Booth, A. N., 1975, Biological threshold levels of soybean trypsin inhibitor by rat bioassay, *Cereal Chem.* **52**:85–93.

Rackis, J. J., Wolf, W. J., and Baker, E. C., 1986, Protease inhibitors in plant foods: Content and inactivation, *Adv. Exp. Med. Biol.* **199**:299–347.

Richter, B. D., and Schneeman, B. O., 1987, Pancreatic response to long-term feeding of soy protein isolate, casein or egg white in rats, *J. Nutr.* **117**:247–252.

Robbins, D. J., Liener, I. E., Spangler, W. M., and de Bruyn, D. B., 1988, The effects of a raw soy protein diet on the pancreas of the chacma baboon, *Nutr. Rep. Int.* **38**:9–16.

Roebuck, B. D., Kaplita, P. V., Edwards, B. R., and Praissman, M., 1987, Effects of dietary fats and soybean protein on azaserine-induced pancreatic carcinogenesis and plasma cholecystokinin in the rat, *Cancer Res.* **47**:1333–1338.

Rossman, T. G., and Troll, W., 1980, Protease inhibitors in carcinogenesis: Possible sites of action, in: *Carcinogenesis: Modifiers of Chemical Carcinogenesis*, Volume 5 (T. J. Slaga, ed.), Raven Press, New York, pp. 127–143.

Rothman, S. S., and Wells, H., 1967, Enhancement of pancreatic enzyme synthesis by pancreozymin, *Am. J. Physiol.* **213**:215–218.

Ryan, C. A., and Kassell, B. 1970, Chymotrypsin inhibitor I from potatoes, *Methods Enzymol.* **19**:883–889.

Ryser, H. J. P., 1971, Chemical carcinogenesis, *N. Engl. J. Med.* **285**:721–734.

St. Clair, W., Billings, P., Carew, J., Keller-McGandy, C., Newberne, P., and Kennedy, A. R., 1990, Suppression of DMH-induced carcinogenesis in mice by dietary addition of the Bowman–Birk protease inhibitor, *Cancer Res.* **50:**580–586.

Sale, J. K., Goldberg, D. M., Fawcett, A. N., and Wormsley, K. G., 1977, Chronic and acute studies indicating absence of exocrine pancreatic feedback inhibition in dogs, *Digestion* **15:**540–555.

Schelp, F.-P., and Pongpaew, P., 1988, Protection against cancer through nutritionally-induced increase in endogenous proteinase inhibitors—A hypothesis, *Int. J. Epidemiol.* **17:**287–292.

Schingoethe, D. J., Aust, S. D., and Thomas, J. W., 1970, Separation of a mouse growth inhibitor in soybeans from trypsin inhibitors, *J. Nutr.* **100:**739–748.

Scrimshaw, N. S., Wayler, A. H., Murray, E., Steinke, F. H., Rand, W. M., and Young, V. R., 1983, Nitrogen balance response in young men given one or two isolated soy proteins or milk proteins, *J. Nutr.* **113:**2492–2497.

Shasby, D. M., 1985, Antioxidant activity of some antiproteases, *Am. Rev. Respir. Dis.* **131:**293–294.

Sheela, S., and Barrett, J. C., 1982, *In vitro* degradation of radiolabelled, intact basement membrane mediated by cellular plasminogen activator, *Carcinogenesis* **3:**363–369.

Silverman, J., and Adams, J. O., 1983, N-Nitrosamines in laboratory animal feed and bedding, *Lab. Anim. Sci.* **33:**161–164.

Slaga, T. J., Klein-Szanto, A. J. P., Fischer, S. M., Weeks, C. E., Nelson, K., and Major, S., 1980, Studies on the mechanism of action of anti-tumor-promoting agents: Their specificity in two-stage promotion. *Proc. Natl. Acad. Sci. USA* **77:**2251–2254.

Smirnoff, P., Khalef, S., Birk, Y., and Applebaum, S. W., 1979, Trypsin and chymotrypsin inhibitor from chick peas, *Int. J. Peptide Protein Res.* **14:**186–192.

Snyder, W. S. (Chairman), Cook, M. J., Karhausen, L. R., Nasset, E. S., Howells, G. P., and Tipton, I. H., 1974, Report of the Task Group on Reference Man, International Commission of Radiological Protection, No. 3, Pergamon Press, Elmsford, N.Y., pp. 348–352.

Solomon, D. H., O'Brian, C. A., and Weinstein, I. B., 1985, N-α-tosyl-L-lysine chloromethyl ketone and N-α-tosyl-L-phenylalanine chloromethyl ketone inhibit protein kinase C, *FEBS Lett.* **190:**342–344.

Soy Protein Council, 1987, Soy protein products: Characteristics, nutritional aspects and utilization, pp. 7–13.

Struthers, B. J., MacDonald, J. R., Dahlgren, R. R., and Hopkins, D. T., 1983, Effects on the monkey, pig and rat pancreas of soy products with varying levels of trypsin inhibitor and comparison with the administration of cholecystokinin, *J. Nutr.* **113:**86–97.

Su, L. N., Toscano, W. A., Jr., and Kennedy, A. R., 1991, Suppression of phorbol ester-enhanced radiation-induced malignancy *in vitro* by protease inhibitors is independent of protein kinase C, *Biochem. Biophys. Res. Commun.* **176:**18–24.

Sugita, H., Ishiura, S., Suzuki, K., and Imahori, K., 1980, Inhibition of epoxide derivatives on chicken calcium-activated neutral protease (CANP) *in vitro* and *in vivo*. *J. Biochem.* **87:**339–341.

Takai, Y., Kishimoto, A., Inoue, M., and Nishizuka, Y., 1977, Studies on a cyclic nucleotide-independent protein kinase and its proenzyme in mammalian tissues, 1. Purification and characterization of an active enzyme from bovine cerebellum, *J. Biol. Chem.* **252:**7603–7609.

Takai, Y., Kishimoto, A., Iwasa, M., Kawahara, Y., Mori, T., and Nishizuka, Y., 1979, Calcium-dependent activation of a multifunctional protein kinase by membrane phospholipid, *J. Biol. Chem.* **254:**3692–3695.

Taylor, A. C., Levy, B. M., and Simpson, T. W. 1970, Collagenolytic activity of sarcoma tissue in culture, *Nature* **228:**366–367.

Torun, B., Pineda, O., Vireti, F. E., and Arrayave, G., 1982, Use of amino acid composition data to predict protein nutritive value for children with specific reference to new estimates for their essential amino acid requirements, in: *Protein Quality in Humans: Assessment and In Vitro Evaluation* (C. E. Bodwell, J. S. Adkins, and D. T. Hopkins, eds.), AVI Publishing, Westport, Conn., pp. 374–393.

Toskes, P. P., 1986, Negative feedback inhibition of pancreatic exocrine secretion in humans, *Adv. Exp. Med. Biol.* **199:**142–152.

Troll, W., 1976, Blocking tumor promotion by protease inhibitors, in: *Fundamentals in Cancer Prevention* (P. N. Magee et al., eds.), University Park Press, Maryland, pp. 41–55.

Troll, W., Klassen, A., and Janoff, A., 1970, Tumorigenesis in mouse skin: Inhibition by synthetic inhibitors of proteases, *Science* **169:**1211–1213.

Troll, W., Belman, S., Weisner, R., and Shellabarger, C. J., 1979a, Protease action in carcinogenesis, in: *Biological Functions of Proteinases* (H. Holtzer and H. Tschesche, eds.), Springer-Verlag, Berlin, pp. 165–170.

Troll, W., Weisner, R., Belman, S., and Shellabarger, C. J., 1979b, Inhibition of carcinogenesis by feeding diets containing soybeans. *Proc. Am. Assoc. Cancer Res.* **20:**265.

Troll, W., Weisner, R., Shellabarger, C. J., Holtzman, S., and Stone, J. P., 1980, Soybean diet lowers breast tumor incidence in irradiated rats, *Carcinogenesis* 1:469–472.

Troll, W., Witz, G., Goldstein, B., Stone, D., and Sugimura, T., 1982, The role of free oxygen radicals in tumor promotion and carcinogenesis, in: *Carcinogenesis: A Comprehensive Survey,* Volume 7 (E. Hecker, N. E. Fusenig, W. Kunz, F. Marks, and H. W. Theilmann, eds.), Raven Press, New York, pp. 593–597.

Umezawa, K., 1972, *Enzyme Inhibitors of Microbial Origin,* University of Tokyo Press, Tokyo, pp. 29–32.

Verloes, R., and Kanarek, L., 1976, Proteolytic activity associated with tumor growth and metastasis. Influence of trypsin inhibitor (soya bean) on Ehrlich ascites tumor growth, *Arch. Int. Physiol. Biochem.* **84:**1119–1120.

von Hofe, E., Brent, R., and Kennedy, A. R., 1990, Inhibition of x-ray induced exencephaly by protease inhibitors, *Radiat. Res.* **123:**108–111.

von Hofe, E., Newberne, P. M., and Kennedy, A. R., 1991, Inhibition of N-nitrosomethylbenzylamine induced esophageal neoplasms by the Bowman–Birk protease inhibitor, *Carcinogenesis* **12:**2147–2150.

Wang, S. Y., and Gudas, L. J., 1990, A retinoic acid-inducible mRNA from F9 teratocarcinoma cells encodes a novel protease inhibitor homologue, *J. Biol. Chem.* **265:**15818–15822.

Watanabe, S., Shiratori, K., Takeuchi, T., and Chey, W. Y., 1986, Intrajejunal administration of a synthetic trypsin inhibitor (camostate) stimulates the release of endogenous secretin but not cholecystokinin in humans, *Gastroenterology* **90:**1685.

Weed, H., McGandy, R. B., and Kennedy, A. R., 1985, Protection against dimethylhydrazine induced adenomatous tumors of the mouse colon by the dietary addition of an extract of soybeans containing the Bowman–Birk protease inhibitor, *Carcinogenesis* **6:**1239–1241.

Weinstein, I. B., 1978, Current concepts on mechanisms of chemical carcinogenesis, *Bull. N.Y. Acad. Med.* **54:**366–383.

Winn, D. M., Ziegler, R. G., Pickle, L. W., Gridley, G., Blot, W. J., and Hoover, R. N., 1984, Diet in the etiology of oral and pharyngeal cancer among women from the southern United States, *Cancer Res.* **44:**1216–1222.

Witschi, H., and Kennedy, A. R., 1989, Modulation of lung tumor development in mice with the soybean-derived Bowman–Birk protease inhibitor, *Carcinogenesis* **10:**2275–2277.

Witz, G., Goldstein, B. D., Amoruso, M., Stone, D. S., and Troll, W., 1980, Retinoid inhibition of superoxide anion radical production by human polymorphonuclear leukocytes stimulated with tumor promoters, *Biochem. Biophys. Res. Commun.* **97:**883–888.

Wolf, W. J., and Cowan, J. C., 1975, *Soybeans as a Food Source,* CRC Press, Boca Raton, Fla., pp. 51–53.

Wynder, E. L., 1975, An epidemiological evaluation of the causes of cancer of the pancreas, *Cancer Res.* **35**:2228–2233.

Yamamoto, R. S., Umezawa, H., Takeuchi, T., Matsushima, T., Hara, K., and Sugimura, T., 1974, Effect of leupeptin on colon carcinogenesis in rats with azoxymethane, *Proc. Am. Assoc. Cancer Res.* **15**:38.

Yamamura, M., Nakamura, N., Fukui, Y., Takamura, C., Yamamoto, M., Minato, Y., Tamura, Y., and Fujii, S., 1978, Inhibition of 7,12 DMBA-induced mammary tumorigenesis by a synthetic protease inhibitor, N,N-dimethylamino (p-p'-guanidino-benzoyloxy) benzilcarbonyloxyglyco-late, *Gann* **69**:749–752.

Yamauchi, Y., Kobayashi, T., and Watanabe, A., 1987, Anticarcinogenic effects of a serine protease inhibitor (FOY-305) through the suppression of neutral serine protease activity during chemical hepatocarcinogenesis in rats, *Hiroshima J. Medical Sciences* **36**:81–87.

Yanatori, Y., and Fujita, T., 1976, Hypertrophy and hyperplasia in the endocrine and exocrine pancreas of rats fed soybean trypsin inhibitor or repeatedly injected with pancreozymin, *Arch. Histol. Jpn.* **39**:67–78.

Yavelow, J., Gidlund, M., and Troll, W., 1982, Protease inhibitors from processed legumes effec-tively inhibit superoxide generation in response to TPA, *Carcinogenesis* **1**:135–138.

Yavelow, J., Finlay, T. H., Kennedy, A. R., and Troll, W., 1983, Bowman–Birk soybean protease inhibitor as an anticarcinogen, *Cancer Res.* **43**:2454–2459.

Yavelow, J., Collins, M., Birk, Y., Troll, W., and Kennedy, A. R., 1985, Nanomolar concentrations of Bowman–Birk soybean protease inhibitor suppress X-ray induced transformation *in vitro*, *Proc. Natl. Acad. Sci. USA* **82**:5395–5399.

Yen, J. T., Jensen, A. H., and Simon, J., 1977, Effect of dietary raw soybean and soybean trypsin inhibitor on trypsin and chymotrypsin activities in the pancreas and in small intestinal juice of growing swine, *J. Nutr.* **107**:156–165.

Young, V. R., Wayler, A., Garza, C., Steinke, F. H., Murray, E., Rand, W. M., and Scrimshaw, N. S., 1984, A long-term metabolic balance study in young men to assess the nutritional quality of an isolated soy protein and beef proteins, *Am. J. Clin. Nutr.* **39**:8–15.

3

In Vitro Studies of Anticarcinogenic Protease Inhibitors

ANN R. KENNEDY

1. Introduction

Several different types of agents have been shown to modify the yield of transformed cells *in vitro*. We have observed that certain protease inhibitors have the
ability to suppress radiation- and chemical-induced malignant transformation *in
vitro* in a highly significant fashion (Kennedy and Little, 1978, 1980a, 1981b;
Little *et al.*, 1979; Kennedy and Weichselbaum, 1981; Kennedy, 1982, 1984a,b,
1985a, 1988, 1990a; Yavelow *et al.*, 1983, 1985; Baturay and Kennedy, 1986;
Billings *et al.*, 1987a, 1989). Several other investigators have also observed that
some protease inhibitors can effectively suppress transformation *in vitro* (Kuroki
and Drevon, 1979; Borek *et al.*, 1979; DiPaolo *et al.*, 1980; Popescu *et al.*,
1980; Sun *et al.* 1988). The studies showing that protease inhibitors suppress
transformation *in vitro* have utilized several different model systems, several
different carcinogens (including x-radiation, UV light, chemical carcinogens,
and steroid hormones as the inducing agents) and several different agents as
promoters (or cocarcinogens) (reviewed in Kennedy, 1984a), as shown in Tables
I and II (culture dishes containing transformed foci/cells are shown in Fig. 1).
These results suggest that protease inhibitors are capable of suppressing similar
processes induced by different carcinogens (with or without promotion or cocarcinogenesis) in several different cell systems. Protease inhibitors have an unusual
ability to suppress information *in vitro* in a highly significant manner, as opposed
to the marginal effects observed for many other classes of possible human cancer

ANN R. KENNEDY • Department of Radiation Oncology, School of Medicine, University of Penn-
sylvania, Philadelphia, Pennsylvania 19104.
Protease Inhibitors as Cancer Chemopreventive Agents, edited by Walter Troll and Ann R. Kennedy.
Plenum Press, New York, 1993.

Table I. Protease Inhibitor Suppression of Transformation *in Vitro* Induced by Several Different Types of Carcinogenic Agents (in Various Cell Systems)

Initiating agent	Inhibiting agent	System used	Authors (year of first publication of authors with inhibitor)
X rays	Protease inhibitors— antipain, etc.	Mouse C3H10T1/2 cells Mouse 3T3 cells	Kennedy and Little (1978)
	Protease inhibitor— antipain	Hamster embryo cells Mouse C3H10T1/2 cells	Borek *et al.* (1979)
3-Methylcholanthrene	Protease inhibitors— antipain, etc.	Mouse C3H10T1/2 cells	Kuroki and Drevon (1979)
N-methyl-*N'*-nitro-*N*-nitrosoguanidine	Protease inhibitor— antipain	Hamster embryo cells	DiPaolo *et al.* (1980)
17-β-estradiol	Protease inhibitors— antipain, etc.	Mouse C3H10T1/2 cells	Kennedy and Weich-selbaum (1981)
UV light	Protease inhibitors— antipain, etc.	Mouse C3H10T1/2 cells	Kennedy (1984b)
X rays	Protease inhibitors— antipain, etc.	Human diploid (1522) cells	Kennedy (1984b)
γ rays	Protease inhibitors— antipain, etc.	Human hybrid (CGL1) cells	Sun *et al.* (1988)

chemopreventive agents which we have studied (Kennedy, 1984a,b, 1985b, 1986; Kennedy *et al.*, 1984b). Not only are many other potential chemopreventive agents marginal in their effectiveness, but most of them need to be added to cultures at toxic or nearly toxic levels to observe any effect [e.g., see the effective levels of vitamin E (Radner and Kennedy, 1986)]. By comparison, protease inhibitors are effective at very low concentrations.

We have reported that several different types of protease inhibitors suppress carcinogen-induced malignant transformation *in vitro,* even when they are added to cells at very long times after carcinogen exposure (Kennedy and Little, 1981b; Kennedy, 1982, 1985). We have observed that inhibitors of a specific protease, chymotrypsin, are the most effective for the suppression of malignant transformation (Kennedy, 1985). Treatment of cells with certain chymotrypsin inhibitors, for short periods of time, will suppress carcinogen-induced transformation effectively at nanomolar or picomolar concentrations in the medium; effective concentrations of protease inhibitors which do not inhibit chymotrypsin are many orders of magnitude higher than this (Kennedy, 1985). [Inhibitors of chymotrypsin are also more effective than other protease inhibitors at the suppression of

Table II. Protease Inhibitors and Other Agents That Inhibit the Enhancement of Transformation *in Vitro* by a Promoting Agent (TPA) or a Cocarcinogen (Pyrene)

Initiating agents	Promoting agent (TPA) or cocarcinogen (pyrene)	Inhibitor of promotion or cocarcinogenesis	Cell system	Authors (year of first publication)
X rays UV light	TPA	Lymphotoxin	Hamster embryo cells	DiPaolo *et al.* (1980)
X rays	TPA	Retinoids	Hamster embryo cells Mouse C3H10T1/2 cells	Miller *et al.* (1981)
3-Methylcholanthrene	TPA	Retinoids	Mouse C3H10T1/2 cells	Mordan *et al.* (1982)
3-Methylcholanthrene 5-Azacytidine	TPA	Dexamethasone Fluocinolone acetonide Indomethacin	Mouse C3H10T1/2 cells	Mondal and Heidelberger (1980)
X rays	TPA	Indomethacin	Mouse C3H10T1/2 cells	Little and Kennedy (1982)
X rays	TPA	Protease inhibitors— antipain, etc.	Mouse C3H10T1/2 cells Mouse 3T3 cells	Kennedy and Little (1978)
N-methyl-N'-nitro-N-nitrosoguanidine	TPA	Protease inhibitor— antipain	Hamster embryo cells	Popescu *et al.* (1980)
γ rays β-Propiolactone Benzo(*a*)pyrene	Pyrene	Protease inhibitor (Bowman–Birk inhibitor)	Mouse BALB/c 3T3 cells	Baturay and Kennedy (1986)

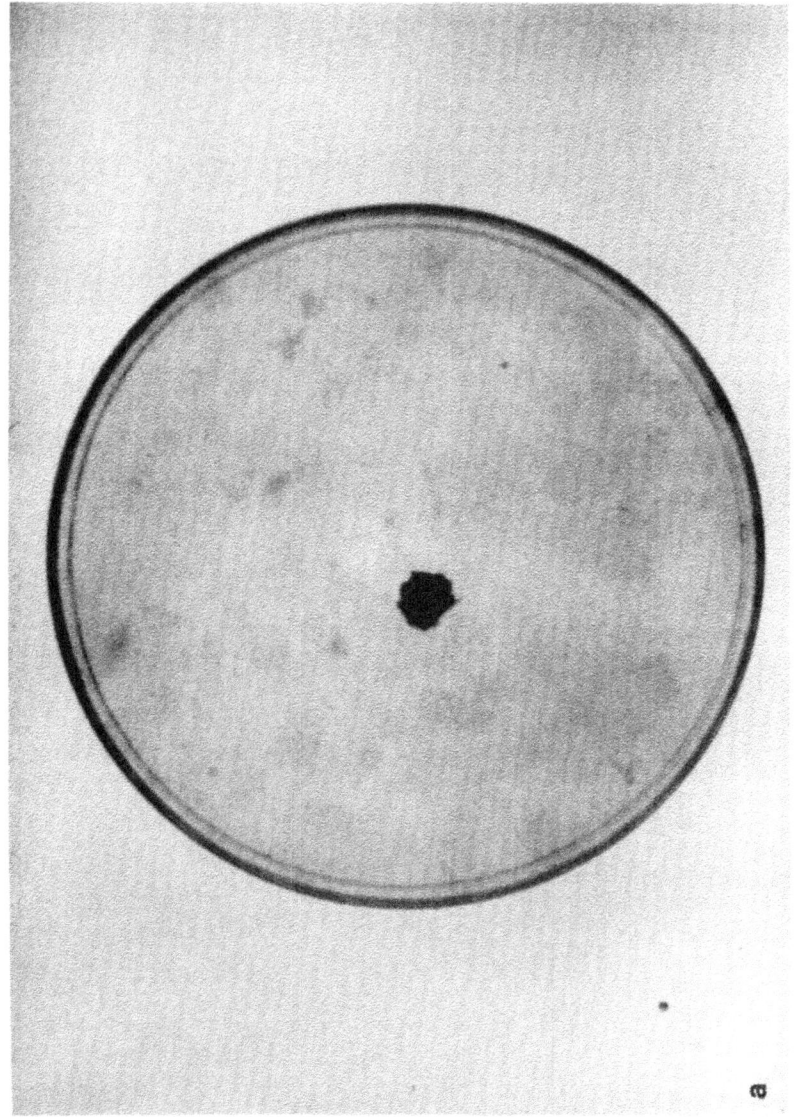

a

Figure 1. (a) Petri dish exhibiting one focus of transformed cells against a background monolayer of nontransformed C3H10T1/2 cells. (b) High-power view of edge of focus of transformed cells. The transformed cells are highly polar and basophilic and exhibit a crisscross pattern of orientation.

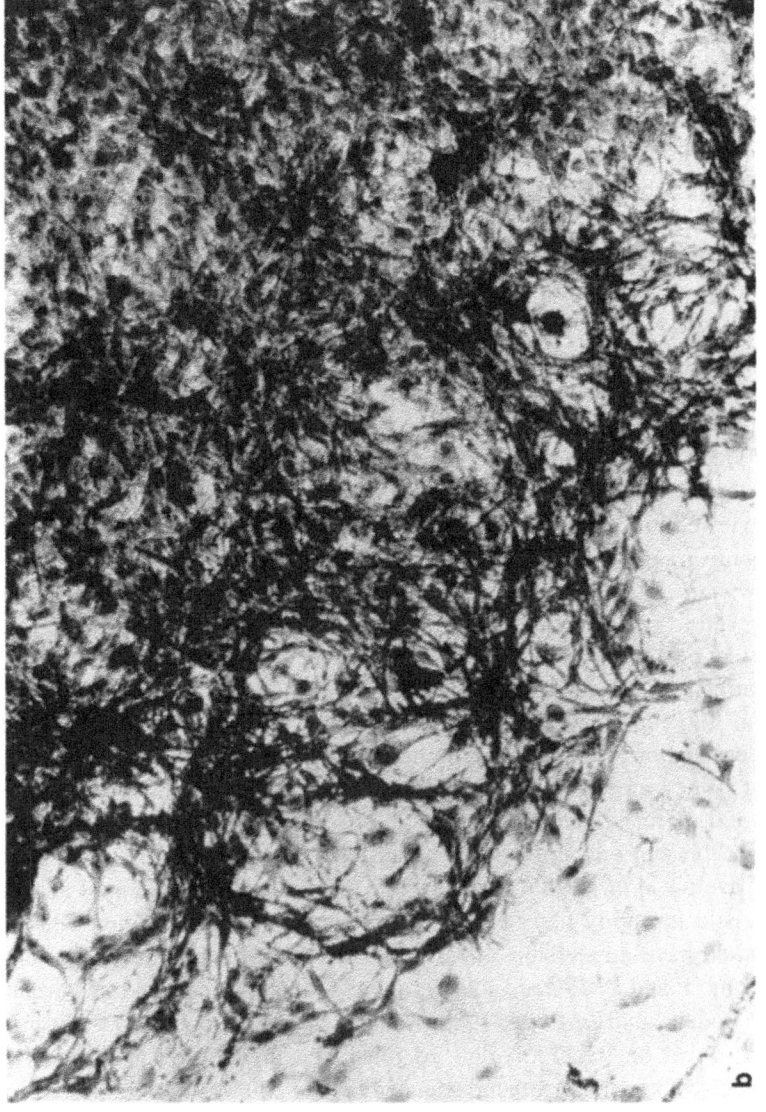

Figure 1. (Continued)

several other phenomena related to carcinogenesis, as has been described else-where (Kennedy, 1985b).] Of particular interest to us have been our studies with chymotrypsin inhibitors naturally present in vegetables—specifically, the soybean-derived Bowman–Birk inhibitor (BBI), the chick pea inhibitor (CPI), and the potato chymotrypsin inhibitor. BBI and CPI inhibit both trypsin and chymotrypsin, but it is only the chymotrypsin inhibitory region (and not the trypsin inhibitory region) of these protease inhibitors that is involved in the suppression of transformation *in vitro* (Yavelow *et al.*, 1985). CPI is more effective than BBI at suppressing transformation (Yavelow *et al.*, 1985) and is a stronger inhibitor of chymotrypsin; CPI contains tyrosine at the chymotrypsin inhibitory site while BBI contains leucine (Smirnoff *et al.*, 1979). The potato chymotrypsin inhibitor does not have a distinct trypsin inhibitory site (discussed in Billings *et al.*, 1987a), but does have the ability to inhibit chymotrypsin. It is not as strong as BBI in its ability to inhibit chymotrypsin or transformation *in vitro* (Billings *et al.*, 1987).

Thus far, our transformation studies with protease inhibitors have indicated that: (1) they can suppress transformation *in vitro* induced by radiation (with and without promoters, such as TPA, or cocarcinogens, such as pyrene or 17-β-estradiol) and the chemical carcinogens, benzo(*a*)pyrene and β-propiolactone (both with and without the cocarcinogen, pyrene), in several different cell systems (reviewed in Kennedy, 1984a), as shown in Fig. 2; (2) they are effective in suppressing transformation when present at extremely low concentrations (Yavelow *et al.*, 1985; Kennedy, 1985a); (3) they can suppress radiation transformation even when added to cultures many days after carcinogen exposure (Yavelow *et al.*, 1985; Kennedy, 1982, 1985), as illustrated in Fig. 3; (4) short-term treatments of protease inhibitors are sufficient for the suppression of transformation [e.g., a 1-day treatment with protease inhibitors, even 5 days after carcinogen treatment, suppresses radiation-induced transformation (Kennedy, 1982)]; (5) they are capable of reversing the initiated state of cells (Kennedy, 1985a); and (6) they have an irreversible effect on the transformation process, even when present only for a short period of time (Kennedy and Little, 1978, 1981b; Yavelow *et al.*, 1985; Kennedy, 1985a), as illustrated in Fig. 4. This last characteristic is highly unusual. Other inhibitors of transformation which we have studied have a reversible effect on the transformation process. For examples, vitamin E and DMSO are able to suppress radiation-induced transformation *in vitro* (Radner and Kennedy, 1986; Kennedy and Symons, 1987), but have a reversible effect on transformation, as illustrated in Fig. 5. These studies are discussed elsewhere in more detail (Kennedy, 1988, 1990a). Our proposed model for the induction of transformation *in vitro* and its suppression by agents such as protease inhibitors, vitamin E, and DMSO is shown schematically in Fig. 6 and discussed elsewhere (Kennedy, 1988).

Not all protease inhibitors can suppress transformation *in vitro;* a summary of those studied for the ability to suppress transformation is given in Table III.

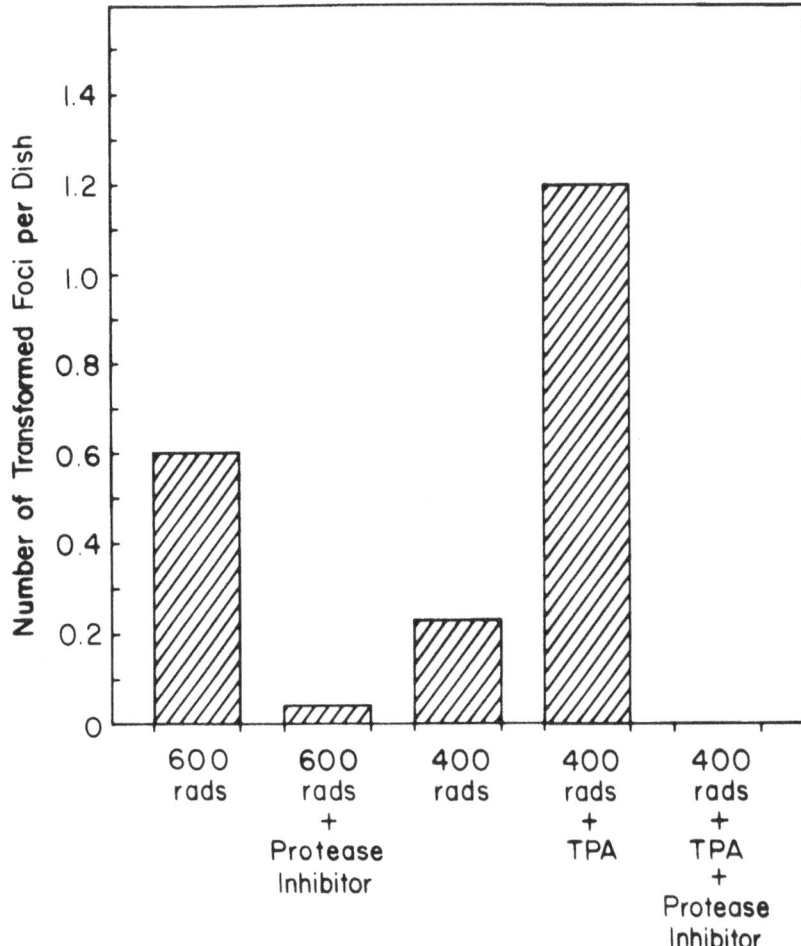

Figure 2. Effects of the protease inhibitor antipain on radiation-induced transformation *in vitro* (Kennedy and Billings, 1987). Protease inhibitors are capable of suppressing the TPA enhancement of radiation transformation as well as the carcinogenic process brought about by a high dose of a complete carcinogen such as x-irradiation, as discussed in Kennedy (1984a).

The results from our laboratory work which are shown in Table III and have not been published elsewhere are given in Table IV. ε-Amino-*n*-caproic acid, Edi Pro A, and FOY-305 were studied by us for their ability to suppress transformation because they had been shown to have anticarcinogenic activity *in vivo*, as reported by Corasanti *et al.* (1982) for ε-amino-*n*-caproic acid, by Becker (1981) for Edi Pro A, and by Ohkoshi and Fujii (1983) for FOY-305 (see Chapter 2 for a review of these studies). Succinylated BBI was prepared by us [according to the methods described by Smirnoff *et al.* (1979)] to remove trypsin inhibitor activity from BBI. As discussed in Chapter 2, trypsin inhibitory activity could have

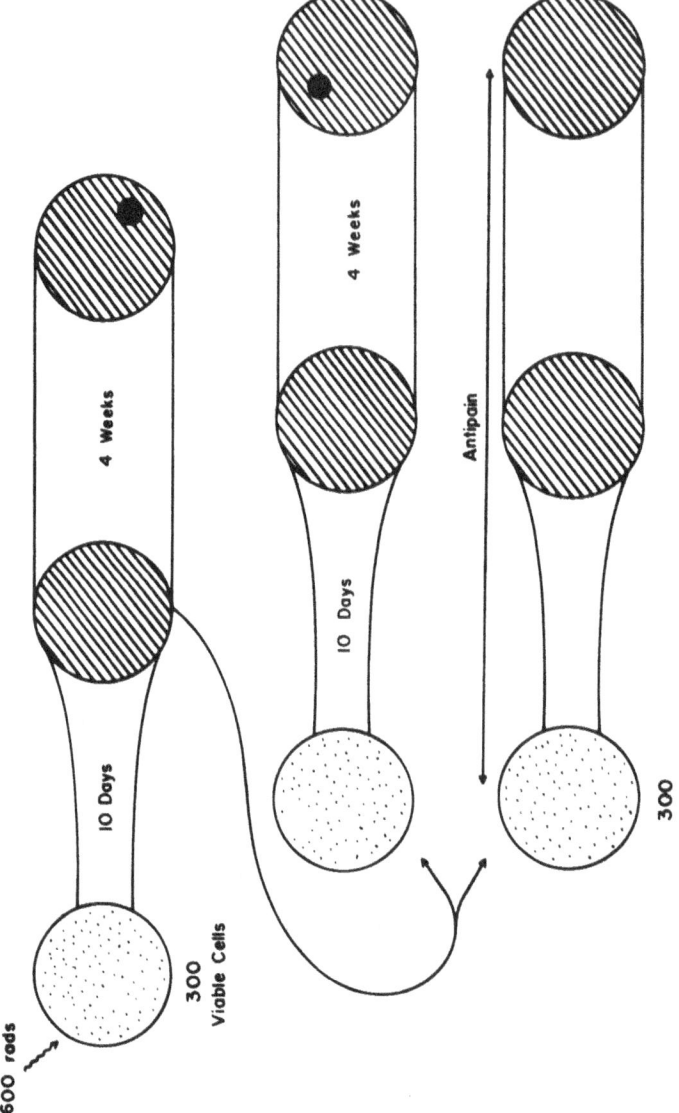

Figure 3. Protease inhibitors can suppress radiation transformation when applied to cultures as late as 10 days and 13 cell divisions after carcinogen exposure. As shown in lines 1 and 2, subculture of the irradiated cells at confluence leads to approximately the same yield of transformed foci as observed for dishes which are not subcultured (e.g., see Kennedy *et al.*, 1980). If protease inhibitors are applied to subcultured dishes, transformed foci do not appear (as shown in line 3); this result is the same as that observed when protease inhibitors are applied to cells soon after carcinogen exposure [as shown in Fig. 4 (line 2)].

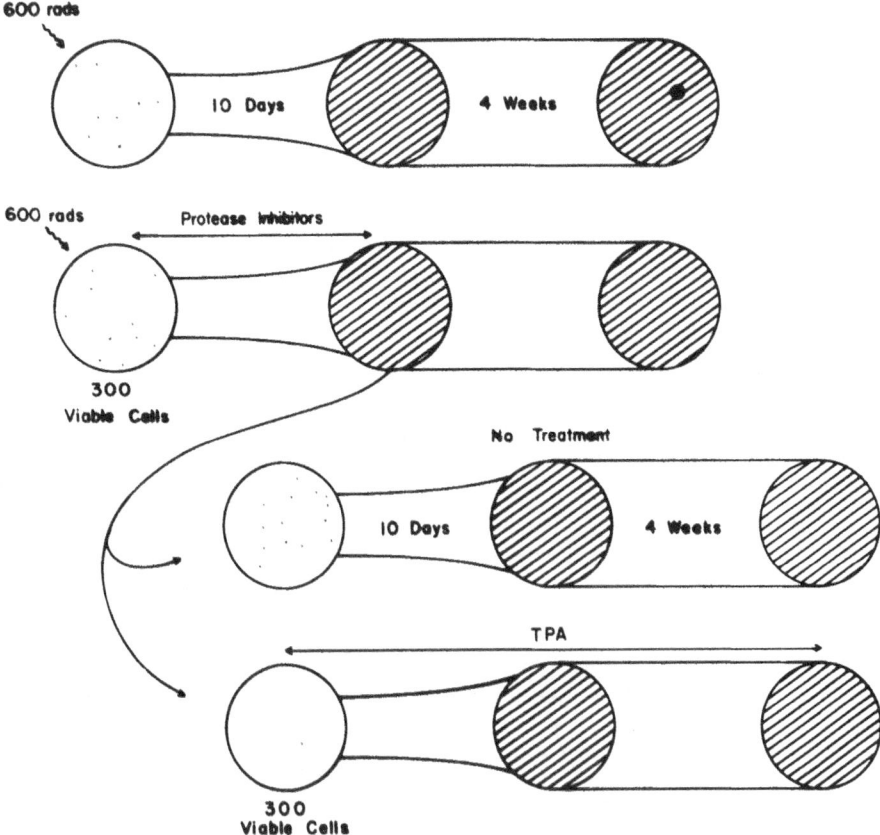

Figure 4. Protease inhibitors affect proliferating initiated cells, and have an irreversible effect on the transformation process. If protease inhibitors are applied to proliferating initiated cells, transformed foci do not occur in the routine transformation assay (as shown in line 2) or in a subculture-type assay in which the carcinogen-treated cells are subcultured and exposed to TPA (or not exposed to TPA) during subsequent growth of the cultures to confluence and maintenance in confluence for the usual 4-week period (lines 3 and 4). These results suggest that protease inhibitors have reversed the initiated state of the carcinogen-treated cells, as discussed in detail in Kennedy (1985a).

deleterious side effects; thus, this activity was removed from BBI in this preparation. Succinylated BBI was prepared by treating pure BBI with succinic anhydride; with this treatment a succinyl group becomes attached to lysine at the trypsin inhibitory site, rendering it inactive while leaving the chymotrypsin inhibitory site intact. For BBI, we have determined that the anticarcinogenic activity is in the chymotrypsin inhibitory portion of the molecule; thus, altering the trypsin inhibitory site does not affect its anticarcinogenic activity *in vitro* (Yavelow *et al.*, 1985).

While many different anticarcinogenic protease inhibitors (or preparations

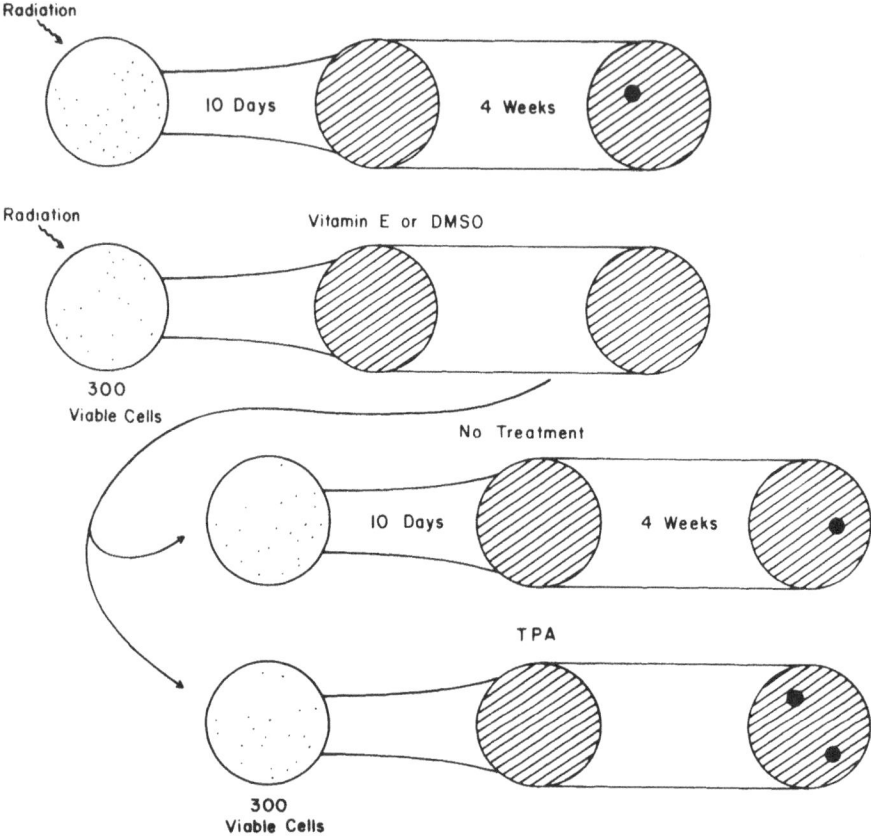

Figure 5. The design of the studies shown schematically here is similar to those described in Figs. 3 and 4. As can be observed in line 2, vitamin E and DMSO have the ability to suppress radiation transformation when present during the entire radiation transformation assay period. If the irradiated cultures are subcultured, however, and maintained without the presence of DMSO or vitamin E (and either with or without TPA), transformed foci appear. These results suggest that vitamin E and DMSO have not reversed the initiated state of the cells. These results are discussed in more detail in Kennedy (1990a).

containing protease inhibitors) are listed in Table III, the concentrations at which these protease inhibitors are able to affect transformation *in vitro* are markedly different. As shown in Table V, effective concentrations of different anticarcinogenic protease inhibitors vary over orders of magnitude. The potency of the protease inhibitor (in terms of its effect on the transformation process) appears to be important as a predictor of anticarcinogenic activity *in vivo*. For example, chymotrypsin inhibitor I from potatoes is relatively weak in its ability to suppress transformation *in vitro* compared with BBI (Billings *et al.*, 1987a) and is a far less effective anticarcinogenic agent than BBI *in vivo* (von Hofe *et al.*, unpublished data; Kennedy *et al.*, unpublished data).

Postulated Scheme for the Induction of Malignant Transformation in vitro

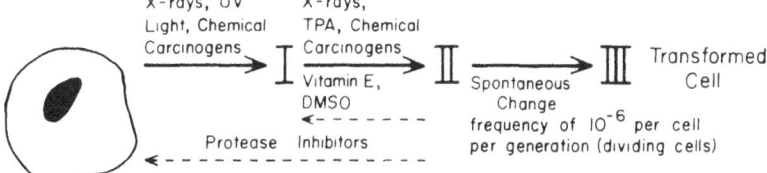

Figure 6. Our current concepts on the steps involved in the induction of transformation in C3H10T1/2 cells. The evidence of each of these postulated steps, and their possible modification by various agents, are discussed elsewhere (Kennedy, 1984a, 1988; Kennedy and Billings, 1987).

Table III. Studies on the Ability of Different Protease Inhibitors to Suppress Transformation *in Vitro* (Induced by Various Carcinogens)

Protease inhibitor	Carcinogen	Carcinogen-induced Yes	Carcinogen-induced No	TPA-enhanced Yes	TPA-enhanced No	Authors (year of first reference utilizing each protease inhibitor)
Antipain	Radiation	+		+		Kennedy and Little (1978)
Leupeptin		+		+		Kennedy and Little (1981b)
Antipain	Radiation	+		ND	ND	Borek *et al.* (1979)
Antipain	3-Methylchol-	+		ND	ND	Kuroki and Drevon
Chymostatin	anthrene	+		ND	ND	(1979)
Elastatinol		+		ND	ND	
Leupeptin		+		ND	ND	
Pepstatin		+		ND	ND	
Antipain	*N*-methyl-*N'*-nitro-*N*-nitrosoguanidine	+		ND	ND	DiPaolo *et al.* (1980)
Soybean trypsin inhibitor	Radiation		+	+		Kennedy and Little (1981)
Antipain	Radiation/17-β-estradiol	+		ND	ND	Kennedy and Weichselbaum (1981)
Leupeptin						
Bowman–Birk inhibitor	Radiation	+			+	Yavelow *et al.* (1983, 1985)
Elastatinol	Radiation		+		+	Kennedy (1984b) (see Table IV)

(continued)

Table III. (*Continued*)

| Protease inhibitor | Carcinogen | Ability to suppress transformation | | | | Authors (year of first reference utilizing each protease inhibitor) |
| | | Carcinogen-induced | | TPA-enhanced | | |
		Yes	No	Yes	No	
Chymostatin	Radiation	+		+		Kennedy (1984b, 1985)
FOY-305 (*N,N*-dimethyl carbamoylmethyl 4-(4-guanidino-benzoyloxy)-phenylacetate methanesulfonate	Radiation		+	+		Kennedy (1984) (see Table IV)
TPCK (tosylamide-2-phenylethyl-chloromethyl-ketone)	Radiation	+		+		Kennedy (1985a)
Bowman–Birk inhibitor (fragment containing chymotrypsin inhibitory site)	Radiation	+		ND	ND	Yavelow *et al.* (1985)
Extract of soybeans containing BBI	Radiation	+		ND	ND	Yavelow *et al.* (1985)
	Radiation, benzo(*a*)pyrene, β-propiolactone (with and without enhancement by pyrene)	+		ND	ND	Baturay and Kennedy (1986)
α₁-antitrypsin "protease inhibitor IV"—trypsin inhibitor from soybeans (from Dr. Donald Foard)	Radiation		+	ND	ND	Yavelow *et al.* (1985)
Chickpea inhibitor	Radiation	+		ND	ND	Yavelow *et al.* (1985)
Chymotrypsin inhibitor I from potatoes	Radiation	+		ND	ND	Billings *et al.* (1987a)

(*continued*)

Table III. (*Continued*)

Protease inhibitor	Carcinogen	Ability to suppress transformation — Carcinogen-induced Yes	Ability to suppress transformation — Carcinogen-induced No	Ability to suppress transformation — TPA-enhanced Yes	Ability to suppress transformation — TPA-enhanced No	Authors (year of first reference utilizing each protease inhibitor)
Carboxypeptidase inhibitor I and inhibitor II from potatoes	Radiation	+		ND	ND	Billings *et al.* (1989)
Aprotinin and N-acetyl-L-tyrosine ethyl ester	Radiation		+	ND	ND	Billings *et al.* (1989)
Pepstatin	Radiation		+	ND	ND	Carew and Kennedy (1990)
Phosphoramidon	Radiation		+	ND	ND	Kennedy (Table IV)
Edi Pro A (soybean extract prepared by Ralston Purina)	Radiation	+		ND	ND	Kennedy (Table IV)
ε-Amino-n-caproic acid	Radiation	+		ND	ND	Kennedy (Table IV)
Succinylated BBI (BBI lacking trypsin inhibitory site)	Radiation	+		ND	ND	Kennedy (Table IV)
BBI–polylysine	Radiation	+		ND	ND	Persiani *et al.* (1991)

BBI proved to be such a potent anticarcinogenic agent in our *in vitro* studies that we began to study it as an anticarcinogenic agent in *in vivo* carcinogenesis systems; our studies which have demonstrated the ability of BBI to prevent or suppress carcinogenesis in animal model systems are discussed in Chapter 2. While pure BBI is highly effective as an anticarcinogenic agent *in vivo*, the cost involved in obtaining a pure preparation would be prohibitive for trials of human cancer prevention. Thus, we have been studying a crude extract of BBI for eventual use in large-scale trials of both animal and human cancer prevention. The crude extract works approximately as well as does the purified inhibitor in C3H10T1/2 cells to inhibit transformation [and the autoclaved crude extract, in which the protease inhibitor activity has been destroyed, has no effect on carcinogen-induced transformation *in vitro* (Yavelow *et al.*, 1985)]. The crude extract works as well as purified BBI in other *in vitro* assay systems as well; for

Table IV. Results of Studies Performed to Determine the Effects of Various Protease Inhibitors (or, in the Case of Edi Pro A, a Preparation Containing Protease Inhibitors) on Radiation Transformation in Vitro[a]

Treatment[b]	Expt No.	P.E.	Total No. of cells	Total No. of transformed foci		Fraction of dishes which contained transformed foci		
				Type 3	Types 2 & 3	Type 3	Types 2 & 3	Total[a]
1. Control (no treatment)	1	32.5	3,575	0	0	0/11	0/11	0/89
	2	53.3	4,800	0	0	0/10	0/10	
	3	58.9	5,300	0	0	0/10	0/10	
	4	50.0	4,500	0	0	0/10	0/10	
	5	25.7	6,168	0	0	0/24	0/24	
	6	22.5	3,150	0	0	0/14	0/14	
	7	28.8	2,880	0	0	0/10	0/10	
2. 600 rads	1	3.1	7,130	3	21	3/23 = 0.13	13/23 = 0.56	50/84 = 0.60
	2	3.6	7,200	4	16	4/20 = 0.20	10/20 = 0.50	
	3	5.1	9,180	9	19	7/18 = 0.39	11/18 = 0.61	
	4	9.2	18,400	11	22	6/20 = 0.30	13/20 = 0.65	
	5	1.5	452	0	7	0/3	3/3 = 1.0	
3. 600 rads + ε-amino-n-caproic acid	1	2.2	5,060	0	5	0/23	5/23 = 0.22	5/23 = 0.22

4. 600 rads + phosphoramidon	2	4.8	4,320	1	5	1/9 = 0.11	5/9 = 0.56	5/9 = 0.56
5. 600 rads + Edi Pro A	3	6.1	12,200	3	4	3/20 = 0.15	4/20 = 0.20	4/20 = 0.20
6. 600 rads + succinylated BBI	3	6.3	5,670	1	4	1/20 = 0.05	4/20 = 0.20	10/40 = 0.25
	4	8.2	16,400	2	8	2/20 = 0.10	6/20 = 0.30	
7. 600 rads + elastatinol	5	2.2	3,300	6	20	6/15 = 0.40	14/15 = 0.93	14/15 = 0.93
8. 600 rads + Foy-305	5	1.9	1,902	2	7	1/6 = 0.17	5/6 = 0.83	5/6 = 0.83
9. 100 rads	5	24.0	10,320	2	4	2/43 = 0.05	4/43 = 0.09	8/86 = 0.09
	6	22.8	5,244	1	2	2/23 = 0.09	2/23 = 0.09	
	7	25.3	5,060	1	2	1/20 = 0.05	2/20 = 0.10	
10. 100 rads + TPA	5	23.4	2,574	2	5	2/11 = 0.18	4/11 = 0.36	9/22 = 0.41
	6	20.7	1,242	1	2	1/6 = 0.17	2/6 = 0.33	
	7	26.0	1,300	2	4	2/5 = 0.40	3/5 = 0.60	
11. 100 rads + TPA + FOY-305	5	23.3	9,087	2	7	2/39 = 0.05	6/39 = 0.15	12/78 = 0.15
	6	17.5	2,975	2	5	2/17 = 0.12	3/17 = 0.18	
	7	29.0	6,380	0	4	0/22	3/22 = 0.14	

[a]The transformation experiments reported here were performed with C3H10T1/2 cells; similar experiments utilizing this cell system are described in detail elsewhere (e.g., see Kennedy, 1985a).
[b]The concentrations and sources of the various compounds used in these studies were: TPA (lot 028, Consolidated Midland Co.) 0.1 μg/ml; FOY-305 (kindly provided by Dr. Tsuyohiko Mori and the ONO Pharmaceutical Co. Ltd., Osaka, Japan) 100 μg/ml; elastinol (kindly provided by Dr. Walter Troll and the U.S. Japan Cooperative Cancer Research Program) 50 μg/ml; ε-amino-n-caproic acic (Sigma Chemical Co., St. Louis, Mo.) 400 μg/ml; Edi Pro A (prepared by Ralston Purina and obtained from Dr. Daniel Medina) 300 μg/ml; succinylated BBI [prepared by Dr. Paul Billings utilizing the procedure described by Smirnoff et al. (1979)] 10 μg/ml (Expt 3) and 0.001 μg/ml (Expt 4); phosphoramidon (Sigma) 10 μg/ml.

Table V. Comparison of Protease
Inhibitors (on a Molar Basis) Regarding
Their Ability to Suppress Radiation
Transformation in Vitro[a]

Protease inhibitor	Concentration[b]
Antipain	1.7×10^{-6} M
Chymostatin	1.7×10^{-12} M
Bowman–Birk inhibitor	1.3×10^{-10} M
TPCK (tosylamide-2-phenyl- ethylchloromethyl ketone)	2.8×10^{-9} M

[a]Data from Kennedy (1985a).
[b]Lowest amount of each protease inhibitor to reduce radiation transformation in vitro to a comparable degree (i.e., to
10% of the dishes containing transformed foci).

example, both pure BBI and the BBI extract are equally capable of reducing the
levels of chromosome abnormalities in the cells of patients with Bloom's syndrome (Kennedy et al., 1984a).

2. Mechanism of Action of the Anticarcinogenic Protease Inhibitors in the Suppression of Transformation in Vitro

As discussed in Chapter 2 and elsewhere in this volume, the mechanism(s)
by which protease inhibitors suppress carcinogenesis is unknown, although many
hypotheses have been discussed by us (e.g., see Kennedy, 1984a) as well as other
investigators (e.g., see Troll et al., 1984, 1987). The major problem in determining the mechanism by which any anticarcinogenic agent is operating is the
fact that the mechanisms involved in carcinogenesis are unknown. When the
causes of cancer become known with certainty, it will become possible to determine the mechanisms involved in cancer prevention and suppression.

From our own previous studies, we believe that the first event in
carcinogen-induced malignant transformation is a high-frequency event occurring in many cells treated with low doses of either chemical or physical carcinogens (Kennedy et al., 1980, 1984; Kennedy and Little, 1981a, 1984; Kennedy,
1984a, 1985c, 1989, 1990b). We believe that the hypothesized high-frequency
initiating event is likely to be caused by a change in gene expression, as it is
known that such changes in gene expression can be caused by carcinogens
(Fahmy and Fahmy, 1980) and can occur in a high proportion (~80%) of
carcinogen-treated cells (e.g., see Scott and Maercklein, 1985). These changes
in gene expression can be thought of as acting like a switch (Kennedy, 1989), and
are well known in radiation biology; such changes have been demonstrated even

in irradiated human cells (Rosen and Klein, 1983). [Other similar inherited epigenetic changes are discussed elsewhere (Kennedy, 1985c, 1989).] We are assuming that a major consequence of the (presumed) carcinogen-induced change in gene expression is that it confers on cells an altered probability that a subsequent event, malignant transformation (i.e., an event which leads directly to the malignant state), will occur (reviewed in Kennedy, 1984a, 1985c). Our past work has suggested that protease inhibitors are able to stop what appears to be an ongoing cellular process begun by the carcinogen exposure, presumably by reversing the carcinogen-induced change in gene expression. Thus, we believe that a cellular process in many cells is begun by carcinogens and that certain "anticarcinogenic" protease inhibitors can turn this process off before a rare, later, mutationlike event (leading directly to the malignant state), can occur (Kennedy, 1982, 1985c).

High-frequency processes which lead to rare genetic events are already known to exist. For example, the SOS repair system in bacteria is known to be turned on in cells exposed to carcinogens; the induction of this system then leads to rare genetic events (mutations) (Witkin, 1976). This is not the likely mechanism to explain carcinogenesis, however. There is little or no effect of protease inhibitors on mammalian DNA repair processes (Borek and Cleaver, 1981; Korbelik *et al.*, 1988). In fact, there is little evidence to support the existence of a mammalian error-prone repair system similar to SOS repair in bacteria, as has been reviewed (Rossman and Klein, 1985). Furthermore, this system is not persistently activated in bacteria, as it would need to be to explain the phenomena involved in carcinogenesis. A system which does have the characteristic of persistent activation is radiation-induced recombination in yeast (Fabre and Roman, 1977). This is a system in which both x rays and UV light have been shown to induce recombinational events which continue to occur for many generations postirradiation. Radiation could induce such a system in mammalian cells which could then produce the transformed cell genotype.

It is reasonable to expect proteases to be involved in the induction of the systems described above. Proteases are known to play a central role in gene regulation (Gottesman, 1987). SOS functions are known to be activated by a protease (Little *et al.*, 1980) and are inhibited by protease inhibitors (Meyn *et al.*, 1977). Radiation-induced recombination in yeast is also suppressed by protease inhibitors, with inhibitors of chymotrypsin being the most effective protease inhibitors studied for suppression of the process (Wintersberger, 1984). We have observed that inhibitors of chymotrypsin are also the most effective protease inhibitors at suppressing radiation-induced transformation *in vitro* (Kennedy, 1985a), a correlation which may suggest a relationship between the process operating in yeast and that involved in the induction of malignancy in mammalian cells.

An ongoing process of the sort we envision as being induced by carcinogens in mammalian cells may be operating in the cells of patients with Bloom's syndrome. It is known that patients with Bloom's syndrome have a higher than normal rate of cancer development, and that the cells of these patients are constantly generating new chromosome abnormalities (reviewed by German, 1983). We have observed that the anticarcinogenic protease inhibitors can reduce the levels of chromosome abnormalities in the cells of patients with Bloom's syndrome (Kennedy et al., 1984a). It is conceivable that the high-frequency cellular process hypothesized by us to be induced by carcinogens is continuously operating in the cells of patients with Bloom's syndrome.

A process of the sort likely to explain our observations on carcinogenesis in mammalian cells has not been identified yet. There are some genes which are likely to play a role in transformation in the systems we have studied, however.

From other in vitro studies, we believe that the expression of the c-myc gene is of importance in the first step of transformation and that the activation of ras is our "later" (hypothesized) genetic event leading directly to the transformed state. Activation of the c-myc gene is often associated with higher levels of expression, or deregulation of this gene (Leder et al., 1983; Campisi et al., 1984), and ras is known to be activated by specific point mutations (reviewed by Balmain, 1985), although both mutation and increased gene expression appear to be necessary in the activation of ras (Spandidos and Wilke, 1984). Some of the evidence that has led to our hypothesis is as follows. (1) There is much evidence to suggest that deregulation of the myc gene and/or the activation of ras occurs in both experimentally induced and human cancers (reviewed by Balmain, 1985; Leder et al., 1983; Hunter, 1981). (2) It is known that carcinogens such as radiation (Sawey et al., 1987; St. Clair et al., 1990), as well as promoting agents such as TPA (e.g., see Kelly et al., 1983) can induce higher levels of expression or amplification of the c-myc gene. Sawey et al. (1987) recently reported that c-myc amplification occurred in 9 out of 12 radiation-induced tumors studied, with ras also activated in 6 of these tumors. (3) It is known that c-myc alone cannot transform normal diploid cells: both myc and ras must be activated (among other changes) for transformation to occur in normal diploid cells (Dotto et al., 1985; Land et al., 1983a,b). Increased c-myc gene expression is considered necessary but not sufficient for cancer development in vivo (Stewart et al., 1984). (4) It has been reported that myc activation must occur first, before ras can transform rodent cells (Connan et al., 1985). (5) It has been shown that the activation of ras occurs in carcinogen-transformed C3H/10T1/2 cells (Parada and Weinberg, 1983; Chen and Herschman, 1989; Smith and Grisham, 1987). (6) The activation of ras occurs as a late step in the malignant transformation of carcinogen-exposed normal diploid rodent cells (e.g., Sukumar et al., 1985), and in many other systems (e.g., Newbold and Overell, 1983), including in vivo carcinogenesis (e.g., Capon et al., 1983; Der and Cooper, 1983; Bos et al., 1987) [although ras activation can occur early in other systems and is considered by some to be consistent with an initiating event (e.g., Brown et al., 1986)]. (7) We have already reported that anticarcinogenic protease inhibitors, including BBI, reduce the levels of c-*myc* expression in carcinogen-treated cells (Chang *et al.*, 1985, 1990; Chang and Kennedy, 1988; Li *et al.*, 1992) and anticarcinogenic protease inhibitors affect the first step of the transformation process (Kennedy, 1985a). While the anticarcinogenic protease inhibitors clearly affect c-*myc* expression in C3H10T1/2 cells, they do not affect c-*myc* expression in C3H10T1/2 cells that have been malignantly transformed (Chang *et al.*, 1990). We believe this aspect of the protease inhibitor effect on c-*myc* expression to be of central importance in our studies, since the development of malignancy involves some phenomenon that can be regulated in normal cells, but is not regulated in cancer cells. c-*myc* expression appears to have these characteristics in our studies; it can be regulated by (anticarcinogenic) protease inhibitors in nontransformed cells and cannot be regulated in the same fashion in transformed cells. Thus, we believe that specific cooperating oncogenes, *myc* and *ras*, may play central roles in carcinogen-induced transformation *in vitro* and carcinogenesis *in vivo*.

Our recent work has shown that c-*myc* is not the only oncogene whose expression is affected by the anticarcinogenic protease inhibitors; c-*fos* expression is also affected, as discussed elsewhere (Caggana and Kennedy, 1989). The particular protease inhibitors which have been studied for their ability to affect c-*myc* and c-*fos* gene expression are shown in Table VI. As seen, there is a general correlation between the ability of a protease inhibitor to affect c-*myc* and/or c-*fos* gene expression and its ability to suppress radiation-induced transformation *in vitro*. Still other oncogenes such as H-*ras* could be affected by the anticarcinogenic protease inhibitors. For example, Garte *et al.* (1987) reported that protease inhibitors could suppress H-*ras*-induced transformation of 3T3 cells; this effect could be mediated through the anticarcinogenic protease inhibitor effect on c-*myc*, however, as *myc* and *ras* are known to interact in transformation (as discussed above). The protease inhibitor suppression of *ras*-induced

Table VI. Suppression of Gene Expression by Protease Inhibitors (in Terms of Effective Molar Concentrations of Protease Inhibitors)

| Protease inhibitor | Actin expression | Ability of protease inhibitors to suppress | | c-*fos* expression | Radiation-induced transformation |
| | | c-*myc* expression | | | |
		Nontransformed cells	Transformed cells		
Bowman–Birk	−	+ +	−	+ + +	+ + +
Antipain	−	+ + +	−	+ +	+ +
Leupeptin	ND	+ +	ND	ND	+ +
α$_1$-antitrypsin	ND	−	ND	−	−
Elastatinol	ND	−	ND	ND	−
Soybean trypsin inhibitor	ND	−	ND	ND	−

transformation is discussed in more detail in Chapter 15. The mechanism(s) by which the anticarcinogenic protease inhibitors affect oncogene expression is unknown. Our own studies suggest that these compounds do not affect the transcription rate of c-*myc* or c-*fos* (Chang *et al.*, 1990; Li *et al.*, 1992).

The most direct approach to determining the mechanism of action of the anticarcinogenic protease inhibitors is to find out what they are interacting with in cells. Although there are many different types of proteases in the cells of the systems we study, very few of them are affected by the anticarcinogenic protease inhibitors. We have studied two different proteolytic activities which could be the "target(s)" of the anticarcinogenic protease inhibitors; the characteristics of these proteases have been described in detail elsewhere (Billings *et al.*, 1987b, 1988, 1990; Kennedy and Billings, 1987; Carew and Kennedy, 1990; Billings, this volume). We believe that these particular proteases are intimately involved in the conversion of a cell to the malignant state, as they cleave particular protease substrates which are themselves able to suppress radiation transformation (presumably these substrates are capable of acting as competitive substrates for the proteases involved in the transformation of cells) (Billings *et al.*, 1990).

The characteristics of one of the proteases studied by us suggest that it may be involved in the processing of a growth factor which is essential for malignant transformation (Billings *et al.*, 1987b; Kennedy and Billings, 1987). Other studies on this activity have shown that it is persistently activated by carcinogen exposure (Billings *et al.*, 1987b), a characteristic we believe to be of great importance for an activity related to malignant transformation. Other work of ours utilizing carboxypeptidase inhibitor I and inhibitor II from potatoes suggests that two different proteolytic activities play a role in transformation—specifically, endopeptidase as well as exopeptidase activities appear to have important functions in the malignant conversion of a cell, as discussed in detail elsewhere (Billings *et al.*, 1989).

The manner in which proteolytic activity and c-*myc* gene expression could be related in the induction of malignant transformation is shown schematically in Figs. 7 and 8. These hypothesized schemes are discussed elsewhere in detail (Kennedy, 1990b). Our model(s) for the protease inhibitor prevention of cancer is based on our data showing that carcinogen treatment increases the level of c-*myc* gene expression as well as the level of proteolytic activity (specifically, the Boc-Val-Pro-Arg-MCA hydrolyzing activity that we have studied) while protease inhibitor (specifically, BBI) treatment brings the carcinogen-induced, elevated levels of c-*myc* gene expression (St. Clair *et al.*, 1990) and proteolytic activity (Messadi *et al.*, 1986) back to "background" levels in the *in vivo* systems we have studied.

While the hypotheses discussed above seem to be the most likely hypotheses to explain the results of our studies at the present time, many other possibilities exist, even in our own studies. For example, we have shown that anticarcinogenic protease inhibitors, including BBI, suppress carcinogen-induced gene

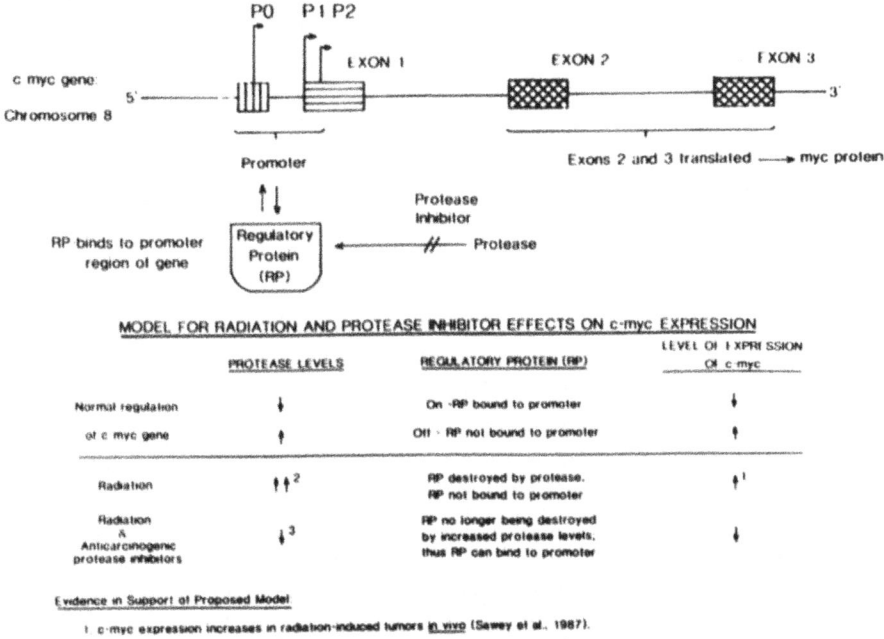

Figure 7. Our postulated model showing interaction between a protease, anticarcinogenic protease inhibitors, and c-*myc* expression. This model is described in more detail in Kennedy (1990b).

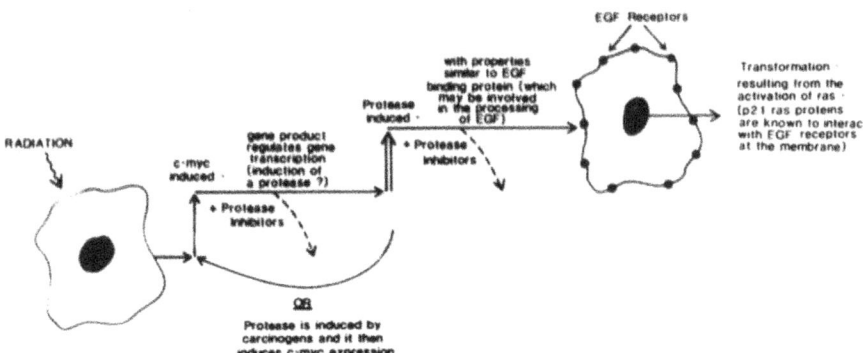

Figure 8. Our postulated model showing interaction between cellular radiation exposure, the expression of c-*myc*, the induction of proteolytic activity, and malignant transformations. Anticarcinogenic protease inhibitors are capable of suppressing c-*myc* expression and elevated levels of proteolytic activity in carcinogen-treated cells. Our model is discussed in more detail in Kennedy (1990b).

amplification (Flick and Kennedy, 1991), an event which is induced in cells by carcinogens in a widespread fashion (Lavi, 1981, 1986). It is known that radiation can induce gene amplification (Lavi, 1986; Tlsty *et al.*, 1984) and that the radiation induction of, or increase in, gene amplification can be further potentiated by tumor-promoting agents such as TPA (Tlsty *et al.*, 1984); thus, the effects of these modifying agents for transformation are well correlated with the effects of these agents on gene amplification. Unfortunately, we will not be able to determine which of the many carcinogen-induced events that protease inhibitors suppress are responsible for the observed anticarcinogenic activity until the mechanism of cancer induction is known.

It may seem to the reader that protease inhibitors have too many effects that could be involved in their anticarcinogenic activity. It is worth pointing out that the effects observed for the anticarcinogenic protease inhibitors are on phenomena altered by carcinogen exposure and that the basal level of each endpoint studied is not affected by the protease inhibitors. For example, normal levels of gene amplification are not affected by protease inhibitors, but the carcinogen-induced, elevated levels of gene amplification are brought to normal levels by the anticarcinogenic protease inhibitors (Flick and Kennedy, 1991). As examples from our own *in vivo* work: (1) c-*myc* expression in normal cells of the colon is not affected by protease inhibitors, while protease inhibitors do affect the radiation-induced, elevated levels of c-*myc* expression by restoring them to normal levels (St. Clair *et al.*, 1990), and (2) protease inhibitors do not affect the endogenous levels of Boc-Val-Pro-Arg-MCA hydrolyzing activity in the hamster cheek pouch, but are capable of restoring the carcinogen-elevated levels of the activity to normal levels (Messadi *et al.*, 1986). In fact, the anticarcinogenic protease inhibitors do not affect any phenomenon which we can measure in normal cells; they have no effect on cell growth, overall DNA synthesis, RNA synthesis, etc. (Kennedy and Little, 1981b). The fact that they do not have detectable effects in normal cell populations is an advantage for compounds we believe will serve as nontoxic cancer chemopreventive agents.

ACKNOWLEDGMENTS. Research performed in the Kennedy laboratory discussed in this report is supported by NIH Grants CA22704, CA46496, and CA34680.

3. References

Balmain, A., 1985, Transforming ras oncogenes and multistage carcinogenesis, *Br. J. Cancer* **51**:1–7.

Baturay, N. Z., and Kennedy, A. R., 1986, Pyrene acts as a cocarcinogen with the carcinogens, benzo(a)pyrene, β-propiolactone and radiation in the induction of malignant transformation of cultured mouse fibroblasts; soybean extract containing the Bowman–Birk inhibitor acts as an anticarcinogen, *Cell Biol. Toxicol.* **2**:21–32.

Becker, F. F., 1981, Inhibition of spontaneous hepatocarcinogenesis in C3H/Hen mice by Edi Pro A, an isolated soy protein, *Carcinogenesis* 2:1213–1214.

Billings, P. C., St. Clair, W., Ryan, C. A., and Kennedy, A. R., 1987a, Inhibition of radiation-induced transformation of C3H/10T1/2 cells by chymotrypsin inhibitor 1 from potatoes, *Carcinogenesis* 8:809–812.

Billings, P. C., Carew, J. A., Keller-McGandy, C. E., Goldberg, A., and Kennedy, A. R., 1987b, A serine protease activity in C3H/10T1/2 cells that is inhibited by anticarcinogenic protease inhibitors, *Proc. Natl. Acad. Sci. USA* 84:4801–4805.

Billings, P. C., St. Clair, W., Owen, A. J., and Kennedy, A. R., 1988, Potential intracellular target proteins of the anticarcinogenic Bowman–Birk protease inhibitor identified by affinity chromatography, *Cancer Res.* 48:1798–1802.

Billings, P. C., Morrow, A. R., Ryan, C. A., and Kennedy, A. R., 1989, Inhibition of radiation-induced transformation of C3H/10T1/2 cells by carboxypeptidase inhibitor I and inhibitor II from potatoes, *Carcinogenesis* 10:687–691.

Billings, P. C., Habres, J. M., and Kennedy, A. R., 1990, Inhibition of radiation-induced transformation of C3H10T1/2 cells by specific protease substrates, *Carcinogenesis* 11:329–332.

Borek, C., and Cleaver, J. E., 1981, Protease inhibitors neither damage DNA nor interfere with DNA repair or replication in human cells, *Mutat. Res.* 82:373–380.

Borek, C., Miller, C., Pain, C., and Troll, W., 1979, Conditions for inhibiting and enhancing effects of the protease inhibitor antipain on x-ray-induced neoplastic transformation in hamster and mouse cells, *Proc. Natl. Acad. Sci. USA* 76:1800–1803; corrections etc. in *Proc. Natl. Acad. Sci. USA* 76:6699.

Bos, J. L., Fearon, E. R., Hamilton, S. R., Verlaan-de Vries, M., van Boom, J. H., van der Eb, A. J., and Vogelstein, B., 1987, Prevalence of ras gene mutations in human colorectal cancers, *Nature* 327:293–297.

Brown, K., Quintanilla, M., Ramsden, M., Kerr, I. B., Young, S., and Balmain, A., 1986, V-ras genes from Harvey and BALB murine sarcoma viruses can act as initiators of two-stage mouse skin carcinogenesis, *Cell* 46:447–456.

Caggana, M., and Kennedy, A. R., 1989, C-fos mRNA levels are reduced in the presence of antipain and the Bowman–Birk inhibitor, *Carcinogenesis* 10:2145–2148.

Campisi, J., Gray, H. E., Pardee, A. B., Dean, M., and Sonenshein, G. E., 1984, Cell cycle control of c-myc but not c-ras expression is lost following chemical transformation, *Cell* 36:241–247.

Capon, D. J., Seeburg, P. H., McGrath, J. P., Hayflick, J. S., Edman, U., Levinson, A. D., and Goeddel, D. V., 1983, Activation of Ki-ras 2 gene in human colon and lung carcinomas by two different point mutations, *Nature* 304:507–513.

Carew, J. A., and Kennedy, A. R., 1990, Identification of a proteolytic activity which responds to anticarcinogenic protease inhibitors in C3H10T1/2 cells, *Cancer Lett.* 49:153–163.

Chang, J. D., and Kennedy, A. R., 1988, Cell cycle progression of C3H10T1/2 and 3T3 cells in the absence of a transient increase in c-myc RNA levels, *Carcinogenesis* 9:17–20.

Chang, J. D., Billings, P., and Kennedy, A. R., 1985, C-myc expression is reduced in antipain-treated proliferating C3H10T1/2 cells, *Biochem. Biophys. Res. Comm.* 133:830–835.

Chang, J. D., Li, J.-H., Billings, P. C., and Kennedy, A. R., 1990, Effects of protease inhibitors on c-myc expression in normal and transformed C3H10T1/2 cells, *Molec. Carc.* 3:226–232.

Chen, A. C., and Herschman, H. R., 1989, Tumorigenic methylcholanthrene transformants of C3H/10T1/2 cells have a common nucleotide alteration in the c-ki-ras gene, *Proc. Natl. Acad. Sci. USA* 86:1608–1611.

Connan, G., Rassoulzadegan, M., and Cuzin, F., 1985, Focus formation in rat fibroblasts exposed to a tumour promoter after transfer of polyoma plt and myc oncogenes, *Nature* 314:277–279.

Corasanti, J. G., Hobika, G. H., and Markus, G., 1982, Interference with dimethylhydrazine induction of colon tumors in mice by ε-aminocaproic acid, *Science* 216:1020–1021.

Der, C. J., and Cooper, G. M., 1983, Altered gene products are associated with activation of cellular ras[k] genes in human lung and colon carcinomas, *Cell* **32**:201–208.

DiPaolo, J. A., Amsbaugh, S. C., and Popescu, N. C., 1980, Antipain inhibits N-methyl-N'-nitro-N-nitrosoguanidine-induced transformation and increases chromosomal aberrations, *Proc. Natl. Acad. Sci. USA* **77**:6649–6653.

Dotto, G. P., Parada, L. F., and Weinberg, R. A., 1985, Specific growth response of ras-transformed embryo fibroblasts to tumor promoters, *Nature* **318**:472–475.

Fabre, F., and Roman, H., 1977, Genetic evidence for inducibility of recombination competence in yeast, *Proc. Natl. Acad. Sci. USA* **74**:1667–1671.

Fahmy, M. J., and Fahmy, O. G., 1980, Intervening DNA insertions and the alteration of gene expression by carcinogens, *Cancer Res.* **40**:3374–3382.

Flick, M. B., and Kennedy, A. R., 1991, Effect of protease inhibitors on DNA amplification in SV40-transformed Chinese hamster embryo cells, *Cancer Lett.* **56**:102–108.

Garte, S. J., Currie, D. C., and Troll, W., 1987, Inhibition of H-ras oncogene transformation of NIH3T3 cells by protease inhibitors, *Cancer Res.* **47**:3159–3162.

German, J., 1983, Bloom's syndrome. X. The cancer proneness points to chromosome mutation as a crucial event in human neoplasia, in: *Chromosome Mutation and Neoplasia* (J. German, ed.), Liss, New York, pp. 347–357.

Gottesman, S., 1987, Regulation by proteolysis, in: *Eschericia coli and Salmonella typhimurium* (F. Neidhardt, ed.), American Society for Microbiology, Washington, D.C., pp. 1308–1312.

Hunter, T., 1981, Oncogenes and proto-oncogenes: How do they differ? *J. Natl. Cancer Inst.* **73**:773–786.

Kelly, K., Cochran, B. H., Stiles, C. D., and Leder, P., 1983, Cell-specific regulation of the c-myc gene by lymphocyte mitogens and platelet-derived growth factor, *Cell* **35**:603–610.

Kennedy, A. R., 1982, Antipain, but not cycloheximide, suppresses radiation transformation when present for only one day at five days post-irradiation, *Carcinogenesis* **3**:1093–1095.

Kennedy, A. R., 1984a, Promotion and other interactions between agents in the induction of transformation *in vitro* in fibroblasts, in: *Mechanisms of Tumor Promotion*, Volume III (T. J. Slaga, ed.), CRC Press, Boca Raton, Fla., pp. 13–55.

Kennedy, A. R., 1984b, Prevention of radiation-induced transformation *in vitro*, in: *Vitamins, Nutrition and Cancer* (K. N. Prasad, ed.), Karger, Basel, pp. 166–179.

Kennedy, A. R., 1985a, The conditions for the modification of radiation transformation *in vitro* by a tumor promoter and protease inhibitors, *Carcinogenesis* **6**:1441–1446.

Kennedy, A. R., 1985b, Effects of antioxidants on the induction of malignant transformation *in vitro*, in: *Vitamins and Cancer—Human Cancer Prevention by Vitamins and Micronutrients* (F. L. Meyskens and K. N. Prasad, eds.), Humana Press, Clifton, N.J., pp. 51–64.

Kennedy, A. R., 1985c, Evidence that the first step leading to carcinogen-induced malignant transformation is a high frequency, common event, in: *Carcinogenesis: A Comprehensive Survey*, Volume 9 (J. C. Barrett and R. W. Tennant, eds.), Raven Press, New York, pp. 355–364.

Kennedy, A. R., 1986, Role of free radicals in the initiation and promotion of radiation-induced and chemical carcinogen induced cell transformation, in: *Oxygen and Sulfur Radicals in Chemistry and Medicine* (A. Breccia, M. A. J. Rodgers, and G. Semerano, eds.), Edizioni Scientifiche, "Lo Scarabeo," Bologna, Italy, pp. 201–209.

Kennedy, A. R., 1988, Implications for mechanisms of tumor promotion and its inhibition by various agents from studies of in vitro transformation, in: *Tumor Promoters, Biological Approaches for Mechanistic Studies and Assay Systems* (R. Langenbach, J. C. Barrett, and E. Elmore, eds.), Raven Press, New York, pp. 201–212.

Kennedy, A. R., 1989, Initiation and promotion of radiation induced transformation *in vitro*: Relevance of *in vitro* studies to radiation induced cancer in human populations, in: *Cell Transformation and Radiation-Induced Cancer* (K. H. Chadwick, C. Seymour and B. Barnhart, eds.), IOP Publishing, Adam Hilger, Bristol and New York, pp. 263–270.

Kennedy, A. R., 1990a, Effects of protease inhibitors and vitamin E in the prevention of cancer, in: *Nutrients and Cancer Prevention* (K. N. Prasad and F. L. Meyskens, Jr., eds.), Humana Press, Clifton, N.J., pp. 79–98.

Kennedy, A. R., 1990b, Is there a critical target gene for the first step in carcinogenesis? *Environ. Health Perspect.* **93:**199–203.

Kennedy, A. R., and Billings, P. C., 1987, Anticarcinogenic actions of protease inhibitors, in: *Anticarcinogenesis and Radiation Protection* (P. A. Cerutti, O. F. Nygaard, and M. G. Simic, eds.), Plenum Press, New York, pp. 285–295.

Kennedy, A. R., and Little, J. B., 1978, Protease inhibitors suppress radiation induced malignant transformation *in vitro, Nature* **276:**825–826.

Kennedy, A. R., and Little, J. B., 1980a, Radiation transformation *in vitro:* Modification by exposure to tumor promoters and protease inhibitors, in: *Radiation Biology in Cancer Research* (R. E. Meyn and H. R. Withers, eds.), Raven Press, New York, pp. 295–307.

Kennedy, A. R., and Little, J. B., 1980b, An investigation of the mechanism for the enhancement of radiation transformation *in vitro* by TPA, *Carcinogenesis* **1:**1039–1047.

Kennedy, A. R., and Little, J. B., 1981a, High efficiency, kinetics and numerology of transformation by radiation *in vitro,* in: *Cancer: Achievements, Challenges and Prospects for the 1980's,* Volume 1 (J. H. Burchenal and J. F. Oettgen, eds.), Grune & Stratton, New York, pp. 491–500.

Kennedy, A. R., and Little, J. B., 1981b, Effects of protease inhibitors on radiation transformation *in vitro, Cancer Res.* **41:**2103–2108.

Kennedy, A. R., and Little, J. B., 1984, Evidence that a second event in x-ray induced oncogenic transformation *in vitro* occurs during cellular proliferation, *Radiat. Res.* **99:**228–248.

Kennedy, A. R., and Symons, M. C. R., 1987, "Water structure" vs "radical scavenger" theories as explanations for the suppressive effects of DMSO and related compounds on radiation induced transformation *in vitro, Carcinogenesis* **8:**683–688.

Kennedy, A. R., and Weichselbaum, R. R., 1981, Effects of 17-β-estradiol on radiation transformation *in vitro;* inhibition of effects by protease inhibitors, *Carcinogenesis* **2:**67–69.

Kennedy, A. R., Radner, B. and Nagasawa, H., 1984a, Protease inhibitors reduce the frequency of spontaneous chromosome abnormalities in cells from patients with Bloom syndrome, *Proc. Natl. Acad. Sci. USA* **81:**1827–1830.

Kennedy, A. R., Troll, W., and Little, J. B., 1984b, Role of free radicals in the initiation and promotion of radiation transformation *in vitro, Carcinogenesis* **5:**1213–1218.

Kennedy, A. R., Cairns, J., and Little, J. B., 1984c, The timing of the steps in transformation of C3H10T1/2 cells by X-irradiation, *Nature* **307:**85–86.

Kennedy, A. R., Fox, M., Murphy, G., and Little, J. B., 1980, Relationship between x-ray exposure and malignant transformation in C3H10T1/2 cells, *Proc. Natl. Acad. Sci. USA* **77:**7262–7266.

Korbelik, M., Osmak, M., Suhar, A., Škrk, J., Turk, V., and Petrovic, D., 1988, Modification of potentially lethal damage repair by some intrinsic intra- and extracellular agents: I. Proteinases and proteinase inhibitors, *Int. J. Radiat. Biol.* **54:**461–474.

Kuroki, T., and Drevon, C., 1979, Inhibition of chemical transformation in C3H10T1/2 cells by protease inhibitors, *Cancer Res.* **39:**2755–2761.

Land, H., Parada, L. F., and Weinberg, R. A., 1983a, Cellular oncogenes and multistep carcinogenesis, *Science* **222:**771–778.

Land, H., Parada, L. F., and Weinberg, R. A., 1983b, Tumorigenic conversion of primary embryo fibroblasts requires at least two cooperating oncogenes, *Nature* **304:**596–602.

Lavi, S., 1981, Carcinogen-mediated amplification of viral DNA sequences in simian virus 40-transformed Chinese hamster embryo cells, *Proc. Natl. Acad. Sci. USA* **78:**6144–6148.

Lavi, S., 1986, Carcinogen-mediated amplification of specific DNA sequences, *J. Cell Biochem.* **18:**149–156.

Leder, P., Battey, J., Lenoir, G., Moulding, C., Murphy, W., Potter, H., Stewart, T., and Taub, R., 1983, Translocations among antibody genes in human cancer, *Science* **222:**765–771.

Li, J.-H., Billings, P. C., and Kennedy, A. R., 1992, Induction of oncogene expression by sodium arsenite in C3H/10T1/2 cells; inhibition of c-myc expression by protease inhibitors, *Cancer J.* **5**:354–358.

Little, J. B., and Kennedy, A. R., 1982, Promotion of X-ray transformation *in vitro,* in: *Carcinogenesis: Cocarcinogenesis and Biological Effects of Tumor Promoters,* Vol. 7 (E. Hecker, N. E. Fusenig, W. Kunz, F. Marks, and H. W. Theilmann, eds.), Raven Press, New York, pp. 243–257.

Little, J. B., Nagasawa, H., and Kennedy, A. R., 1979, DNA repair and malignant transformation: Effect of X-irradiation, TPA and protease inhibitors on transformation and sister chromatid exchanges in mouse 10T1/2 cells, *Radiat. Res.* **79**:241–255.

Little, J. W., Edmiston, S. H., Pacelli, L. Z., and Mount, D. W., 1980, Cleavage of the *Escherichia coli* lex A protein by the rec A protease, *Proc. Natl. Acad. Sci. USA* **77**:3225–3229.

Messadi, P. V., Billings, P., Shklar, G., and Kennedy, A. R., 1986, Inhibition of oral carcinogenesis by a protease inhibitor, *J. Natl. Cancer Inst.* **76**:447–452.

Meyn, M. S., Rossman, T., and Troll, W., 1977, A protease inhibitor blocks SOS functions in *Escherichia coli;* antipain prevents λ repressor inactivation, ultraviolet mutagenesis and filamentous growth, *Proc. Natl. Acad. Sci. USA* **74**:1152–1156.

Miller, R. C., Geard, C. R., Osmak, R. S., Rutlege-Freeman, M., Ong, A., Mason, H., Napholz, A., Perez, N., Harisiadis, L., and Borek, C., 1981, Modification of sister chromatid exchanges and radiation-induced transformation in rodent cells by the tumor promoter 12-O-tetradecanoylphorbol-13-acetate and two retinoids, *Cancer Res.* **41**:655–659.

Mondal, S., and Heidelberger, C., 1980, Inhibition of induced differentiation of C3H/10T1/2 clone 8 mouse embryo cells by tumor promoters, *Cancer Res.* **40**:334–338.

Mordan, L. J., Bergin, L. M., Budnick, J. E., Meegan, R. R., and Bertran, J. S., 1982, Isolation of methylcholanthrene-"initiated" C3H/10T1/2 cells by inhibiting neoplastic progression with retinyl acetate, *Carcinogenesis* **3**:279–285.

Newbold, R. F., and Overell, R. W., 1983, Fibroblast immortality is a prerequisite for transformation by EJ c-Ha-ras oncogene, *Nature* **304**:648–651.

Ohkoshi, M., and Fujii, S., 1983, Effect of the synthetic protease inhibitor [N,N-dimethylcarbamoylmethyl 4-(4-guanidinobenzoyloxy)-phenyl acetate] methanesulfate on carcinogenesis by 3-methylcholanthrene in mouse skin, *J. Natl. Cancer Inst.* **71**:1053–1057.

Parada, L. F., and Weinberg, R. A., 1983, Presence of a Kirsten murine sarcoma virus ras oncogene in cells transformed by 3-methylcholanthrene, *Mol. Cell Biol.* **3**:2298–2301.

Persiani, S., Yeung, A., Shen, W.-C., and Kennedy, A. R., 1991, Polylysine conjugates of Bowman–Birk protease inhibitor as targeted anticarcinogenic agents, *Carcinogenesis* **12**:1149–1152.

Popescu, N. C., Amsbaugh, S. C., and DiPaolo, J. A., 1980, Enhancement of N-methyl-N-nitro-N-nitrosoguanidine transformation of Syrian hamster embryo cells by a phorbol diester is independent of sister chromatid exchanges and chromosome aberrations, *Proc. Natl. Acad. Sci. USA* **77**:7282–7286.

Radner, B. S., and Kennedy, A. R., 1986, Suppression of x-ray induced transformation by vitamin E in mouse C3H/10T1/2 cells, *Cancer Lett.* **32**:25–32.

Rosen, A., and Klein, G., 1983, UV light-induced immunoglobulin heavy-chain class switch in a human lymphoblastoid cell line, *Nature* **306**:189–190.

Rossman, T. G., and Klein, C. B., 1985, Mammalian SOS system: A case of misplaced analogies, *Cancer Invest.* **3**(2):175–187.

St. Clair, W. H., Billings, P. C., and Kennedy, A. R., 1990, The effects of the Bowman–Birk protease inhibitor on c-myc expression and cell proliferation in the unirradiated and irradiated mouse colon, *Cancer Lett.* **52**:145–152.

Sawey, M. J., Hood, A. T., Burns, F. J., and Garte, S. J., 1987, Activation of myc and ras oncogenes in primary rat tumors induced by ionizing radiation, *Mol. Cell Biol.* **7**:932–935.

Scott, R. E., and Maercklein, P. B., 1985, An initiator of carcinogenesis selectively and stably inhibits stem cell differentiation: A concept that initiation of carcinogenesis involves multiple phases, *Proc. Natl. Acad. Sci. USA* **82:**2995–2999.

Smirnoff, P., Khalef, S., Birk, Y., and Applebaum, S. W., 1979, Trypsin and chymotrypsin inhibitor from chickpeas, *Int. J. Peptide Protein Res.* **14:**186–192.

Smith, G. J., and Grisham, J. W., 1987, Activation of the Ha-*ras* gene in C3H/10T1/2 cells transformed by exposure to N-methyl-N'-nitro-N-nitrosoguanidine, *Biochem. Biophys. Res. Commun.* **147:**1194–1199.

Spandidos, D. A., and Wilkie, N. M., 1984, Malignant transformation of early passage rodent cells by a single mutated human oncogene, *Nature* **310:**469–475.

Stewart, T. A., Pattengale, P. K., and Leder, P., 1984, Spontaneous mammary adenocarcinomas in transgenic mice that carry and express MTV/myc fusion genes, *Cell* **38:**627–637.

Sukumar, S., Pulciani, S., Doniger, J., DiPaolo, J. A., Evans, C. H., Zarbl, B., and Barbacid, M., 1985, A transforming ras gene in tumorigenic guinea pig cell lines initiated by diverse chemical carcinogens, *Science* **223:**1197–1199.

Sun, C., Colman, M., and Redpath, J. L., 1988, Suppression of the radiation-induced expression of a tumor-associated antigen in human cell hybrids by the protease inhibitor antipain, *Carcinogenesis* **9:**2333–2335.

Tlsty, T. O., Brown, P. C., and Schimke, R. T., 1984, Ultraviolet radiation facilitates methotrexate resistance and amplification of the dihydrofolate reductase gene in cultured 3T6 mouse cells, *Mol. Cell Biol.* **4:**1050–1056.

Troll, W., Frenkel, K., and Wiesner, R., 1984, Protease inhibitors as anticarcinogens, *J. Natl. Cancer Inst.* **73:**1245–1250.

Troll, W., Wiesner, R., and Frenkel, K., 1987, Anticarcinogenic action of protease inhibitors, *Adv. Cancer Res.* **49:**265–283.

Wintersberger, U., 1984, The selective advantage of cancer cells: A consequence of genome mobilization in the course of the induction of DNA repair processes? (model studies of yeast) *Adv. Enzyme Regul.* **22:**311–323.

Witkin, E. M., 1976, Ultraviolet mutagenesis and inducible DNA repair in Escherichia coli, *Bacteriol. Rev.* **40:**869–907.

Yavelow, J., Finlay, T. H., Kennedy, A. R., and Troll, W., 1983, Bowman–Birk soybean protease inhibitor as an anticarcinogen, *Cancer Res.* **43:**2454–2459.

Yavelow, J., Collins, M., Birk, Y., Troll, W., and Kennedy, A. R., 1985, Nanomolar concentrations of Bowman–Birk soybean protease inhibitor suppress X-ray induced transformation *in vitro*, *Proc. Natl. Acad. Sci. USA* **82:**5395–5399.

4

Discovery and Background of the Bowman–Birk Protease Inhibitors

DONALD E. BOWMAN

1. Origin of Interest in Legumes

This is an account of the initial work on a protease inhibitor now generally and appropriately designated simply as BBI. It is also appropriate that this account be brief. It is the work of other investigators that provides whatever significance inhibitors of this type possess.

This study began in 1941 when the dean of the Indiana University School of Medicine, Willis D. Gatch, asked the most junior member of his faculty to conduct investigations that hopefully would provide some information about postoperative abdominal discomfort. The dean thought that some legumes might provide insight.

2. Unexpected Protease Inhibition by Amylase Inhibition Preparations

In pursuing this assignment, attention was first given to the remarkable resistance of navy bean starch to the action of pancreatic amylase *in vitro*. It was found that common store yeast improved the action of amylase on aged complexes consisting of the ether-soluble fraction of navy beans and reagent-soluble starch. However, heating the beans themselves in dilute acid was an effective and more direct method of improving the digestion of the bean starch (Bowman, 1943). Furthermore, grinding the dry navy beans to a fine powder before cooking

DONALD E. BOWMAN • Departments of Biochemistry and Molecular Biology, School of Medicine, Indiana University, Indianapolis, Indiana 46202-5122.

Protease Inhibitors as Cancer Chemopreventive Agents, edited by Walter Troll and Ann R. Kennedy. Plenum Press, New York, 1993.

(presumably to disrupt starch granules) served as well as heating the beans in dilute acid (Bowman, 1944a).

In a final approach to the starch question, it was found that an amylase inhibitor could bé prepared from an extract of navy beans by discarding inert proteins at pH 4 and recovering the active material by alcohol precipitation. However, such preparations also inhibited trypsin. An abstract was published (Bowman, 1945a) but interest in the starch problem had been lost. Nothing more was done with the amylase inhibitor by the author. (But others have used it more recently in the experimental treatment of some types of diabetes mellitus to slow the rate of carbohydrate absorption.) In the meantime, in the original study, attention had been given to trypsin inhibition by factors especially in soybeans and navy beans (Bowman, 1944b). For quite some time a number of investigators had devoted attention to the proteins of the legumes and their nutritional value.

The predominant protein(s) had been identified and studied as globulin(s) in white and kidney beans (Osborne and Clapp, 1907), in jack beans (Jones and Johns, 1916–17), in peanuts (Johns and Jones, 1916–17), in Chinese velvet beans (Johns and Finks, 1918), and in Georgia velvet beans (Johns and Waterman, 1920). The velvet beans were of interest as feed for cattle.

In nutritional studies, Mendel and Fine (1911–12) had found that soybeans and their crude proteins, when heated in water, provided generous positive nitrogen balances in man and dogs, but such positive balances were less than with meat. Osborne and Mendel (1917) had observed little growth in rats with raw soy meal in spite of addition of known essential factors other than protein. However, when the meal was heated on a steam bath for 3 hr, normal growth rate resulted. The difference seemed to be associated with failure of the rats to eat the raw meal readily. In any case, when the salt mixture (consisting of 13 different salts) was removed from the diet, it was found that the salt mixture constituted a limiting factor in growth that no amount of cooking could rectify. Johns and Finks (1920) had found that cooked phaseolin, a globulin of navy beans, produced normal growth in rats if a cystine supplement was provided.

Perhaps it was natural that many of these early nutritional studies, as well as later investigations, were conducted mainly with rats. But we now know that investigators have warned against extrapolating all aspects of rat studies to other species when dealing with legume components. Nevertheless, these and many other early studies of the legumes stimulated research in various ways. In reporting on the *in vitro* peptic–tryptic digestion of phaseolin, Waterman and Jones (1921) had referred to Fisher and Abderhalden who had pointed out that some polypeptides are hydrolyzed by trypsin while others consisting of the same amino acids arranged in a different order are not attacked at all.

Having been freed of the starch problem (without really answering the original question) and having found evidence for a trypsin inhibitor as an unexpected component of an amylase inhibitor extract, attention was devoted to protease inhibition. Simple aqueous extracts of navy beans, soybeans, wheat, and corn (Bowman, 1944b) were added to buffered solutions of casein and pancreatin. Following incubation and precipitation of the undigested protein with trichloroacetic acid, the marked visual differences between the legumes on the one hand and the grains on the other were quantitated by nitrogen determination.

To concentrate with the trypsin-inhibiting material of a navy bean aqueous extract, inert proteins were removed at pH 4 and the active material precipitated with 90% acetone or ethyl alcohol. But in parallel experiments, part of the soybean trypsin-inhibiting fraction was lost with alcohol precipitation. Nevertheless, the alcohol-insoluble trypsin-inhibiting fraction of soybeans could be precipitated repeatedly with alcohol (Bowman, 1945b). Both acetone and alcohol precipitates of aqueous extracts of Georgia velvet beans and Chinese velvet beans exhibited antitryptic activity.

Kunitz (1945) soon reported the crystallization of a globulin trypsin inhibitor of soybeans and extended the details of the crystallization (Kunitz, 1946). Later that year, Bowman (1946) described a preferred method of preparing an acetone-insoluble inhibitor from soybeans and compared it with the crystalline globulin trypsin inhibitor kindly provided by Kunitz. While the crystalline inhibitor was insoluble in 40% saturated ammonium sulfate, 2.5% trichloroacetic acid as well as 60% alcohol, the acetone-insoluble inhibitor was soluble in such solutions.

In continuing his landmark studies of crystalline soybean inhibitor, Kunitz (1947a) dealt with its isoelectric point, stability, denaturation, release of trypsin, combining weight with trypsin, and other properties. Kunitz (1947b) defined other physical and chemical properties of the crystalline inhibitor and found that it inhibited slightly the proteolytic action of chymotrypsin in a loose reversible manner in keeping with the law of mass action.

Evidence was presented (Bowman, 1948) indicating that there is more than one soybean inhibitor that shares properties with the acetone-insoluble inhibitor. But we now know that there are many BBI-type inhibitors.

Starting with an extract of the acetone-insoluble inhibitor of soybeans prepared by the author, neither Kunitz nor the author succeeded in obtaining a crystalline inhibitor. And there the BBI study remained—essentially dormant until Dr. Yehudith Birk breathed lasting life into it, with the farseeing work by her group continuing today.

3. References

Bowman, D. E., 1943, The ether-soluble fraction of navy beans and the digestion of starch, *Science* **98**:308–309.

Bowman, D. E., 1944a, Digestive availability of bean starch, *Science* **99**:280–281.

Bowman, D. E., 1944b, Fractions derived from soybeans and navy beans which retard tryptic digestion of casein, *Proc. Soc. Exp. Biol. Med.* **57**:139–140.

Bowman, D. E., 1945a, Amylase inhibitor of navy beans, *Science* **102**:358–359.

96

DONALD E. BOWMAN

Bowman, D. E., 1945b, Further observations on the trypsin-retarding fractions of navy and other beans, *Fed. Proc.* **4**:84.

Bowman, D. E., 1946, Differentiation of soy bean antitryptic factors, *Proc. Soc. Exp. Biol. Med.* **63**:547–550.

Bowman, D. E., 1948, Further differentiation of bean trypsin inhibiting factors, *Arch. Biochem. Biophys.* **16**:109–113.

Johns, C. O., and Finks, A. J., 1918, Stizolobin, the globulin of the Chinese velvet bean, Stizolobium niveum, *J. Biol. Chem.* **34**:429–438.

Johns, C. O., and Finks, A. J., 1920, Studies on nutrition. II. The role of cystine in nutrition as exemplified by nutrition experiments with proteins of the navy bean, Phaseolus vulgaris, *J. Biol. Chem.* **41**:379–389.

Johns, C. O., and Jones, D. B., 1916–17, The proteins of the peanut, Arachis hypogaea. I. The globulins arachin and conarachin, *J. Biol. Chem.* **28**:77–87.

Johns, C. O., and Waterman, H. C., 1920, Some proteins from Georgia velvet bean, Stizolobium derringianun, *J. Biol. Chem.* **42**:59–69.

Jones, D. B., and Johns, C. O., 1916–17, Some proteins from the jack bean, Canavalia ensiformis, *J. Biol. Chem.* **28**:67–75.

Kunitz, M., 1945, Crystallization of a trypsin inhibitor from soybean, *Science* **101**:668–669.

Kunitz, M., 1946, Crystalline soybean trypsin inhibitor, *J. Gen. Physiol.* **29**:149–154.

Kunitz, M., 1947a, Crystalline soybean trypsin inhibitor, *J. Gen. Physiol.* **30**:291–310.

Kunitz, M., 1947b, Isolation of a crystalline protein compound of trypsin and of soybean trypsin inhibitor, *J. Gen. Physiol.* **30**:311–320.

Mendel, L. B., and Fine, M. S., 1911–12, Studies in nutrition. IV. The utilization of the proteins of the legumes, *J. Biol. Chem.* **10**:433–458.

Osborne, T. B., and Clapp, S. H., 1907, Hydrolysis of phaseolin, *Am. J. Physiol.* **18**:295–308.

Osborne, T. B., and Mendel, L. B., 1917, The use of soy bean as food, *J. Biol. Chem.* **32**:369–387.

Waterman, H. C., and Jones, D. B., 1921, Studies on the digestibility of proteins *in vitro*. II. The relative digestibility of various preparations of the proteins from the Chinese and Georgia velvet beans, *J. Biol. Chem.* **47**:285–295.

5

Protease Inhibitors of Plant Origin and Role of Protease Inhibitors in Human Nutrition
Overview

YEHUDITH BIRK

1. Introduction

Protein protease inhibitors are widely distributed among different botanical families in the plant kingdom (reviewed by Liener and Kakade, 1980). Their common source is the seed but they are also present in tubers and leaves. Most of them are proteins with M_r values in the range of 8000–10,000 but there are a few notable exceptions. The inhibitors differ in specificities, most of them inhibit trypsin and many inhibit chymotrypsin. They are frequently multiheaded as a consequence of gene elongation via gene multiplication. Different kinds of inhibitors can be present in a single tissue as exemplified in barley grains, soybeans, and potato tubers (reviewed by Birk, 1987). Their presence in valuable plant foods and their possible involvement in nutritive and physiological properties have attracted the attention of nutritionists. The nutritional significance of protease inhibitors in foods has recently been discussed (Friedman, 1986). The physiological significance of plant protease inhibitors *in situ* has been questioned for a long time. The hypothesis that the inhibitors may have evolved as a defense mechanism of plants toward insects has been supported by various studies (reviewed by Birk, 1987). The extensively studied inhibitors of serine proteases have been classified into

YEHUDITH BIRK • Department of Biochemistry and Human Nutrition, Faculty of Agriculture, The Hebrew University of Jerusalem, Rehovot 76100, Israel.

Protease Inhibitors as Cancer Chemopreventive Agents, edited by Walter Troll and Ann R. Kennedy. Plenum Press, New York, 1993.

inhibitor families on the basis of sequence homology, assignment of the inhibitory site(s), and interaction with the protease(s) according to a standard mechanism (Laskowski and Kato, 1980; Laskowski, 1986). Since the inhibitory capacities are usually evaluated on bovine pancreatic proteases, the validity and relevance of nutritional and clinical uses of the inhibitors in other species should be questioned.

2. Protease Inhibitors from Legume Seeds

The first plant protease inhibitor was isolated from soybeans and characterized in 1947 (Kunitz, 1947a,b). By now, the presence of protein protease inhibitors in all legume seeds is a well-established fact. They are grouped in two inhibitor families and are represented by the two predominant inhibitors from soybeans: the Kunitz soybean trypsin inhibitor (STI) and the Bowman–Birk trypsin and chymotrypsin inhibitor (BBI).

2.1. STI

STI ($M_r \sim 22,000$) includes two disulfide bridges (Fig. 1) and is primarily an inhibitor of trypsin but also weakly inhibits chymotrypsin. It is inactivated by heat and by gastric juice. STI has been thoroughly studied in numerous laboratories and its characteristics such as specificity, stability, assay procedures, and kinetic properties have been determined (Kassell, 1970; Birk, 1976). STI served also as the model for the establishment of the standard mechanism as well as for the development of reactive site replacement techniques (Laskowski and Kato, 1980). Enzymatic mutation of STI, via replacement of Arg-63 at the inhibitory site by Trp, converts the trypsin inhibitor into a chymotrypsin inhibitor. However, only a few inhibitors homologous to STI have been found in common legume seeds and in other plant sources.

2.2. BBI

The predominant type of inhibitor in legume seeds is BBI. It has an M_r of about 8000 with a high content of cystine, forming seven disulfide bridges. The inhibitor consists of two tandem homology regions on the same polypeptide chain, each with a reactive, inhibitory site (Fig. 2). It forms a 1:1 complex with either trypsin or chymotrypsin and a ternary complex with both enzymes. In aqueous solutions, BBI undergoes self-association which is concentration dependent. BBI inhibits human trypsin and chymotrypsin, it is highly active against dog trypsin and chymotrypsin, and it is a potent inhibitor of trypsins and chymotrypsins from the digestive tracts of insects. BBI has also shown a strong

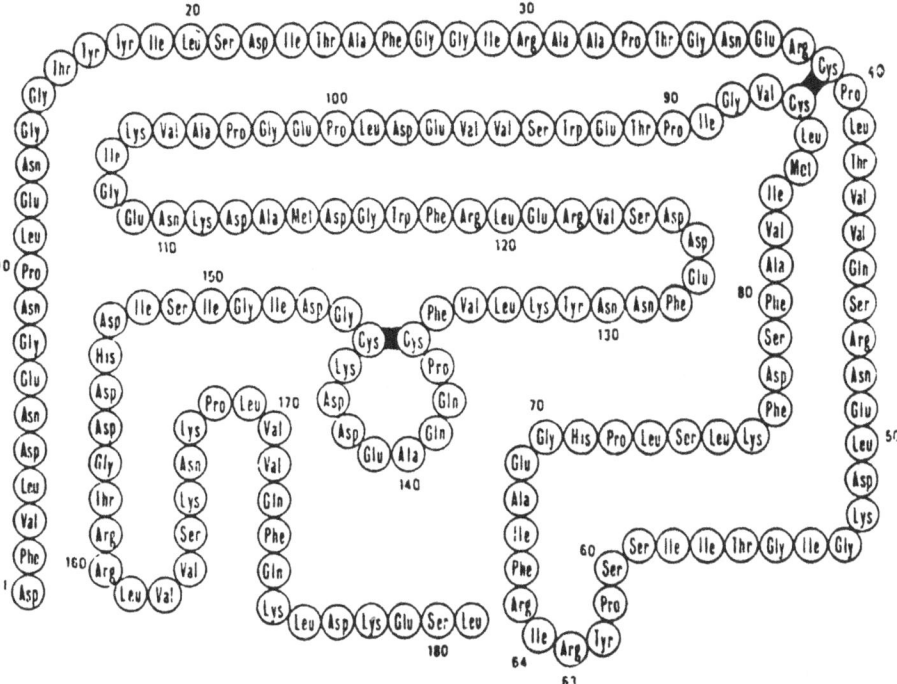

Figure 1. Covalent structure of Kunitz soybean trypsin inhibitor (STI). (From Koide and Ikenaka, 1973, as revised by Kim *et al.*, 1985.)

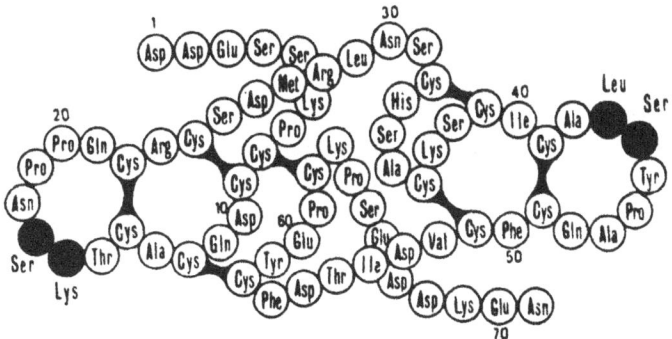

Figure 2. Covalent structure of Bowman–Birk soybean trypsin–chymotrypsin inhibitor (BBI). Residues at the two reactive sites are shown as black circles. (From Odani and Ikenaka, 1973a.)

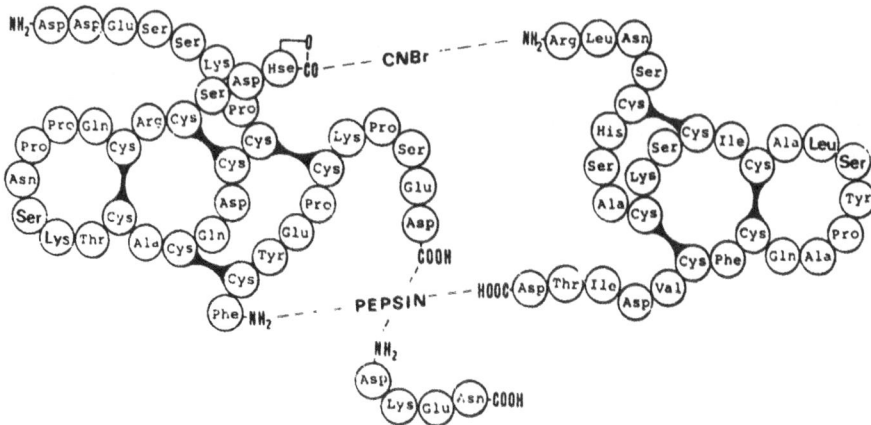

Figure 3. Sites of peptide bond cleavage by cyanogen bromide followed by pepsin and the structure of BBI fragments. (From Odani and Ikenaka, 1973b.)

interaction with elastases from human and dog granulocytes (summarized by Birk, 1985, 1987).

The inhibitor is relatively stable to heat and to gastric juice and has an unusual resistance to various proteolytic enzymes, including pepsin and pronase. However, highly specific limited proteolysis under acid conditions by either of its target enzymes, or chemical modifications at either of the inhibitory sites may be utilized to modify the "double-headed" BBI into a "single-headed" inhibitor that inhibits solely either trypsin or chymotrypsin (Birk, 1985), or to alter the specificity of inhibition (Kurokawa *et al.*, 1987a,b). The scission of BBI with cyanogen bromide followed by pepsin resulted in two active fragments, one with trypsin inhibitory activity and the other with chymotrypsin inhibitory activity (Fig. 3).

Inhibitors homologous to BBI have been found in lima beans, garden beans, azuki beans, mung beans, ground nuts, chick-peas and recently also in plant sources other than legume seeds, such as wheat germ and rice (Odani *et al.*, 1986; Tashiro *et al.*, 1987). The inhibitors may possess inhibitory sites with different steric orientations. Thus, in Cl, the double-headed trypsin–chymotrypsin inhibitor from chick-peas, the two inhibitory sites seem to be close to each other, allowing the formation of stoichiometric complexes with either trypsin or chymotrypsin, but not with both. However, similarly to BBI from soybeans, scission of Cl with cyanogen bromide followed by pepsin yields two active, independent fragments (Smirnoff *et al.*, 1979). Attempts to synthesize cyclic peptides modeled after the disulfide loops that include the inhibitory sites of BBI resulted in poor inhibitors (Terada *et al.*, 1980). *In vitro* synthesis of BBI has been achieved with the aid of mRNA isolated from immature soybean embryos (Hammond *et al.*, 1984).

3. Protease Inhibitors from Other Plant Sources

3.1. Potato Protease Inhibitors

A large number of protease inhibitors have been isolated from potatoes and related plants and have been extensively studied by C. A. Ryan and associates (reviewed by Ryan, 1973, 1981). They comprise a variety of inhibitors of serine endopeptidases, metallocarboxypeptidases, papain, microbial proteinases, and kallikreins. The inhibitors account for up to 25% of the soluble proteins of potato tuber with M_r values in the range 4200–40,000. They fall into three main categories: inhibitor I (primarily a chymotrypsin inhibitor which is also a weak inhibitor of trypsin), inhibitor II, and the carboxypeptidase inhibitor. The latter is a thermostable polypeptide of M_r 4300 that is a potent inhibitor of mammalian pancreatic carboxypeptidase A and B (Pearce and Ryan, 1983). In addition, several other potato polypeptide inhibitors of serine proteinases have recently been isolated and characterized.

3.2. Squash Protease Inhibitors

The newly defined squash inhibitor family consists of potent inhibitors of trypsin isolated from squash, zucchini, summer squash, and cucumber seeds. Their M_r is about 3000, they are cross-linked by three disulfide bridges and their reactive site is the Arg-5-Ile-6 peptide bond (Wieczorek et al., 1985).

3.3. Protease Inhibitors in Cereals

Numerous protease inhibitors have been found in cereal grains such as barley, rye, wheat, maize (corn), rice sorghum, and oats. However, only a few reports have addressed their nutritional influence, probably due to the significantly lower inhibitor activity in cereal seeds compared with legume seeds (surveyed by Boisen, 1983). The highly homologous trypsin inhibitors from barley, rye, and maize, as well as the bifunctional amylase–trypsin inhibitor from seeds of ragi, contain an Arg-Leu reactive site peptide bond in positions corresponding to the Arg-33-Leu-34 in the sequence of the barley inhibitor (Lyons et al., 1987). The latter, a single polypeptide chain of $M_r \sim 13,000$ with five disulfide bridges, serves as a prototype for this group (Odani et al., 1983). A corn inhibitor of trypsin and activated Hageman factor with a reactive site peptide bond at Arg-36-Leu-37 also belongs to this group (Mahoney et al., 1984). Recently, single- and double-headed trypsin inhibitors of the BBI family have been isolated from wheat germ (Odani et al., 1986) and the presence, in rice bran, of a double-headed trypsin inhibitor that has a duplicated structure of the BBI-type inhibitor has been reported (Tashiro et al., 1987). A thermostable, multifunctional inhibitor of trypsin, chymotrypsin, and *Tribolium* midgut proteinases, isolated from the seeds of amaranth, appears not to belong to any of the established inhibitor families (Tamir *et al.*, 1988).

In addition, many unassigned plant protease inhibitors have been isolated and characterized.

4. Role in Nutrition

4.1. Effect on Growth

The wide distribution of protease inhibitors in the human diet questioned their possible nutritive properties, but most of the information on the nutritional effects of the inhibitors has come from experiments with animals. The discovery of a heat-labile, proteinaceous, trypsin inhibitor in raw soybeans suggested that the trypsin inhibitor was the major cause of the poor utilization of the protein in raw soybeans, and that the improved nutritional quality of the heat-processed soybeans was due to the inactivation of the inhibitors. Feeding experiments of rats and chicks carried out on properly heated soybean meal diets supplemented with STI, BBI, or both, resulted in an insignificant depression of animal growth rate, but the inhibitors were responsible for pancreatic enlargement (Gertler *et al.*, 1967). In addition, feeding of rats with raw soybean protein isolates that had a very low trypsin inhibitor content resulted in remarkable growth depression (Naim *et al.*, 1982). The failure of soybean trypsin inhibitors to cause growth depression was also demonstrated in calves (Kakade *et al.*, 1976). It is of interest to point out that the thermostable pancreatic carboxypeptidase inhibitor from potatoes had no significant effect on growth when ingested by chicks (Pearce *et al.*, 1983).

4.2. Effects on the Pancreas

Ingestion of raw soybean meal or trypsin inhibitors caused pancreatic enlargement in rats, chicks, mice, and young guinea pigs. It failed to occur in adult guinea pigs, dogs, growing swine, calves, and, presumably, humans (reviewed by Gallaher and Schneeman, 1986), and it has not been noted in primates even after 5 years of feeding on soybean-based protein diets containing trypsin inhibitors (Harwood *et al.*, 1985). The pancreata of rats and chicks adapted to raw soybean meal synthesized more trypsinogen and chymotrypsinogen and less amylase than pancreata of rats adapted to heated soybean meal (Konijn *et al.*, 1970). Ingestion of diets supplemented with BBI, modified or masked at the trypsin inhibitory site, did not cause pancreatic enlargement and had no significant effect on the amount of pancreatic proteinases. This has indicated that the trypsin inhibitory site, rather than the chymotrypsin inhibitory site of BBI, is involved in the enlargement of the pancreas and in the increase of pancreatic proteolytic activity (Madar *et al.*, 1974).

The pancreatic enlargement and increased proteolytic enzyme concentrations caused by trypsin inhibitors are explained in terms of the mechanism of regulation of pancreatic secretion. The free intestinal trypsin and chymotrypsin regulate the level of pancreatic secretions and pancreas size by a negative feedback inhibition mediated by the humoral agent, cholecystokinin–pancreozymin (CCK-PZ), which is known for its ability to stimulate pancreatic secretion and cause both pancreatic hypertrophy and hyperplasia. The free enzymes present in the upper intestine suppress release of CCK-PZ whereas the trypsin inhibitors, which form the "inert" enzyme–inhibitor complexes, stimulate the release of CCK-PZ-like activity. The negative feedback mechanism of pancreatic enzyme secretion found in the rat exists also in the pig and calf, which do not develop pancreatic enlargement (reviewed by Gallaher and Schneeman, 1986). A recent study has confirmed the existence of feedback control in humans (Liener et al., 1988).

The finding that prolonged feeding of male Wistar rats on raw soybean meal enhanced the action of the pancreatic carcinogen azaserine (Morgan et al., 1977) triggered a series of investigations on the effects of ingested trypsin inhibitors, as "unheated soy protein," on the pancreas of various animal species. In the "USDA trypsin inhibitor study," male Wistar rats, which had been fed raw soybean meal or experimental unheated soy protein isolates for 2 years, developed pancreatic nodular hyperplasia and acinar adenoma in a dose-dependent manner (Gumbmann et al., 1985). However, similar long-term feeding of mice and hamsters on raw soybean meal, in the presence or absence of chemical carcinogens, failed to induce carcinogenic changes in their pancreata. Moreover, the raw soybean meal seems to have exerted a protective effect on the chemical induction of tumors in the hamster (Liener and Hasdai, 1986).

In view of the difference in species response to the presence of inhibitors in the diet, the relevance of the above pancreatic effects in humans remains unknown.

5. Therapeutic Potential of Protease Inhibitors

Epidemiological studies have identified legumes as possible protective agents in the decreased occurrence of breast, colon, and prostatic cancers in vegetarian populations. Synthetic and natural protease inhibitors have been shown to inhibit tumor promotion *in vivo* and *in vitro* (reviewed by Troll et al., 1986). It has been suggested that the mechanism of anticarcinogenesis of ingested protease inhibitors may involve the indirect effect of partially blocking protein absorption (Yavelow et al., 1983). Yavelow et al. (1985) have also shown that nanomolar concentrations of BBI suppress the x-ray-induced transformation *in vitro*, and that the chymotrypsin inhibitory domain of BBI is responsible for this effect. A similar inhibition of transformation in cell culture was achieved by chymotrypsin inhibitor I from potatoes (Billings et al., 1987). Several successful attempts have been made recently to identify potential intracellular target enzymes and proteins of the anticarcinogenic protease inhibitors BBI (summarized by Billings *et al.*, 1988).

In conclusion, the possible contribution of dietary protease inhibitors to the prevention of various types of cancer opens a new era in the research of native, modified, or synthetic inhibitors.

ACKNOWLEDGMENTS. The support of a grant from the National Council for Research and Development, Ministry of Science and Development, Israel, is appreciated.

6. References

Billings, P. C., St. Clair, W., Ryan, C. A., and Kennedy, A. R., 1987, Inhibition of radiation-induced transformation of C3H/10T1/2 cells by chymotrypsin inhibitor from potatoes, *Carcinogenesis* **8**:809–812.

Billings, P. C., St. Clair, W., Owen, A. J., and Kennedy, A. R., 1988, Potential intracellular target proteins of the anticarcinogenic Bowman–Birk protease inhibitor identified by affinity chromatography, *Cancer Res.* **48**:1798–1802.

Birk, Y., 1976, Proteinase inhibitors from plant sources, *Methods Enzymol.* **45**:695–739.

Birk, Y., 1985, The Bowman–Birk inhibitor: Trypsin- and chymotrypsin-inhibitor from soybeans, *Int. J. Peptide Protein Res.* **25**:113–131.

Birk, Y., 1987, Protease inhibitors, in: *Hydrolytic Enzymes* (A. Neuberger and K. Brocklehurst, eds.), Elsevier, Amsterdam, pp. 257–305.

Boisen, S., 1983, Protease inhibitors in cereals, *Acta Agric. Scand.* **33**:369–381.

Friedman, M. (ed.), 1986, *Nutritional and Toxicological Significance of Enzyme Inhibitors in Foods*, Plenum Press, New York.

Gallaher, D., and Schneeman, B. O., 1986, Nutritional and metabolic response to plant inhibitors of digestive enzymes, in: *Nutritional and Toxicological Significance of Enzyme Inhibitors in Foods* (M. Friedman, ed.), Plenum Press, New York, pp. 167–184.

Gertler, A., Birk, Y., and Bondi, A., 1967, A comparative study of the nutritional and physiological significance of pure soybean trypsin inhibitors and of ethanol-extracted soybean meals in chicks and rats, *J. Nutr.* **91**:358–370.

Gumbmann, M. R., Spangler, W. L., Dugan, G. M., Rackis, J. J., and Liener, I. E., 1985, The USDA trypsin inhibitor study. IV. The chronic effects of soyflour and soy protein isolate in rats after two years, *Qual. Plant. Plant Foods Hum. Nutr.* **35**:275–314.

Hammond, R. W., Foard, D. E., and Larkins, B. A., 1984, Molecular cloning and analysis of a gene coding for the Bowman–Birk protease inhibitor in soybeans, *J. Biol. Chem.* **259**:9883–9890.

Harwood, J. P., Ausman, L. M., King, N. W., Sehgal, P. K., Nicolosi, R. J., Liener, I. E., Donatucci, D., and Tarcza, J., 1985, Effect of long-term feeding of soy-based diets on the pancreas of cebus monkeys, *Fed. Proc.* **44**:1496.

Kakade, M. L., Thompson, R. D., Engelstad, W. E., Behrens, G. C., Yoder, R. D., and Crane, F. M., 1976, Failure of soybean trypsin inhibitor to exert deleterious effects in calves, *J. Dairy Sci.* **59**:1484–1489.

Kassell, B., 1970, Naturally-occurring inhibitors of proteolytic enzymes, *Methods Enzymol.* **19**:839–906.

Koide, T., and Ikenaka, T., 1973, Studies on soybean trypsin inhibitors. 3. Amino-acid sequence of the carboxyl-terminal region and the complete amino-acid sequence of soybean trypsin inhibitor

(Kunitz), *Eur. J. Biochem.* **32**:417–431 (as revised by Kim, S. H., Hara, S., Hase, S., Ikenaka, T., Toda, H., Kitamura, K., and Kaizuma, N., 1985, *J. Biochem.* **98**:435–448).

Konijn, A. M., Birk, Y., and Guggenheim, K., 1970, *In vitro* synthesis of pancreatic enzymes: Effects of soybean trypsin inhibitor, *Am. J. Physiol.* **218**:1113–1117.

Kunitz, M., 1947a, Crystalline soybean trypsin inhibitor, *J. Gen. Physiol.* **30**:291–310.

Kunitz, M., 1947b, Isolation of a crystalline protein compound of trypsin and of soybean trypsin-inhibitor, *J. Gen. Physiol.* **30**:311–320.

Kurokawa, T., Hara, S., Takahara, H., Sugawara, K., and Ikenaka, T., 1987a, Conversion of peanut trypsin–chymotrypsin inhibitor B-III to a chymotrypsin inhibitor by deimination of the P′₁ arginine residues in two reactive sites, *J. Biochem.* **101**:1361–1367.

Kurokawa, T., Hara, S., Teshima, T., and Ikenaka, T., 1987b, Chemical replacement of P′₁ serine residue at the second reactive site of soybean protease inhibitor C-II, *J. Biochem.* **102**:621–626.

Laskowski, M., Jr., 1986, Protein inhibitors of serine proteinases—Mechanism and classification, in: *Nutritional and Toxicological Significance of Enzyme Inhibitors in Foods* (M. Friedman, ed.), Plenum Press, New York, pp. 1–17.

Laskowski, M., Jr., and Kato, I., 1980, Protein inhibitors of proteinases, *Annu. Rev. Biochem.* **49**:593–626.

Liener, I. E., and Hasdai, A., 1986, The effect of the long-term feeding of raw soyflour on the pancreas of the mouse and hamster, in: *Nutritional and Toxicological Significance of Enzyme Inhibitors in Foods* (M. Friedman, ed.), Plenum Press, New York, pp. 189–197.

Liener, I. E., and Kakade, M. L., 1980, Protease inhibitors, in: *Toxic Constituents of Plant Foodstuffs* (I. E. Liener, ed.), Academic Press, New York, pp. 7–71.

Liener, I. E., Goodale, R. L., Deshmukh, A., Satterberg, T. L., Ward, G., DiPietro, C. M., Bankey, P. E., and Borner, J. W., 1988, Effect of a trypsin inhibitor from soybeans (Bowman–Birk) on the secretory activity of the human pancreas, *Gastroenterology* **94**:419–427.

Lyons, A., Richardson, M., Tatham, A. S., and Shewry, P. R., 1987, Characterization of homologous inhibitors of trypsin and alpha-amylase from seeds of rye (*Secale cereale* L.), *Biochim. Biophys. Acta* **915**:305–313.

Madar, Z., Birk, Y., and Gertler, A., 1974, Native and modified Bowman–Birk trypsin inhibitor—Comparative effect on pancreatic enzymes upon ingestion by quails (*Coturnix coturnix japonica*), *Comp. Biochem. Physiol.* **48B**:251–256.

Mahoney, W. C., Hermondson, M. A., Jones, B., Powers, D. D., Corfman, R. S., and Reeck, G. R., 1984, Amino acid sequence and secondary structural analysis of the corn inhibitor of trypsin and activated Hageman factor, *J. Biol. Chem.* **259**:8412–8416.

Morgan, R. G. H., Levinson, D. A., Hopwood, D., Saunders, J. H. B., and Wormsley, K. G., 1977, Potentiation of the action of azaserine on the rat pancreas by raw soyabean flour, *Cancer Lett.* **3**:87–90.

Naim, M., Gertler, A., and Birk, Y., 1982, The effect of dietary raw and autoclaved soya-bean protein fractions on growth, pancreatic enlargement and pancreatic enzymes in rats, *J. Nutr.* **47**:281–288.

Odani, S., and Ikenaka, T., 1973a, Studies on soybean trypsin inhibitors. VIII. Disulphide bridges in soybean Bowman–Birk proteinase inhibitor, *J. Biochem.* **74**:697–715.

Odani, S., and Ikenaka, T., 1973b, Scission of soybean Bowman–Birk proteinase inhibitor into two small fragments having either trypsin or chymotrypsin inhibitory activity, *J. Biochem.* **74**:857–860.

Odani, S., Koide, T., and Ono, T., 1983, The complete amino acid sequence of barley trypsin inhibitor, *J. Biol. Chem.* **258**:7998–8003.

Odani, A., Koide, T., and Ono, T., 1986, Wheat germ trypsin inhibitors. Isolation and structural characterization of single-headed and double-headed inhibitors of the Bowman–Birk type, *J. Biochem.* **100**:975–983.

Pearce, G., and Ryan, C. A., 1983, A rapid, large-scale method for purification of the metallocarboxypeptidase inhibitor from potato tubers, *Anal. Biochem.* **130**:223–225.

Pearce, G., McGinnis, J., and Ryan, C. A., 1983, Effects of feeding a carboxypeptidase inhibitor from potatoes to newly hatched chicks, *Proc. Soc. Exp. Biol. Med.* **173:**447–452.

Ryan, C. A., 1973, Proteolytic enzymes and their inhibitors in plants, *Annu. Rev. Plant Physiol.* **24:**173–196.

Ryan, C. A., 1981, Proteinase inhibitors, in: *The Biochemistry of Plants: A Comprehensive Treatise*, Volume 6 (P. K. Stumpf and E. E. Conn, eds.), Academic Press, New York, pp. 351–371.

Smirnoff, P., Khalef, S., Birk, Y., and Applebaum, S. W., 1979, Trypsin and chymotrypsin inhibitor from chick peas. Selective chemical modifications of the inhibitor and isolation of two isoinhibitors, *Int. J. Peptide Protein Res.* **14:**186–192.

Tamir, S., Smirnoff, P., Yonah, N., and Birk, Y., 1988, Isolation and characterization of a proteinase inhibitor from the seeds of amaranth (unpublished results).

Tashiro, M., Hashino, K., Shiozaki, M., Ibuki, F., and Maki, Z., 1987, The complete amino acid sequence of rice bran trypsin inhibitor, *J. Biochem.* **102:**297–306.

Terada, S., Sato, K., Kato, T., and Izumiya, N., 1980, Studies on the synthesis of proteinase inhibitors. II. Synthesis of cyclic nonapeptide fragments and analogs related to the reactive sites of soybean Bowman–Birk inhibitor, *Int. J. Peptide Protein Res.* **15:**441–454.

Troll, W., Frenkel, K., and Wiesner, R., 1986, Protease inhibitors: Their role as modifiers of carcinogenic processes, in: *Nutritional and Toxicological Significance of Enzyme Inhibitors in Foods* (M. Friedman, ed.), Plenum Press, New York, pp. 153–165.

Wieczorek, M., Otlewski, J., Cook, J., Parks, K., Leluk, J., Wilimowska-Pelc, A., Polanowski, A., Wilusz, T., and Lawkowski, M., Jr., 1985, The squash family of serine proteinase inhibitors. Amino acid sequences and association equilibrium constants of inhibitors from squash, summer squash, zucchini, and cucumber seeds, *Biochem. Biophys. Res. Commun.* **126:**646–652.

Yavelow, J., Finlay, T. H., Kennedy, A. R., and Troll, W., 1983, Bowman–Birk soybean protease inhibitor as an anticarcinogen, *Cancer Res.* **43:**2454–2459.

Yavelow, J., Collins, M., Birk, Y., and Troll, W., 1985, Nanomolar concentrations of Bowman–Birk soybean protease inhibitor suppress x-ray induced transformation *in vitro*, *Proc. Natl. Acad. Sci. USA* **82:**5395–5399.

6

Antigenicity of Soybean Protease Inhibitors

DAVID L. BRANDON, ANNE H. BATES, and
MENDEL FRIEDMAN

1. Introduction

Trypsin inhibitors (TIs) constitute at least 6% of the protein of soybeans (Ryan, 1973). In addition to their beneficial effects elaborated upon in this volume, high levels of protease inhibitors have both antinutritional and toxicological effects (reviewed by Gallaher and Schneeman, 1984; Rackis and Gumbmann, 1981). In the rat, dietary protease inhibitors can induce the development of pancreatic acinar cell adenoma, but the mechanistic basis, involving cholecystokinin, appears not to operate in other species, including humans (see Chapter 18). Accurate measurement of specific protease inhibitors will be important to define the human dietary exposure to protease inhibitors in epidemiological studies. Such studies should elucidate the role of protease inhibitors in preventing breast, colon, and prostatic cancer, as well as their potential contribution to human pancreatic cancer (see Chapters 1 and 18).

The standard methods of measuring protease inhibitors in foods, enzyme inhibition assays, do not accurately quantitate specific protease inhibitors. In addition, most soy foods are derived from thermally processed flours or low-inhibitor isolates, and have low residual inhibitory activities (Rackis *et al.*, 1986). Enzyme assays often give inaccurate results with processed samples having low residual activity (Lehnhardt and Dills, 1984; DiPietro and Liener, 1989).

DAVID L. BRANDON, ANNE H. BATES, and MENDEL FRIEDMAN • Western Regional Research Center, Agricultural Research Service, U.S. Department of Agriculture, Albany, California 94710. *Protease Inhibitors as Cancer Chemopreventive Agents*, edited by Walter Troll and Ann R. Kennedy. Plenum Press, New York, 1993.

Moreover, these low activities must be assessed in the presence of nonspecific inhibitors of proteases.

A further complexity is the existence of multiple protease inhibitors. In addition to the two major soybean TIs, the Kunitz trypsin inhibitor (KTI) and the double-headed Bowman–Birk trypsin and chymotrypsin inhibitor (BBI), the glycine-rich inhibitor (Tan-Wilson *et al.*, 1987) and several double-headed TIs related to BBI are present. Both KTI and BBI exist as several isoforms, derived from different genes or produced by proteolysis (Hwang *et al.*, 1977; Orf and Hymowitz, 1979; Freed and Ryan, 1980; Tan-Wilson *et al.*, 1985; Hartl *et al.*, 1986). Thus, it is impossible to establish the exact protease inhibitor composition of a sample through enzymatic assay.

Enzyme immunoassays, or enzyme-linked immunosorbent assays (ELISAs), have had widespread utility for quantitation of proteins as well as other molecules. Extensively used for clinical diagnostics and for research purposes, ELISAs and related immunoassays have potential for monitoring nutritional and toxicological properties of foods which may be altered during processing (Brandon *et al.*, 1986a, 1987a, 1991a; Friedman *et al.*, 1988). Thus, ELISA seemed an appropriate choice for assaying protease inhibitors in processed food samples. The development of monoclonal antibodies to the inhibitors was undertaken because we thought that immunoassays would offer the specificity and sensitivity lacking in enzymatic assays. These features are necessary for analysis of complex mixtures such as foods containing heat-treated soy flour or low-TI soy isolates. In this chapter, we present data on the immunoassays which enable the measurement of residual levels of soybean protease inhibitors in complex samples such as infant formulas.

2. Kunitz Trypsin Inhibitor

KTI was characterized by Kunitz (1947) and the primary structure of isoform a (Ti[a]) was reported by the Ikenaka group (Koide and Ikenaka, 1973a,b; Koide *et al.*, 1973; Kim *et al.*, 1985). Ti[a] has 181 amino acids and two disulfide bonds. There are three closely related isoforms of KTI, encoded by codominant alleles in a multiple allelic system at one locus (Hymowitz and Hadley, 1972; Orf and Hymowitz, 1977). The *Ti[c]* gene product, KTI isoform c (Ti[c]), differs from the *Ti[a]* product (Ti[a]) in only one amino acid residue, a change from glycine to glutamic acid at residue 55. Although Ti[b] retains glycine at position 55, it differs at eight other positions from Ti[a]. KTI is also modified, apparently proteolytically, upon germination of the soybean (see Section 2.1).

2.1. Immunochemistry of KTI

Until recently, immunochemical analysis of soybean TIs utilized polyclonal antibodies from rabbit antisera. Catsimpoolas and Leuthner (1969) described a radial immunodiffusion assay, sensitive to 30 μg/ml. Catsimpoolas *et al.* (1969) also reported a microcomplement fixation method. These procedures have not become standard methods of food analysis. They are relatively insensitive, and complement is an unstable mixture of serum proteins, subject to interference from a variety of compounds. Offir *et al.* (1971) reported in an abstract that antibodies to KTI can prevent its interaction with trypsin. Rossebo and Nordal (1972) made similar findings, and used the antibodies to determine the soybean protein content of raw meat products containing added soy protein.

In addition to their use in food analysis, antibodies to KTI have been utilized by plant physiologists. Freed and Ryan (1978a,b) used rocket immunoelectrophoresis to quantitate KTI in soybean seeds and to confirm the results of Orf *et al.* (1977) concerning the appearance of germination forms. Tan-Wilson *et al.* (1982) and Hartl *et al.* (1986) extended these studies to the quantitation of KTI in seedlings. These investigators found that the electrophoretic mobility of KTI changes quickly upon germination, consistent with proteolysis. Antigenic changes occur later, coincident with substantial degradation of the protein. There was no indication of the isoform specificity of these antibodies. Horisberger and Tacchini-Vonlanthen (1983a) used immunocytochemical methods and rabbit antisera to localize KTI in the protein bodies, cell wall, nucleus, and cytoplasm of soybean cotyledon cells. However, there appeared to be a considerable amount of nonspecific staining as well, since a Ti-null line exhibited weaker, but distinct staining. KTI immunogenicity is not limited to the rabbit or to parenteral administration. Moroz and Yang (1980) reported the presence of KTI-specific IgE in the serum of a patient allergic to soybeans. In addition, since 1985, we have prepared and used mouse monoclonal antibodies to KTI (Brandon *et al.*, 1986b, 1987b, 1988, 1990, 1991a; Brandon and Bates, 1988; Friedman *et al.*, 1989; Oste *et al.*, 1990). The methodology is described in detail in these references. Salient features of the immunochemistry of KTI are summarized below.

2.2. Specificities of Monoclonal Antibodies to KTI

Antibody specificities were determined by ELISA, using one of several formats:

1. Direct binding of antibody to solid-phase KTI
2. Inhibition ELISA, in which liquid-phase sample inhibits binding of antibody to the solid-phase KTI
3. Competition ELISA, in which liquid-phase sample and enzyme-labeled KTI compete for solid-phase antibody binding sites
4. Epitope mapping, in which labeled and unlabeled monoclonal antibodies compete for solid-phase KTI epitopes

Studies were performed using purified KTI isoforms as well as isolines of soybeans which express only a single isoform (Hymowitz, 1986). All of the results were reproduced in several ELISA formats, so we are confident that artifacts

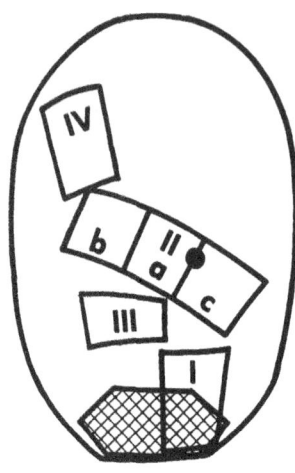

Figure 1. Schematic diagram of antibody-binding epitopes in relation to the trypsin- binding site (cross-hatched area; surrounding residues 63 and 64). Roman numerals I–IV refer to epitopes, with epitope II further divided into sites a–c. The solid circle represents the region of the molecular surface of KTI altered in isoform c due to the substitution of glutamic acid for glycine at residue 55. (◉ , Trypsin binding site.)

which can result from adsorption of protein onto plastic (Dierks *et al.*, 1986) were not significant. The results from these studies led us to conceptualize the immunochemistry of KTI as shown in Fig. 1.

There appear to be six epitopes, denoted by roman numerals and lowercase letters, corresponding to antibody groups as follows:

- *Group 1* (epitope I). These antibodies bind poorly to the KTI–trypsin complex. Thus, epitope I is assumed to overlap the trypsin-binding site or be affected by allosteric changes which occur when KTI binds trypsin.
- *Group 2* (epitopes IIa, b, and c). These antibodies bind to several closely associated sites, denoted by the subdivision of epitope II into three sites. Epitopes IIa and IIc are altered when the glycine as position 55 of isoform a is replaced by glutamic acid (as in isoform c). Epitope IIc is further distinguished from IIa and IIb by its sensitivity to heat and its proximity to epitope I.
- *Group 3* (epitope III). These antibodies bind to a site which is distinct from epitope IIc, but close to epitopes IIa and IIb. Epitope III is moderately sensitive to heat and to substitution at residue 55, but not as sensitive as epitope IIc.
- *Group 4* (epitope IV). These antibodies bind to a site which is highly conserved among the three isoforms of KTI. Epitope IV is unaffected by the binding of trypsin and its topographically close to epitope IIb.

This conceptual model of KTI as an antigen is based partly on the data shown in Fig. 2, which illustrates the competitive ELISA analysis of KTI isoforms using six antibodies. Antibody 171 binds equally to the different isoforms, as illustrated by nearly identical assay curves. Antigenic activity of samples was calculated by using the midpoint of the ELISA curve used to determine the

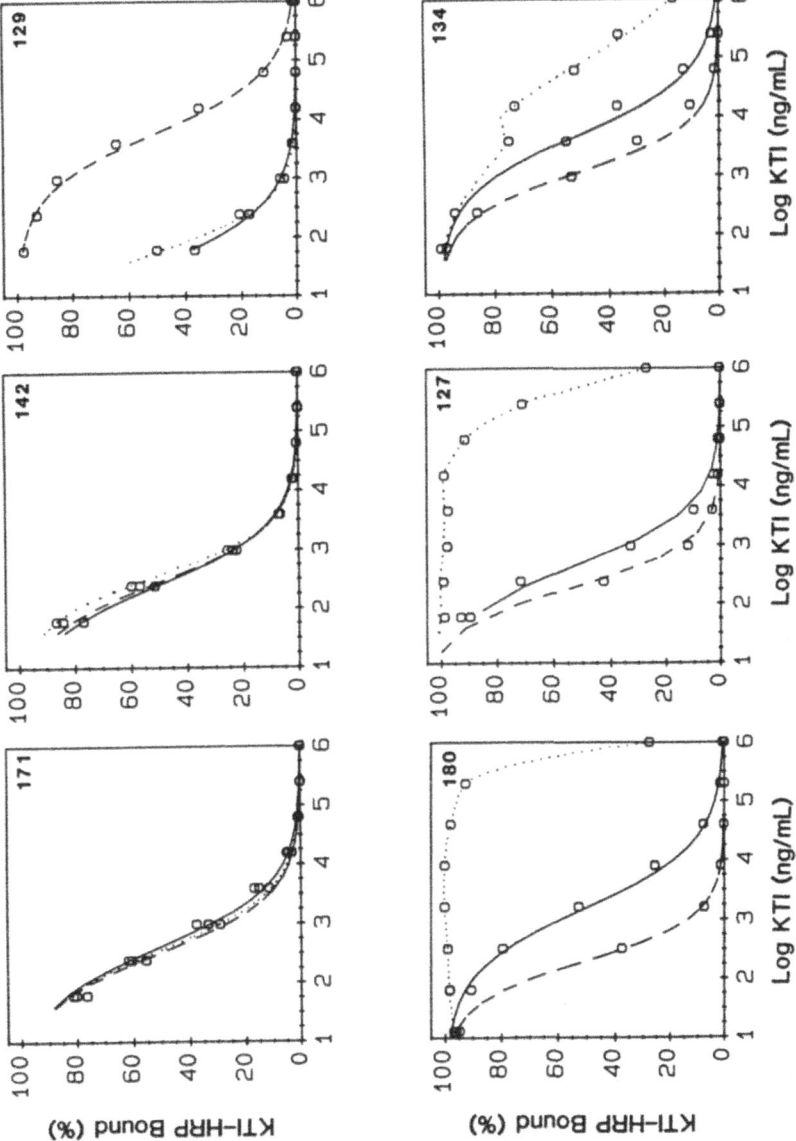

Figure 2. Competitive binding of KTI isoforms to solid-phase monoclonal antibodies: ——, Ti[a]; ——, Ti[b]; ·····, Ti[c].

concentration of sample that inhibits antibody binding by 50% (I_{50}). Relative antigenic activity was calculated as follows:

$$Relative\ antigenic\ activity = I_{50}(control)/I_{50}(sample)$$

The relative binding of two different antibodies to the same sample can be calculated by the same method. Antibody 129 binds equally well to isoforms a and c, but not to isoform b (I_{50} = 78-fold greater than the I_{50} for isoform a). Antibody 180 binds better to isoform b than to isoform a. It does not bind to isoform c.

Based on these results, the antibodies have been utilized as follows:

- *Active KTI*. We have used antibody 180 to measure *active* KTI isoforms a and b in soy-derived foods which may contain significant amounts of partially heat-denatured forms. Commercial samples contain predominantly isoform a, with some isoform b. Although antibody 180 is a relatively low-affinity antibody, it binds to epitope III which is labile to mild heat treatment. ELISA's using antibody 180 correlates very well with enzymatic estimations of trypsin inhibitory activity (Fig. 3).

  Since antibody 180 is a relatively low-affinity antibody, we have used high-affinity antibodies such as 129 for samples very low in KTI, such as those containing toasted soy flour or low-TI soy isolates. Antibody 129 is the highest-affinity antibody (I_{50} = 0.067 µg/ml) in our collection, and is most useful for quantitation of very low concentrations of isoforms a and c.

  If the isoform composition of a sample is not known or if it is important for the assay to be isoform-independent, antibodies of group 4 should be used (e.g., 142 or 171).

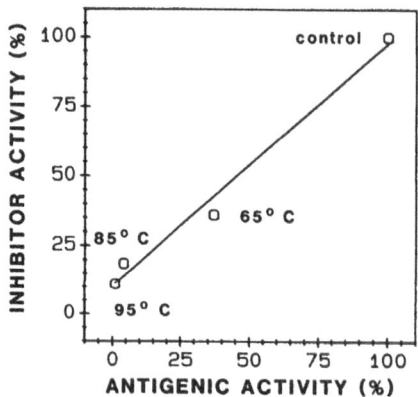

Figure 3. Correlation of antigenicity with the inhibitory activity of heat-treated KTI (r = 0.99).

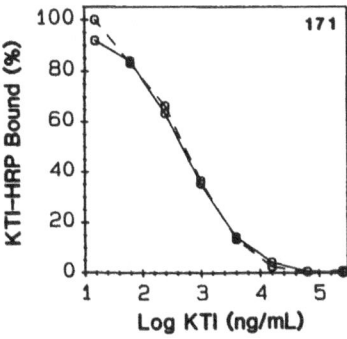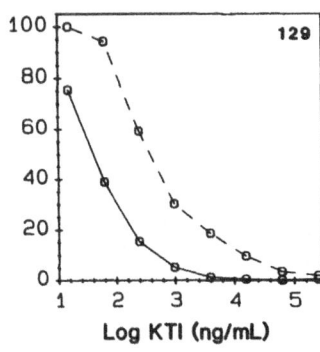

Figure 4. Competition ELISA on solid phases coated with antibody 171 or 129. KTI-HRP is the labeled analyte, with KTI (——) and KTI–trypsin (— —) as samples.

- *Isoform analysis*. A combination of antibodies can be used to estimate the isoform content of a sample. In this procedure, antibody 142 or 171 is used to measure all isoforms, with other antibodies (such as 180 and 129) measuring two of the three.
- *KTI complexed with trypsin*. Antibody 171 binds equally well to KTI or its trypsin complex, but antibody 129 binds only weakly to the trypsin complex of isoform a (Fig. 4). Thus, the difference in KTI detected by these two antibodies indicates the amount of uncomplexed KTI isoform a.

3. Immunochemistry of the Bowman–Birk Inhibitor

The second major protease inhibitor in soybeans is the low-molecular-weight BBI, reviewed by Birk (1985) and discussed in detail elsewhere in this volume. Although antibodies to BBI have been reported by several groups (Offir *et al.*, 1971; Hwang *et al.*, 1977; Tan-Wilson *et al.*, 1982; Horisberger and Tacchini-Vonlanthen, 1983b), the native molecule was thought to be insufficiently immunogenic to elicit usable antisera. To increase its immunogenicity, these workers cross-linked BBI with glutaraldehyde and elicited antibodies in rabbits. However, these polyclonal antibodies were low in affinity and the resulting immunoassays (e.g., Hwang *et al.*, 1977) were not sensitive enough for complex samples such as processed foods. The problems with polyclonal anti-BBI in food analysis have been well documented in a dissertation (DiPietro, 1987). In contrast to these previous findings, we found that non-cross-linked BBI is sufficiently immunogenic in mice and was used to generate high-affinity monoclonal antibodies (Brandon *et al.*, 1989). Immunochemical methods for BBI complement those for KTI and enable characterization of the major protease inhibitors in soybean cultivars and processed foods (Brandon *et al.*, 1991a,b). As the evidence for both the toxicity and beneficial effects of TIs accumulates, these methods should become increasingly useful.

3.1. Sources and Treatment of Protease Inhibitors

BBI (Birk, 1985) and chick pea inhibitor (Smirnoff *et al.*, 1976) were kindly provided by Professor Y. Birk (Faculty of Agriculture, The Hebrew University of Jerusalem, Rehovot, Israel). Lima bean inhibitor (LBI) and KTI were obtained from Sigma Chemical Co. (St. Louis, Mo.). Treatment of inhibitors at elevated temperatures and with disulfide-modifying reagents (*N*-acetylcysteine, sodium sulfite) was described and TI units were defined previously (Friedman *et al.*, 1982; Friedman and Gumbmann, 1986; Brandon *et al.*, 1989).

3.2. Polyclonal Antibodies

Antisera were prepared from blood drawn 1 week after two intraperitoneal inoculations of BALB/c mice with 50 μg of either native BBI or glutaraldehyde-treated BBI emulsified with complete Freund's adjuvant. All mice inoculated with either native or glutaraldehyde-treated BBI produced anti-BBI antibodies. In contrast to previous reports, there was no indication that glutaraldehyde-treated BBI elicited a better response than native BBI, as measured by ELISA using assay wells coated with the native form. The specificity of the antisera was confirmed by inhibition ELISA. A typical assay curve obtained with these polyclonal antibodies is presented in Fig. 5. All subsequent studies were performed using antibodies derived from mice inoculated with native BBI.

3.3. Monoclonal Antibodies to BBI

Monoclonal antibodies were derived from the fusion of the myeloma cell line P3-X65-Ag8.653 with splenocytes from mice inoculated with native BBI. Antibodies were purified by ammonium sulfate fractionation and ion-exchange chromatography from ascitic fluid obtained from BALB/c mice previously inoculated intraperitoneally with the appropriate hybridoma cell line. Antibody 238 was selected for further characterization and determined to be IgG_1. The high affinity of this monoclonal antibody resulted in an ELISA sensitivity 100-fold greater than could be obtained with polyclonal antibodies (Fig. 5). The affinity (as estimated by ELISA) was reduced by 97% for BBI denatured by treatment with sodium sulfite at 85°C for 2 hr (Fig. 6). The antibody did not bind to LBI measurably, and its cross-reaction with KTI was about 0.1%. This cross-

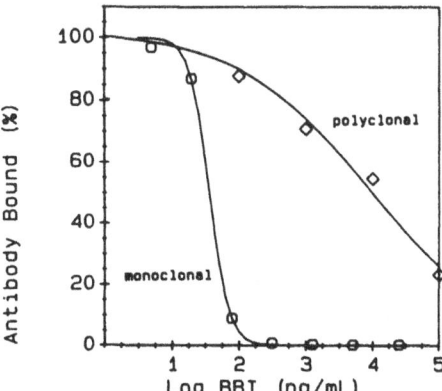

Figure 5. Inhibition ELISA of BBI using polyclonal antibodies or monoclonal antibody 238. The assays were conducted using antiserum at 1:500 dilution or antibody 238 at 0.4 μg/ml.

reactivity with commercial preparations of KTI varied from lot to lot and was reduced following further purification of the KTI by gel filtration. Thus, the binding is due to impurities—presumably BBI—which contaminate samples of KTI. The antibody did not bind to the BBI-like inhibitor from chick peas (not shown).

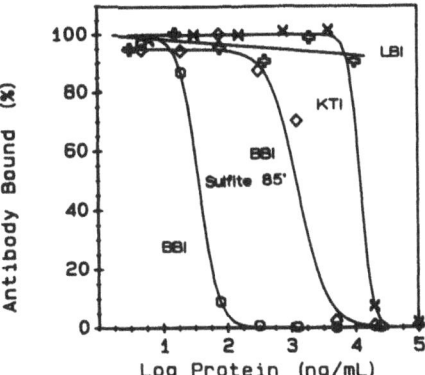

Figure 6. Inhibition ELISA to determine specificity of antibody 238. The reactivity of antibody with BBI was compared with its binding to LBI, KTI, and BBI previously treated with sodium sulfite at 85°C for 2 hr.

Table 1. Epitopes of BBI

Epitope	Steric hindrance by		Heat stability[a]
	Trypsin	Chymotrypsin	
I	+	−	1.0
II	−	−	0.012

[a]The relative antigenic activity of BBI treated at 95°C for 1 hr in solution compared with native BBI.

Our results indicate the presence of two epitopes on BBI (see Table I). Antibody 238 binds to epitope I, which is altered by heat in parallel to the protease-reactive sites (see next section). A second BBI-specific monoclonal antibody, antibody 217, binds to epitope II, which is very heat-labile and is altered even under relatively mild conditions which do not affect the trypsin- and chymotrypsin-reactive sites.

3.4. Relationship of Inhibitory Activities and Antigenicity

The relationship among the enzyme inhibitory activities and ELISA was further studied using BBI treated at 85°C in buffer only, or in the presence of N-acetylcysteine or sodium sulfite. The resulting samples were assayed for trypsin and chymotrypsin inhibition and for activity in the inhibition ELISA, using antibody 238. The I_{50} values were computed for the samples and a control, and the antigenic activity calculated as described above (Section 2.2).

Figure 7 shows that there is excellent agreement among the ELISA results and the enzymatic assays, especially in the area of low residual activity. Loss of activities was progressive over the 3-hr time course of the experiment. The

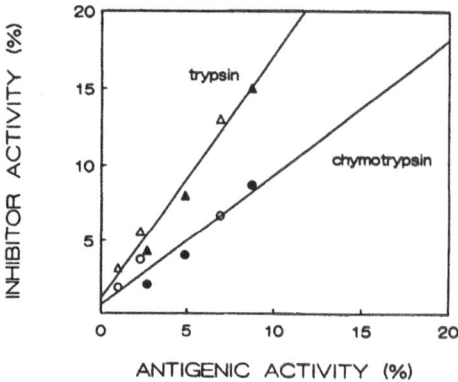

Figure 7. Correlation of BBI antigenic activity determined by ELISA and enzymatic activity determined by inhibition of chymotrypsin ($r = 0.96$) and trypsin ($r = 0.98$). Solid symbols refer to N-acetylcysteine-treated samples, and open symbols to samples treated with sodium sulfite.

N-acetylcysteine- and sodium sulfite-treated samples lost 85–90% of their inhibitory activities within 1 hr. Samples treated at 85°C without a disulfide-modifying reagent (not shown) retained 69–87% of trypsin inhibitory activity, 60–75% of chymotrypsin inhibitory activity, and 100% of antigenic activity. It thus appears that the antibody recognizes the native structure of BBI, which is most affected by disruption of disulfides.

4. Immunoassays of KTI and BBI

4.1. Antibody Titrations, Inhibition ELISA, and Competition ELISA

These immunoassays were conducted as described previously (Brandon *et al.*, 1987b, 1988, 1989, 1991a). Assays requiring KTI-coated plates were performed using polystyrene plates, since KTI did not bind well to some lots of polyvinylchloride plates. However, either kind of plastic ELISA plate could be coated with BBI or mouse monoclonal IgG antibody.

KTI and BBI can be labeled with biotin or enzymes. Biotinylation is conveniently performed using the N-hydroxysuccinimide ester (Guesdon *et al.*, 1979). Unreacted ester is readily removed by dialysis. A second useful label is horseradish peroxidase (HRP). HRP is conjugated to KTI or BBI by adaptation of the method of Nakane and Kawaoi (1974). Unconjugated protease inhibitor is removed by gel filtration using Sephadex G-100. The resulting conjugate is stored refrigerated in PBS containing 10 mg/ml bovine serum albumin (BSA) and 0.1% merthiolate.

4.2. Sandwich ELISA

The inhibition and competition ELISAs cited above provide convenient assays of soy protease inhibitors in foods. However, accurate pipetting and sample preparation are needed in order to achieve reproducible results. Most experienced laboratory workers would require no further training to be able to perform such assays. However, simpler techniques which do not demand precise pipetting would be appropriate for less skilled workers or for qualitative assays. A format which offers this advantage is the sandwich assay.

In the typical sandwich format, one monoclonal antibody is coated onto the solid phase and binds active inhibitor in the sample extract. This antibody is sometimes referred to as the "capture antibody." A second, labeled antibody is used to detect the immobilized or "captured" inhibitor. The second antibody is tagged by biotinylation or conjugation with HRP, for example. If biotinylated antibody is used, a suitably labeled biotin-binding antibody or avidin-like protein is used in the next step.

In the sandwich ELISA of BBI, antibody 217 proved very useful as detection antibody, in combination with antibody 238 as capture antibody. A note of caution is that BBI-specific monoclonal antibody 217 binds to a heat-labile epitope (epitope II, Table I), and the sandwich assay employing this antibody could give erroneous results for heat-treated samples. For KTI, a variety of combinations of monoclonal antibodies can be used, or a combination of polyclonal capture antibody, with labeled monoclonal antibody for detection. Judicious selection of capture and labeled antibodies permits the sandwich ELISAs to be optimized for particular applications.

4.2.1. Advantages of Sandwich ELISA

The following factors may lead some investigators to prefer the sandwich ELISA format over other formats:

1. The analyte dilution is less critical, since it is made in diluent not containing antibody or enzyme conjugate. Assay precision is thus improved.
2. Interference with the assay is minimized, because sample components (other than bound analyte) are washed away prior to application of second antibody and enzyme.
3. Positive samples (containing analyte) give a positive signal in the assay, unlike assays dependent on inhibition or competition.
4. Sandwich assays are well suited for qualitative screening tests, but can be made into sensitive, quantitative methods as well.
5. The sandwich format is generally faster than the inhibition assay, and takes about the same time as the competition assay.

4.2.2. Procedure for Sandwich Assay

The assay of BBI using HRP-labeled second antibody is conducted as follows:

1. Antibody 238 is coated on a polyvinylchloride assay plate, as described above (5 μg/ml, 50 μl/well, for 4–16 hr, followed by blocking uncoated "sticky" sites with BSA). Volumes in all steps are doubled for the larger wells of typical polystyrene plates.
2. A dilution series of sample is prepared, using BSA–PBS–Tween as diluent (150 mM NaCl, 5 mM Na phosphate, 0.05% Tween 20, and 10 mg/ml BSA, pH 7.0).
3. Diluted samples are applied to the assay wells (50 μl/well) and incubated with shaking for 1 hr.
4. The assay wells are then washed and rinsed, and HRP-labeled antibody is applied (50 μl/well) and incubated with shaking for 1 hr.

5. The assay plate is again washed and rinsed, and substrate is applied.
6. The absorbance is determined using a microplate reader, and values are computed with reference to a standard curve. Assay curves are generally fit to a logistic model (Finney, 1964). Typical software packages for ELISA readers offer this option.

4.3. Availability of Cell Lines

Cell lines producing antibodies 171, 129, 180, and 238 are available to researchers from the American Type Culture Collection (Rockville, Md.) as HB 9515, HB 9516, HB 9517, and HB 9657. Interested readers should contact the Agricultural Research Service for technology transfer information.

5. Examples of Use of Monoclonal Antibodies to Analyze Soy Foods and Germ Plasm

The development of monoclonal antibody-based assays was motivated by concerns for the safety of soy-derived foods. Of particular interest because of their consumption by humans are soy flours and soy-based infant formulas.

5.1. Autoclaved Soy Meal

Soy flours are commercially toasted, a process we model in the laboratory using an autoclave. In order to assess the protease inhibitor content of toasted flours, and to distinguish between KTI and other TIs, we studied soy meal prepared from two isolines of soybeans. The L81-4590 variety (Hymowitz, 1986) lacks KTI, while the Williams 82 cultivar contains the Ti^a isoform. The results of the autoclave treatment on KTI and BBI analysis are shown in Table II. The enzymatic assays indicate that nearly 20% of chymotrypsin inhibitory activity and trypsin inhibitory activity remained in the Williams sample after 30 min of autoclaving. The ELISA analysis, however, indicates that only about 1% of the BBI activity remained in this sample, while 24% of KTI activity could still be measured by ELISA. The relative stability of KTI under these processing conditions was surprising, and was not apparent from consideration of the enzymatic data alone. These results confirmed and extended the findings by Liener and Tomlinson (1981). We postulate that much of the residual chymotrypsin inhibitory activity is due to nonspecific inhibitors such as phytate and fat. Some of the residual TI activity is probably due to other minor protease inhibitors (Tan-Wilson et al., 1985, 1987), in addition to nonspecific inhibitors. More recent studies in our laboratory suggest that the rate of heating may influence the stability of BBI.

Using the Ti-null isoline, toasted flours with near-zero TI levels could be

Table II. Chymotrypsin and Trypsin Inhibition by Enzymatic Assays and BBI Content by ELISA in Autoclaved Meal from Two Soybean Cultivars

Variety[b]	Autoclaving time (min)	% activity remaining[a]				$TI_{non-KTI}$[c] (units/g)
		ChTI	TI	BBI	KTI	
Williams	10	83	64	84	46	2014
(*Ti*[a] *Ti*[a])	20	38	26	1.9	34	466
	30	18	17	1.4	24	264
L81-4590	10	40	83	59	—	2075
(*ti ti*)	20	10	9.3	1.7	—	233
	30	7.0	2.3	0.09	—	58

[a]Chymotrypsin inhibition (ChTI) and trypsin inhibition (TI) were measured enzymatically, while BBI and KTI were measured by ELISA.
[b]The Williams control sample inhibited 150 chymotrypsin units and 4800 trypsin units/g and contained 2.9 mg BBI/g by ELISA. L81-4590 meal inhibited 143 chymotrypsin units and 2500 trypsin units/g and contained 3.0 mg BBI/g by ELISA.
[c]For the Williams sample, KTI activity calculated from the ELISA was subtracted from the total TI units. For the L81-4590 sample, the total TI activity is indicated.

prepared with less heating than required for currently used varieties. Most strikingly, despite the greater heat stability of purified BBI relative to KTI (e.g., Obara and Watanabe, 1971), it is KTI that is responsible for the heat-stable TI activity of toasted soy products. Thus, the matrix in which protease inhibitors are found appears to influence their stability (Friedman *et al.*, 1991), a conclusion also reached by DiPietro and Liener (1989).

5.2. Infant Formula

Because infant formula may provide most or all of an infant's nutrition, the impacts of soy protease inhibitors, positive or negative, are likely to be most pronounced on infants receiving soy-based formula. In addition, the infant's lower gastric acidity and increased intestinal permeability could affect the fate of dietary protease inhibitors in the digestive tract. Some results of analysis of infant formulas are shown in Table III. (More complete data, including comparison with enzymatic assays, form the basis of a manuscript in preparation.)

Table III. Analysis of Soy Infant Formula by ELISA[a]

Method	BBI (μg/ml)	KTI (μg/ml)
Sandwich ELISA	6.3 ± 0.46 (*n* = 4)	6.6 ± 1.9 (*n* = 5)
Competition ELISA	7.4 ± 1.7 (*n* = 3)	7.2 ± 1.6 (*n* = 3)

[a]Analyte was Isomil Concentrated Liquid (Ross Laboratories, Columbus, Ohio). All assays used antibody 238 for binding BBI, with antibody 217 used as second antibody in the sandwich assay. Assay of KTI used antibody 129 in the competition ELISA and various combinations of antibodies in the sandwich ELISA (Brandon *et al.*, 1991a).

Based on these data and similar results obtained with other samples, we conclude that soy formula contains active KTI and BBI at about 0.1% of the levels found in raw soy flour. An infant obtaining 100% nutrition from soy formula would consume about 10 mg of active KTI plus BBI per day. The health significance of these concentrations remains to be determined (Hathcock, 1991).

5.3. Immunoaffinity Methods

Monoclonal anti-BBI also proved effective for immunoaffinity isolation of BBI from extracts of soybeans (Brandon *et al.*, 1989). Soy isolate was applied to a matrix of antibody 238 coupled to agarose. Retained proteins were eluted with 0.1 M acetic acid. Column fractions were dialyzed against water and analyzed by electrophoresis in a polyacrylamide gel (12% acrylamide, 0.3% methylenebisacrylamide, 0.4 M Tris-Cl, pH 8.8, containing 4 M urea). Amido black was used to stain the proteins. Figure 8 illustrates typical results. The retained fractions had one component with the mobility and antigenicity of native BBI.

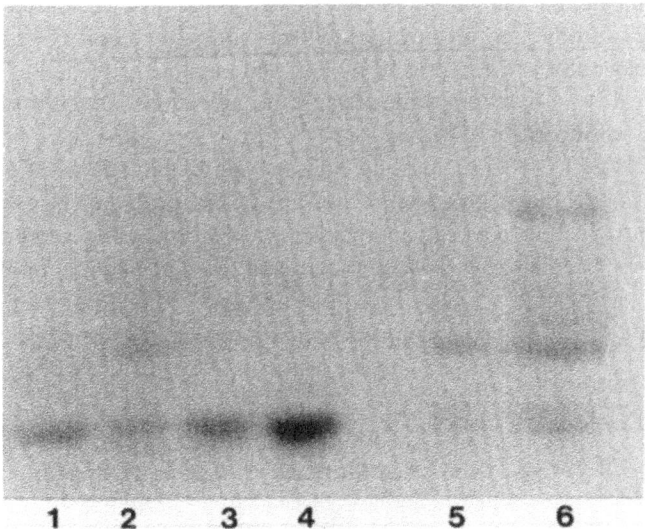

Figure 8. Electrophoretic analysis of soy isolate fractionated by immunoaffinity chromatography on antibody 238 coupled to agarose. The samples were as follows. 1, BBI; 2, soy isolate; 3, retained fraction (experiment 1); 4, retained fraction (experiment 2); 5, flow-through (experiment 1); 6, flow-through (experiment 2).

5.4. Screening the Genus Glycine

A preliminary immunochemical study indicated considerable variation of BBI content among varieties of soybeans (Friedman *et al.*, 1991). Soybeans with reduced amounts of protease inhibitors could have enhanced value, especially for animal feed, since much of the heat processing could possibly be eliminated. As a first step toward developing soybean cultivars lacking both major protease inhibitors, Domagalski *et al.* (1992) screened each accession from the USDA Northern and Southern Soybean Germplasm Collections and additional lines of wild perennial species. The competition ELISA with antibody 238 was used to identify lines lacking BBI, with confirmation by immunoblotting and sandwich ELISA. To prepare extracts, a 30- to 40-mg seed chip from each accession was crushed, homogenized in buffer, and clarified by centrifugation. This procedure retained seed viability, so presumptive BBI variants could be propagated.

All of the 12,370 accessions of the USDA collections were positive for BBI. However, 126 presumptive BBI nulls were identified among the 260 samples from wild perennial species. Figure 9 shows the results of the sandwich ELISA used to confirm the competition ELISA. Assays of trypsin and chymotrypsin inhibitory activities were also performed on some of the accessions. All samples, including the presumptive nulls, had considerable enzymatic inhibitory activities, which could possibly be attributed to other inhibitors (KTI, the glycine-rich inhibitor, isoforms of BBI) and to nonprotein inhibitors such as phytate. Recent results reported by the Hymowitz laboratory at the University of Illinois indicate that the wild perennial species could provide source material for the genetic introduction of the BBI null trait into commercially grown *Glycine max* soybean cultivars (Singh *et al.*, 1990, and unpublished results). In addition, the practicality of screening the germplasm collections for accessions high in BBI is demonstrated by this study.

Double-null soybeans, lacking KTI as well as the major lectin, have been produced (Prischmann and Hymowitz, 1988). A triple-null also lacking BBI would be an excellent soybean not requiring costly processing for animal feed. In contrast, we speculate that the double-null trait, combined with high BBI content (probably having a particularly high content of sulfur-containing amino acids as well), could result in a soybean exceptionally well suited for a healthful human diet.

6. Other Effects of Food Processing on Antigenicity of KTI

6.1. Chemical Changes during Food Processing

As part of a study of the effects of food processing conditions on the antigenicity of food proteins, we investigated the reactions of alkali and carbohydrates with KTI. Treatment of plant proteins such as corn or soy storage proteins

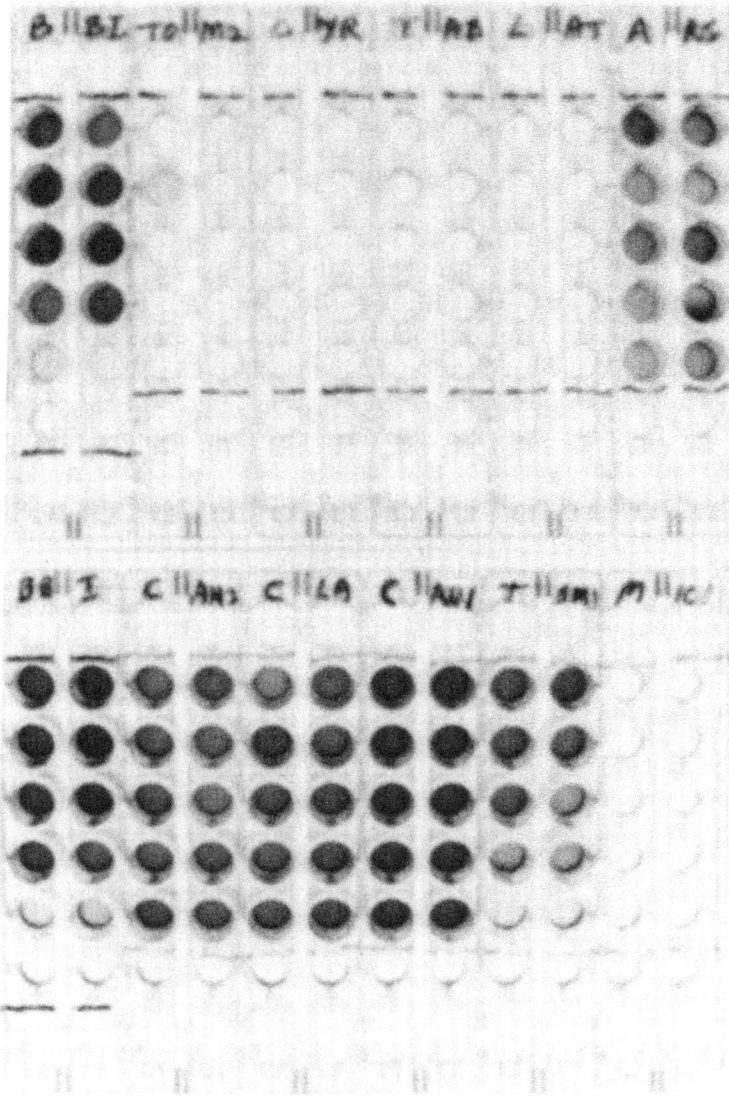

Figure 9. Quantitative sandwich ELISA of wild perennial accessions and BBI standards. Dilution series of extracts or standards were assayed in duplicate. For both plates, columns 1 and 2 contain BBI standards. Columns 3–10 in the top plate and columns 11 and 12 in the bottom plate contain extracts from presumptive nulls, indicated by the absence of color.

or animal protein such as casein with alkali brings about desirable changes in flavor, texture, and solubility and is used by the food industry to prepare protein isolates. Chemical changes which may accompany such treatment include cross-linking, degradation, browning reactions, and racemization. While these treatments may inactivate undesirable proteins such as lectins, they can also lower the nutritional quality of the protein and induce the formation of potentially toxic components such as lysinoalanine (LAL). The biological effects of alkali-treated protein were discussed by Gould and MacGregor (1977).

6.2. Effects of Alkali

Alkali, especially at elevated temperatures, can inactivate KTI, as determined by enzymatic assay and by ELISA (Brandon et al., 1988). Most likely, several mechanisms are involved in this inactivation. We considered whether the antigenic changes could be related to the formation of LAL, one of the several kinds of cross-links which are induced by alkali. Figure 10 shows the antigenicity of KTI treated with alkali at 75°C (relative to the control at pH 7) plotted versus the predicted number of LAL cross-links (based on the study of soy protein by Friedman et al., 1984). Over 90% of the antigenic change occurred under conditions expected to induce cross-linking of essentially all KTI molecules (0.5 cross-link per molecule). The possibility that LAL or other cross-links contribute significantly to the altered antigenicity of KTI or other proteins remains to be tested directly.

6.3. Effects of Carbohydrates

Carbohydrates react with proteins to form nonenzymatically browned products, especially under conditions of high temperature and low moisture content,

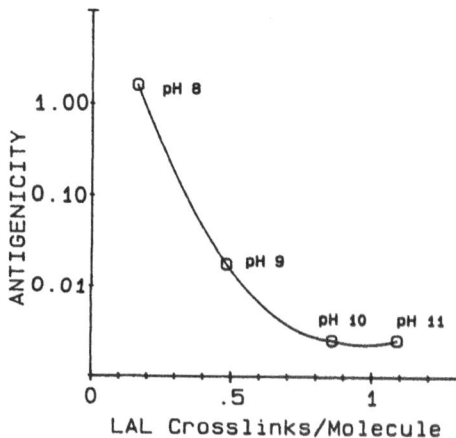

Figure 10. Effects of alkali on KTI at 75°C. Antigenicity determined by ELISA with antibody 180 is plotted against the expected degree of lysinoalanine (LAL) cross-linking.

which occur during food processing. The reactions include the Maillard reaction of reducing carbohydrates as well as reactions of nonreducing carbohydrates such as sucrose (Smith and Friedman, 1984). Oste *et al.* (1990) studied the effects of carbohydrate–protein reactions on the antigenicity of KTI, using two monoclonal antibodies. Heating KTI as a dry powder in the presence of reducing carbohydrates for 50 min at 120°C reduced the antigenicity of KTI up to 90% compared with control samples lacking carbohydrate. Nonreducing carbohydrate had a lesser effect. Analysis of the protein by gel electrophoresis showed that the KTI, in the presence of reducing carbohydrate, underwent a small mobility change within 10 min of heating.

The results indicate that an initial rapid reaction of carbohydrate with protein (probably lysine residues) to form an early Maillard product produces antigenic changes. Further rearrangement of protein-bound carbohydrate appears to increase the browning of the protein (change in absorbance at 420 nm) without significant further change in antigenicity. These experiments suggest that food processing strategies might be developed to exploit the beneficial effects of mild nonenzymatic browning, for example, to selectively inactive KTI. Further work is needed to evaluate the positive as well as negative consequences of such an approach.

7. Conclusions

The results demonstrate that monoclonal antibody-based enzyme immunoassays can be effective in measuring levels of active protease inhibitors in a variety of processed soy food products. These immunoassays could be provided as a kit for use by nonspecialists with modest laboratory facilities. The enzyme conjugates are remarkably stable in antigenic and enzymatic activities and can be stored in the refrigerator, or, with cryoprotectant, in the freezer. In addition to the analysis of foods, the assays and related immunohistochemical techniques could be used to screen soybean germplasm or to monitor the fate of inhibitors in nutritional or pharmacological studies. The methods have already proved effective in determining the level of BBI in soybean varieties and in identifying varieties lacking KTI and BBI (Friedman *et al.*, 1991; Domagalski *et al.*, 1992).

The immunochemical study of BBI demonstrated that native BBI is immunogenic in mice. Earlier studies (Hwang *et al.*, 1977; Tan-Wilson *et al.*, 1982; Horisberger and Tacchini-Vonlanthen, 1983b) utilized glutaraldehyde-treated BBI for enhanced immunogenicity. Use of ELISA may have permitted us to detect antibodies overlooked by precipitation techniques such as immunodiffusion. In addition, the BALB/c mouse may respond particularly well to this antigen. The antigenicity of BBI must be explored further if pharmaceutical uses of this molecule are to be developed.

The demonstration that anti-BBI is effective for affinity purification of BBI suggests a potential pharmaceutical application. Anti-BBI could be used as part of a cellular delivery system directing BBI to specific tissues and cells. For example, a bispecific antibody—with one site specific for a cellular antigen and one site identical with that of antibody 238—would provide a well-defined cross-linking agent.

The use of specific monoclonal antibody-based assays of soy protease inhibitors revealed an unexpected effect of food processing. Table II illustrates the relative stability of KTI, compared with BBI, in autoclaved soy flour. While the precise numbers have varied, we have consistently found that about 20–30% of the KTI activity remains after this processing which is similar to the commercial toasting of soy flour. Under these conditions, the stable, highly disulfide-bonded BBI is 100% inactivated. Assays of enzyme inhibitory activity agree with the ELISA results, but the ELISAs put the picture in sharper focus.

Clearly, food processing strategies could be designed to optimize soy products with regard to protease inhibitor content. These strategies should take into account the nutritional, toxicological, and potentially beneficial pharmacological effects of these naturally occurring compounds (Hathcock, 1991). Genetic approaches for modifying the protease inhibitor content of soybeans combined with food processing research could help provide more nutritious, healthful soy products for human and animal consumption.

Note Added in Proof

A third epitope of BBI was reported by S. Sørensen and H. Frøkiaer (Dept. of Biochemistry and Nutrition, Technical University of Denmark, DK-2800 Lyngby, Denmark) in a poster, "Comparison of experimentally elucidated antigenic determinants of soybean trypsin inhibitors with antigenic determinants predicted from the primary sequences," Prediction and Recognition of Antigenic Determinants, Budapest, Hungary, August 29–31, 1992.

8. References

Birk, Y., 1985, The Bowman–Birk inhibitor, *Int. J. Peptide Protein Res.* **25:**113–131.

Brandon, D. L., and Bates, A. H., 1988, Definition of functional and antibody-binding sites on Kunitz soybean trypsin inhibitor isoforms using monoclonal antibodies, *J. Agric. Food Chem.* **36:**1336–1341.

Brandon, D. L., Bates, A. H., Friedman, M., and Corse, J. W., 1986a, Monitoring nutritional and toxicological changes in processed foods using monoclonal antibodies, in: *Food Processing,* Online International, New York, pp. 27–37.

Brandon, D. L., Haque, S., and Friedman, M., 1986b, Antigenicity of native and modified Kunitz soybean trypsin inhibitors, in: *Nutritional and Toxicological Significance of Enzyme Inhibitors in Foods* (M. Friedman, ed.), Plenum Press, New York, pp. 449–467.

Brandon, D. L., Bates, A. H., and Friedman, M., 1987a, Immunoassays for measuring beneficial and adverse changes in food proteins, in: *Biotech USA 1987*, Online International, New York, pp. 308–317.

Brandon, D. L., Haque, S., and Friedman, M., 1987b, Interaction of monoclonal antibodies with soybean trypsin inhibitors, *J. Agric. Food Chem.* **35**:195–200.

Brandon, D. L., Bates, A. H., and Friedman, M., 1988, Enzyme-linked immunoassay of soybean Kunitz trypsin inhibitor using monoclonal antibodies, *J. Food Sci.* **53**:97–101.

Brandon, D. L., Bates, A. H., and Friedman, M., 1989, Monoclonal antibody-based enzyme immunoassay of the Bowman–Birk protease inhibitor of soybeans, *J. Agric. Food Chem.* **37**:1192–1196.

Brandon, D. L., Bates, A. H., and Friedman, M., 1990, Monoclonal antibodies to soybean Kunitz trypsin inhibitor and immunoassay methods, U.S. Patent No. 4,959,310.

Brandon, D. L., Bates, A. H., and Friedman, M., 1991a, ELISA analysis of soybean trypsin inhibitors in processed foods, in: *Nutritional and Toxicological Consequences of Food Processing* (M. Friedman, ed.), Plenum Press, New York, pp. 321–337.

Brandon, D. L., Bates, A. H., and Friedman, M., 1991b, High affinity monoclonal antibodies to Bowman–Birk inhibitor and immunoassay methods, U.S. Patent No. 5,053,327.

Catsimpoolas, N., and Leuthner, E., 1969, Immunochemical methods for detection and quantitation of Kunitz soybean trypsin inhibitor, *Anal. Biochem.* **31**:437–447.

Catsimpoolas, N., Rogers, D. A., and Meyer, E. W., 1969, Immunochemical and disc electrophoresis study of soybean trypsin inhibitor SBTIA-2, *Cereal Chem.* **46**:136–144.

Dierks, S. E., Butler, J. E., and Richerson, H. B., 1986, Altered recognition of surface adsorbed compared to antigen-bound antibodies in the ELISA, *Mol. Immunol.* **23**:403–411.

DiPietro, C. M., 1987, Heat stability and occurrence of the Kunitz and Bowman–Birk soybean protease inhibitors in soybean products: Quantitation with enzymatic and immunochemical techniques, Dissertation, University of Minnesota.

DiPietro, C. M., and Liener, I. E., 1989, Heat inactivation of the Kunitz and Bowman–Birk soybean protease inhibitors, *J. Agric. Food Chem.* **37**:39–44.

Domagalski, J. M., Kollipara, K. P., Bates, A. H., Brandon, D. L., Friedman, M., and Hymowitz, T., 1992, Nulls for the major soybean Bowman–Birk protease inhibitor in the genus *Glycine*, *Crop Sci.* 32:1502–1505.

Finney, D. J., 1964, *Statistical Method in Biological Assay*, Hafner, New York.

Freed, R. C., and Ryan, D. S., 1978a, Changes in Kunitz trypsin inhibitors during germination of soybeans: An immunoelectrophoresis assay system, *J. Food Sci.* **43**:1316–1319.

Freed, R. C., and Ryan, D. S., 1978b, Note on modification of the Kunitz soybean trypsin inhibitor during seed germination, *Cereal Chem.* **55**:534–538.

Freed, R. C., and Ryan, D. S., 1980, Isolation and characterization of genetic variants of the Kunitz soybean trypsin inhibitor, *Biochim. Biophys. Acta* **624**:562–572.

Friedman, M., and Gumbmann, M. R., 1986, Nutritional improvement of legumes through disulfide interchange, in: *Nutritional and Toxicological Significance of Enzyme Inhibitors in Foods* (M. Friedman, ed.), Plenum Press, New York, pp. 357–389.

Friedman, M., Grosjean, O. K., and Zahnley, J. C., 1982, Inactivation of soya bean trypsin inhibitor by thiols, *J. Sci. Food Agric.* **33**:165–172.

Friedman, M., Levin, C. E., and Noma, A. T., 1984, Factors governing lysinoalanine formation in soy proteins, *J. Food Sci.* **49**:1282–1288.

Friedman, M., Gumbmann, M. R., and Brandon, D. L., 1988, Nutritional, toxicological, and immunological consequences of food processing, *Front. Gastrointest. Res.* **14**:79–90.

Friedman, M., Gumbmann, M. R., Brandon, D. L., and Bates, A. H., 1989, Inactivation and analysis of soybean inhibitors of digestive enzymes, in: *Food Proteins* (J. E. Kinsella and W. G. Soucie, eds.), American Oil Chemists' Society, Champaign, Ill., pp. 296–328.

Friedman, M., Brandon, D. L., Bates, A. H., and Hymowitz, T., 1991, Comparison of a commercial soybean cultivar and an isoline lacking the Kunitz trypsin inhibitor: Composition, nutritional value, and effects of heating, *J. Agric. Food Chem.* **39**:327–335.

Gallaher, D., and Schneeman, B. O., 1984, Nutritional and metabolic response to plant inhibitors of digestive enzymes, in: *Nutritional and Toxicological Aspects of Food Safety* (M. Friedman, ed.), Plenum Press, New York, pp. 299–320.

Gould, D. H., and MacGregor, J. T., 1977, Biological effects of alkali-treated protein and lysinoalanine: An overview, in: *Protein Crosslinking: Nutritional and Medical Consequences* (M. Friedman, ed.), Plenum Press, New York, pp. 29–48.

Guesdon, J. L., Ternynck, T., and Avrameas, S., 1979, The use of avidin–biotin interaction in immunoenzymatic techniques, *J. Histochem. Cytochem.* **27**:1131–1139.

Hartl, P. N., Tan-Wilson, A. L., and Wilson, K. A., 1986, Proteolysis of Kunitz soybean trypsin inhibitor during germination, *Phytochemistry* **25**:23–26.

Hathcock, J. N., 1991, Residue trypsin inhibitor: Data needs for risk assessment, in: *Nutritional and Toxicological Consequences of Food Processing* (M. Friedman, ed.), Plenum Press, New York, pp. 273–279.

Horisberger, M., and Tacchini-Vonlanthen, M., 1983a, Ultrastructural localization of Kunitz inhibitors on thin sections of *Glycine max* (soybean) cv. Maple Arrow by the gold method, *Histochemistry* **77**:37–50.

Horisberger, M., and Tacchini-Vonlanthen, M., 1983b, Ultrastructural localization of Bowman–Birk inhibitor on thin sections of *Glycine max* (soybean) cv. Maple Arrow by the gold method, *Histochemistry* **77**:313–321.

Hwang, D. L. R., Lin, K. T. D., Yang, W. K., and Foard, D. E., 1977, Purification, partial characterization, and immunological relationships of multiple low molecular weight protease inhibitors of soybean, *Biochim. Biophys. Acta* **495**:369–382.

Hymowitz, T., 1986, Genetics and breeding of soybeans lacking the Kunitz trypsin inhibitor, in: *Nutritional and Toxicological Significance of Enzyme Inhibitors in Foods* (M. Friedman, ed.), Plenum Press, New York, pp. 291–298.

Hymowitz, T., and Hadley, H. H., 1972, Inheritance of a trypsin inhibitor variant in seed protein of soybeans, *Crop Sci.* **12**:197–198.

Kim, S., Hara, S., Hase, S., Ikenaka, T., Toda, H., Kitamura, K., and Kaizuma, N., 1985, Comparative study on amino acid sequences of Kunitz-type soybean trypsin inhibitors, Ti[a], Ti[b], and Ti[c], *J. Biochem.* **98**:435–448.

Koide, T., and Ikenaka, T., 1973a, Studies on soybean trypsin inhibitors. 1. Fragmentation of soybean trypsin inhibitor (Kunitz) by limited proteolysis and by chemical cleavage, *Eur. J. Biochem.* **32**:401–407.

Koide, T., and Ikenaka, T., 1973b, Studies on soybean trypsin inhibitors. 3. Amino-acid sequence of the carboxyl-terminal region and the complete amino-acid sequence of soybean trypsin inhibitor (Kunitz), *Eur. J. Biochem.* **32**:417–431.

Koide, T., Tsunasawa, S., and Ikenaka, T., 1973, Studies on soybean trypsin inhibitors. 2. Amino-acid sequence around the reactive site of soybean trypsin inhibitor (Kunitz), *Eur. J. Biochem.* **32**:408–416.

Kunitz, M., 1947, Crystalline soybean trypsin inhibitor. II. General properties, *J. Exp. Med.* **30**:291–310.

Lehnhardt, W. L., and Dills, H. G., 1984, Analysis of trypsin inhibitors in soy products, *J. Am. Oil Chem. Soc.* **61**:691.

Liener, E. I., and Tomlinson, S., 1981, Heat inactivation of protease inhibitors in a soybean line lacking Kunitz trypsin inhibitor, *J. Food Sci.* **46**:1354–1356.

Moroz, L. A., and Yang, W. H., 1980, A specific allergen in food anaphylaxis, *N. Engl. J. Med.* **302**:1126–1128.

Nakane, P. K., and Kawaoi, A., 1974, Peroxidase-labeled antibody. A new method of conjugation, *J. Histochem. Cytochem.* **22**:1084–1091.

Obara, T., and Watanabe, Y., 1971, Heterogeneity of soybean trypsin inhibitors. II. Heat inactivation, *Cereal Chem.* **48**:523–527.

Offir, E., Trop, M., and Birk, Y., 1971, Studies on the antigenicity of trypsin inhibitors from soybeans and lima beans, *Isr. J. Chem.* **9**:17BC–18BC.

Orf, J. H., and Hymowitz, T., 1977, Inheritance of a second trypsin inhibitor variant in seed protein of soybeans, *Crop Sci.* **17**:811–813.

Orf, J. H., and Hymowitz, T., 1979, Genetics of the Kunitz trypsin inhibitor: An antinutritional factor in soybeans, *J. Am. Oil Chem. Soc.* **56**:722–726.

Orf, J. H., Mies, D. W., and Hymowitz, T., 1977, Qualitative changes of the Kunitz trypsin inhibitor in soybean seeds during germination as detected by electrophoresis, *Bot. Gaz.* **138**:255–260.

Oste, R. E., Brandon, D. L., Bates, A. H., and Friedman, M., 1990, Effects of nonenzymatic browning reactions of the Kunitz soybean trypsin inhibitor on its interaction with monoclonal antibodies, *J. Agric. Food Chem.* **38**:258–261.

Prischmann, J. A., and Hymowitz, T., 1988, Inheritance of double nulls for protein components of soybean seeds, *Crop Sci.* **28**:1010–1012.

Rackis, J. J., and Gumbmann, M. R., 1981, Protease inhibitors: Physiological properties and nutritional significance, in: *Antinutrients and Natural Toxicants in Foods* (R. L. Ory, ed.), Food and Nutrition Press, Westport, CT, pp. 203–237.

Rackis, J. J., Wolf, W. J., and Baker, E. C., 1986, Protease inhibitors in plant foods: Content and inactivation, in: *Nutritional and Toxicological Significance of Enzyme Inhibitors in Foods* (M. Friedman, ed.), Plenum Press, New York, pp. 299–347.

Rossebo, L., and Nordal, J., 1972, A serological method for the detection of trypsin inhibitor in commercial soy proteins and its use in detecting soy protein addition to raw meat, *Z. Lebenst. Unters. Forsch.* **147**:335–338.

Ryan, C. A., 1973, Proteolytic enzymes and their inhibitors in plants, *Annu. Rev. Plant Physiol.* **24**:173–196.

Singh, R. J., Kollipara, K. P., and Hymowitz, T., 1990, Backcross-derived progeny from soybean and *Glycine tomentella* Hayata intersubgeneric hybrids, *Crop Sci.* **30**:871–874.

Smirnoff, P., Khalef, S., and Birk, Y., 1976, A trypsin and chymotrypsin inhibitor from chick peas *Cicer arietinum, Biochem. J.* **157**:745–751.

Smith, G. A., and Friedman, M., 1984, Effect of carbohydrates and heat on the amino acid composition and chemically available lysine content of casein, *J. Food Sci.* **49**:817–820, 843.

Tan-Wilson, A. L., Rightmire, B. R., and Wilson, K. A., 1982, Different rates of metabolism of soybean proteinase inhibitors during germination, *Plant Physiol.* **70**:493–497.

Tan-Wilson, A. L., Cosgriff, S. E., Duggan, M. C., Obach, R. S., and Wilson, K., 1985, Bowman–Birk proteinase isoinhibitor complements of soybean strains, *J. Agric. Food Chem.* **33**:389–393.

Tan-Wilson, A. L., Chen, J. C., Duggan, M. C., Chapman, C., Obach, R. S., and Wilson, K. A., 1987, Soybean Bowman–Birk trypsin isoinhibitors: Classification and report of a glycine-rich trypsin inhibitor class, *J. Agric. Food Chem.* **35**:974–980.

Low-Molecular-Weight Protease Inhibitors of Microbial Origin

KAZUO UMEZAWA, TAKAAKI AOYAGI, WATARU TANAKA, and TOMIO TAKEUCHI

1. Introduction

Various protease inhibitors are contained in plants used for human consumption. For example, soybeans contain a specific trypsin inhibitor. Such inhibitors may play a role in controlling carcinogenesis in the digestive tract. Others are found in the bloodstream and tissues of animals, and it is possible that they function to suppress carcinogenesis in the body. These protease inhibitors from plants and animals are all proteins.

The role of proteases and their inhibitors in carcinogenesis has been demonstrated in cell culture and animal experiment studies. However, more precise mechanisms remain to be unraveled, especially in relation to oncogene functions. Cell culture experiments are most useful for these mechanistic studies. However, protease inhibitors from plants and animals may not be suitable because of their high molecular weight, which might prevent their penetration into the cells.

Microorganisms such as *Streptomyces*, mushrooms, and fungi produce antibiotics, antitumor agents, and other bioactive compounds as secondary metabolites. They have been shown to also produce many specific protease inhibitors. These protease inhibitors of microbial origin are of low molecular weight and are particularly useful for cell culture experiments.

KAZUO UMEZAWA • Department of Applied Chemistry, Faculty of Science and Technology, Keio University, Kohoku-ku, Yokohama 223, Japan.   TAKAAKI AOYAGI, WATARU TANAKA, and TOMIO TAKEUCHI • Institute of Microbial Chemistry, Shinagawa-ku, Tokyo 141, Japan.
Protease Inhibitors as Cancer Chemopreventive Agents, edited by Walter Troll and Ann R. Kennedy. Plenum Press, New York, 1993.

In the present review are shown the structure and activity of microbial protease inhibitors including very recently discovered ones. Previously, microbial protease inhibitors were reviewed by Umezawa (Umezawa, 1989) and Aoyagi (Aoyagi, 1989).

2. Endopeptidase Inhibitors

Most endopeptidase inhibitors were isolated from microorganisms in the 1960s and 1970s. They are classic protease inhibitors, but are still being widely used in biochemical experiments. They are specific inhibitors and are especially useful for protease typing.

Leupeptin isolated from *Streptomyces roseus* (Aoyagi *et al.*, 1969) inhibits serine proteases such as plasmin, trypsin, and thrombokinase and thiol proteases such as papain and cathepsin B. It is readily soluble in water, methanol, and dimethyl sulfoxide (DMSO), but poorly soluble in ethyl acetate, acetone, and chloroform. Leupeptin does not inhibit either thrombin or urokinase; but its derivatives, dansyl-L-leucyl-L-argininal and pyroglutamyl-L-leucyl-L-argininal, inhibit thrombin and urokinase, respectively (Saino *et al.*, 1988). Leupeptin was shown to inhibit radiation-induced malignant transformation *in vitro* (Kennedy and Little, 1978).

Antipain was isolated from *Streptomyces michigaensis* (Suda *et al.*, 1972). It also inhibits serine and thiol proteases such as trypsin, papain, and cathepsin B, but does not inhibit plasmin. Antipain is soluble in water and methanol and was shown to inhibit TIF-induced mutagenesis in *E. coli* (Meyn *et al.*, 1977).

Chymostatin isolated from *Streptomyces testaceus* (Umezawa *et al.*, 1970) inhibits α-, β-, γ-, and δ-chymotrypsins. It inhibits thiol proteases such as papain and cathepsin B weakly. This inhibitor is soluble in DMSO, slightly soluble in water and methanol, and insoluble in ethyl acetate and chloroform. It is recommended that chymostatin be dissolved in DMSO at 10 mg/ml and diluted with medium for use in cell culture. The inhibitor was shown to inhibit chromatin-associated alkaline protease of tumorous rat tissues (Hagiwara *et al.*, 1981).

Elastatinal isolated from *Streptomyces griseoruber* (Umezawa *et al.*, 1973a) inhibits pancreatic elastase, but not granulocyte elastase. It is soluble in water and methanol. Elastatinal was shown to inhibit chemical carcinogen-induced mutagenesis in *Salmonella typhimurium* (K. Umezawa *et al.*, 1977). Elasnin was isolated from *Streptomyces noboritoensis* as an inhibitor of granulocyte elastase (Ohno *et al.*, 1978).

Pepstatin isolated from *Streptomyces testaceus* inhibits acid proteases such as pepsin, cathepsin D, renin, and human immunodeficiency virus-produced protease (Morishima *et al.*, 1970). It is hardly soluble in water, and thus should be dissolved in DMSO and diluted with medium. Hydroxypepstatin (Umezawa *et al.*, 1973b) and pepstanone (Miyano *et al.*, 1972) were also isolated from *Streptomyces testaceus* and act as acid protease inhibitors.

Other inhibitors of nonmetallo-endopeptidase include the following. E-64 (Hanada *et al.*, 1978) isolated from *Aspergillus japonica* is often used as an inhibitor of thiol proteases. It inhibits papain, calpain, ficin, and bromelain. Streptin isolated from *Streptomyces tanabeensis* inhibits trypsin, calpain, and papain (Ogura *et al.*, 1985). β-MAPI (Murao and Watanabe, 1977) is an inhibi-

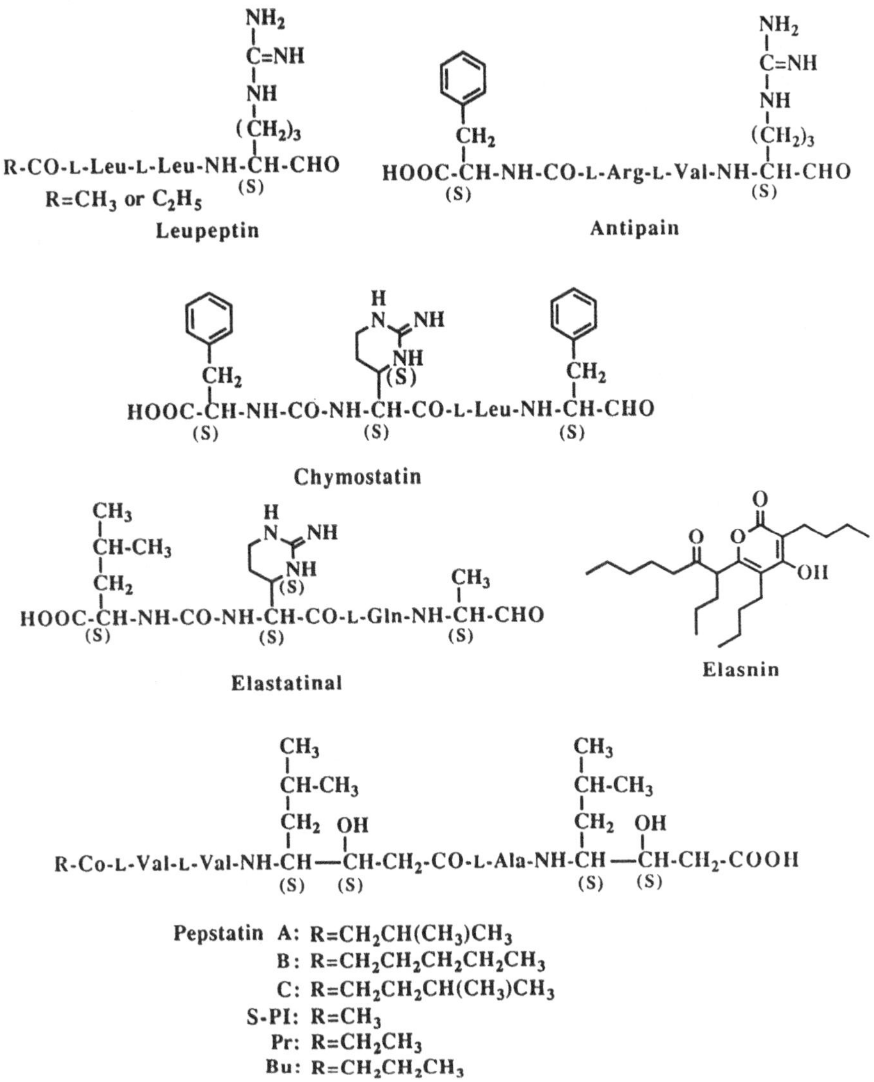

Figure 1. Endopeptidase inhibitors I.

tor of subtilisin, α-chymotrypsin, papain, cathepsin B, ficin, and bromelain. It was isolated from *Streptomyces nigrescens*. Thiolstatin isolated from *Bacillus cereus* inhibits papain, ficin, and trypsin (Murao *et al.*, 1985). K76 is an inhibitor of complement-associated proteases isolated from *Stachybotrys complementi* (Kaise *et al.*, 1979). Marinostatins were isolated from a marine microorganism, *Alteromonas*, and are active against subtilisin and chymotrypsin (Imada *et al.*, 1986).

Inhibitors of metallo-endopeptidases include phosphoramidon, talopeptin, and steffimycins. Phosphoramidon (Suda *et al.*, 1973) and talopeptin (Fukuhara *et al.*, 1982) were isolated from *Streptomyces transhiensis* and *S. mozunensis*, respectively. They both inhibit thermolysin. Phosphoramidon is soluble in water, methanol, and DMSO. Phosphoryl-L-leucyl-L-tryptophan, which is obtained by mild hydrolysis of phosphoramidon, is more active than phosphoramidon. Stef-

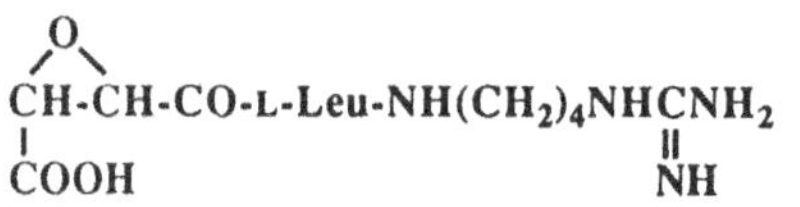

E64

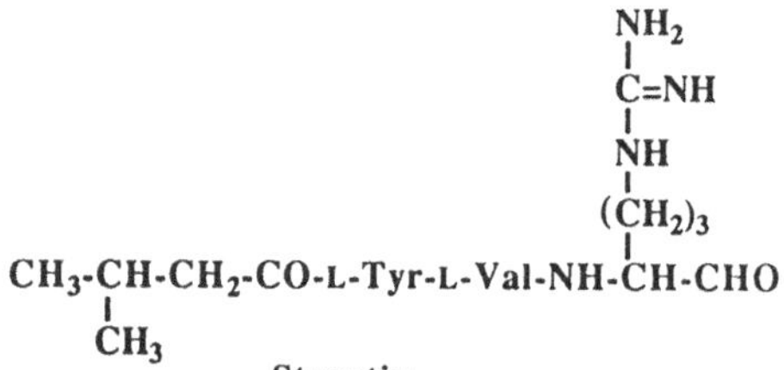

Streptin

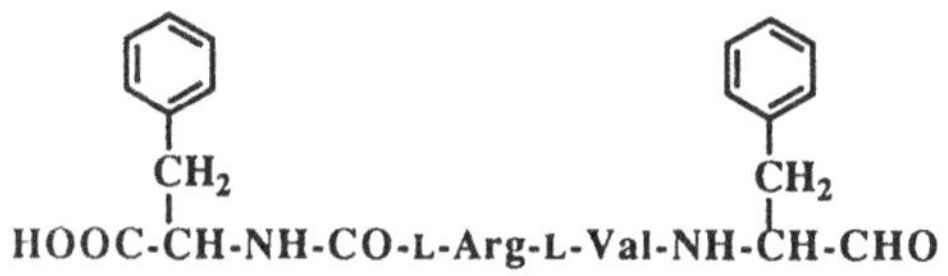

β-MAPI

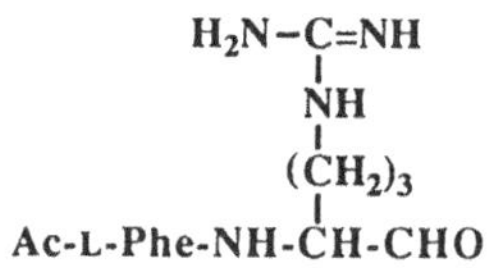

Thiolstatin

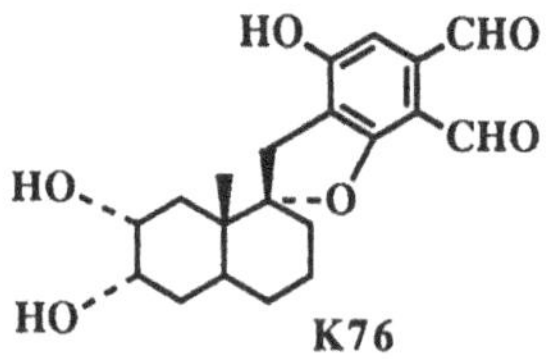

K76

C-I: Phe-Ala-Thr-Met-Arg-Tyr-Pro-Ser-Asp-Asp-Ser-Glu
C-II: Thr-Met-Arg-Tyr-Pro-Ser-Asp-Asp-Ser-Glu

Marinostatins

Figure 2. Endopeptidase inhibitors II.

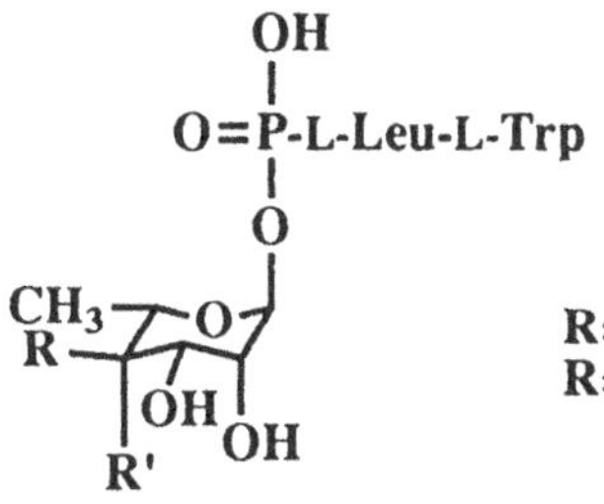

OH
|
O=P-L-Leu-L-Trp
|
O

R=OH, R'=H: Phosphoramidon
R=H, R'=OH: Talopeptin

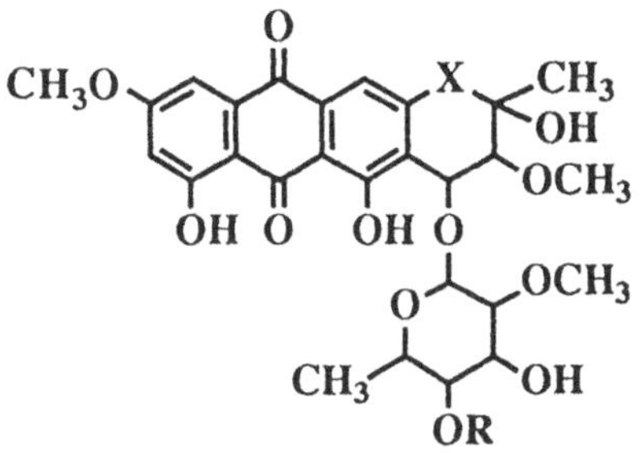

	X	R
Steffimycin	C=O	H
Steffimycin B	C=O	CH_3
Steffimycin C	CH_2	CH_3
Steffimycin D	CH_2	H

Figure 3. Endopeptidase inhibitors III.

fimycins (Aoyagi, 1989) have been isolated from *Streptomyces* as inhibitors of collagenase, toward which phosphoramidon is inactive. Steffimycins have a unique anthracycline structure. A steffimycin analogue, 2-deoxysteffimycin D, was shown to inhibit *ras* oncogene functions, possibly by inhibiting fast turnover of the ras protein (K. Yamazaki, M.A. thesis, Showa College of Pharmaceutical Sciences).

Structures of these microbial endopeptidase inhibitors are shown in Figs. 1–3.

3. Exopeptidase Inhibitors

Aminopeptidase and carboxypeptidase activities have been found on the surface of lymphocytes, macrophages, and normal or transformed cell lines. T. Aoyagi and H. Umezawa have isolated various specific inhibitors for these exopeptidases from microorganisms. Many of them modulated immunological functions in cell culture or in animals. The effects of exopeptidase inhibitors on tumor cells have not been studied extensively. The structures of various microbial exopeptidase inhibitors are shown in Figs. 4–6.

Bestatin (Umezawa *et al.*, 1976) inhibits aminopeptidase B (AP-B), leucine aminopeptidase (Leu-AP), alanine aminopeptidase (Ala-AP), and tripeptidyl and tetrapeptidyl aminopeptidases. It enhances delayed-type hypersensitivity in mice

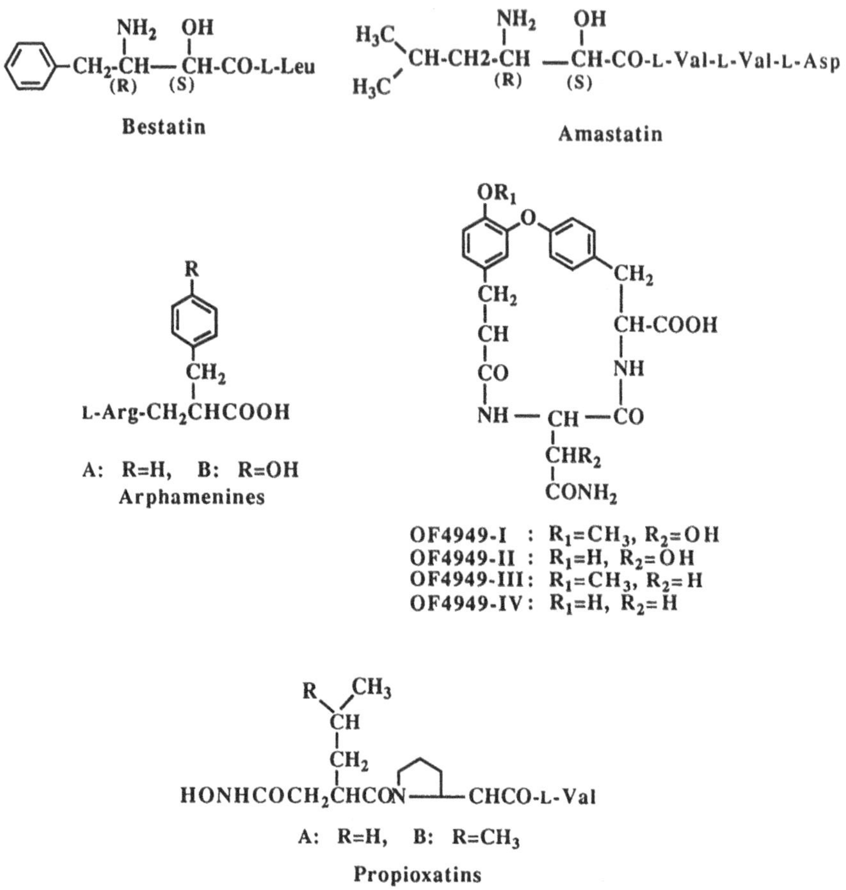

$$NH_2 \quad OH$$

⟨benzene⟩-CH$_2$-CH—CH-CO-L-Leu
         (R)   (S)

Bestatin

$$H_3C \quad\quad NH_2 \quad OH$$
$$CH-CH2-CH —CH-CO-L-Val-L-Val-L-Asp$$
$$H_3C \quad\quad\quad\quad (R) \quad\quad (S)$$

Amastatin

OR$_1$

⟨benzene⟩-O-⟨benzene⟩

CH$_2$ CH$_2$
CH   CH-COOH
CO   NH
NH — CH — CO
       CHR$_2$
       CONH$_2$

L-Arg-CH$_2$CHCOOH

A: R=H, B: R=OH
Arphamenines

OF4949-I   : R$_1$=CH$_3$, R$_2$=OH
OF4949-II : R$_1$=H, R$_2$=OH
OF4949-III : R$_1$=CH$_3$, R$_2$=H
OF4949-IV : R$_1$=H, R$_2$=H

$$R \quad CH_3$$
$$CH$$
$$CH_2$$

HONHCOCH$_2$CHCON——CHCO-L-Val

A: R=H, B: R=CH$_3$

Propioxatins

Figure 4. Aminopeptidase inhibitors (of AP-A, AP-B, Leu-AP).

and thymidine incorporation into mouse spleen cells. Bestatin is now being used as an immunopotentiating agent in leukemia patients. It has also been shown to reversibly inhibit epidermal growth factor-induced DNA synthesis in rat hepatocytes (Takahashi et al., 1989).

Amastatin (Aoyagi et al., 1978) is an inhibitor of aminopeptidase A (AP-A), Leu-AP, tyrosine aminopeptidase (Tyr-AP), and tripeptidyl and tetrapeptidyl aminopeptidases. Arphamenines A and B were isolated as specific inhibitors of AP-B (Umezawa et al., 1983). They do not inhibit Leu-AP. OF4949 compounds isolated from Penicillium rugulosum OF4949 inhibit AP-A (Sano et al., 1986). Propioxatin isolated from Kitasatoporiasetae SANK60684 inhibits aminopeptidase I and II, Leu-AP, and enkephalinase B (Inaoka et al., 1986).

Aminopeptidase M (AP-M) activity is found in the microsomal fraction of brush borders of mammalian renal tubules, while N-formylmethionine aminopeptidase (fMet-AP) is located on the cell surface and has been shown to play

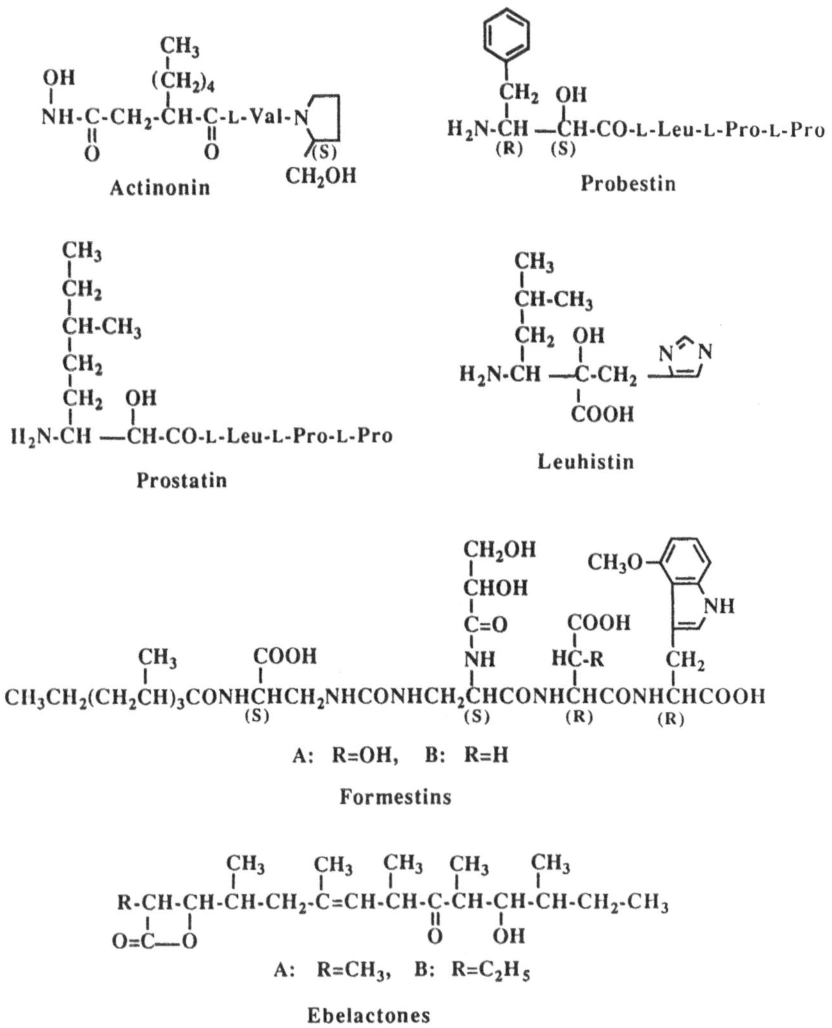

Actinonin

Probestin

Prostatin

Leuhistin

Formestins

A: R=OH, B: R=H

Ebelactones

A: R=CH$_3$, B: R=C$_2$H$_5$

Figure 5. Aminopeptidase inhibitors (of AP-M, fMet-AP).

a role in chemotaxis. Aoyagi and co-workers isolated inhibitors of these exopeptidases from microorganisms. Actinonin, previously isolated as an antibiotic, is a specific inhibitor of AP-M (Umezawa *et al.*, 1985). Probestin (Aoyagi *et al.*, 1990) and prostatin (Aoyagi, 1989) are inhibitors of AP-M and Leu-AP. Leuhistin (Yoshida *et al.*, 1991) specifically inhibits AP-M. Formestins (Aoyagi, 1989) are novel microbial metabolites that inhibit fMet-AP. Ebelactones have been isolated as esterase inhibitors, but they also inhibit fMet-AP.

Dipeptidylpeptidase-IV (DPP-IV) releases NH$_2$-terminal dipeptide (X-Pro) from appropriate peptides. The serum level of DPP-IV is known to be elevated in liver disease patients, especially hepatocarcinoma patients, while it is decreased

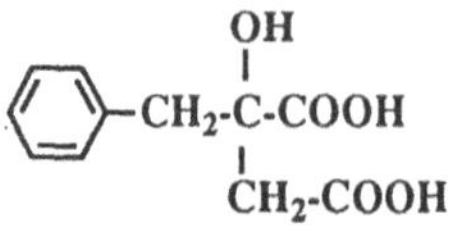

Figure 6. Carboxypeptidase inhibitors.

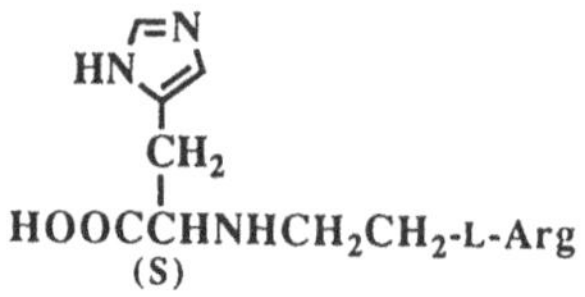

in stomach carcinoma, lung carcinoma, lymphoma, and systemic lupus erythematosus patients. DPP-IV activity is found on the surface of cultured T cells, L cells, FM3A cells, and Ehrlich carcinoma cells. Diprotin A (L-Ile-L-Pro-L-Ile) and B (L-Val-L-Pro-L-Leu) were isolated from *Bacillus cereus* as DPP-IV inhibitors (Umezawa *et al.*, 1984a).

As an inhibitor of carboxypeptidase A, (S)-α-benzylmalic acid was isolated from *Streptomyces hydroscopicus* MG368-CF16 (Tanaka *et al.*, 1984). It weakly inhibits carboxypeptidase B. Histargin isolated from *Streptomyces roseoviridus* MF118-A5 also inhibits carboxypeptidase B (Umezawa *et al.*, 1984b).

Angiotensin-converting enzyme releases a COOH-terminal dipeptide from angiotensin I. It is located in plasma and various tissues, and also inactivates bradykinin and enkephalin. Its inhibitors from microorganisms include ancovenin, L-681, 176, muraceins, I5B2, K-4, phenacein, A58365A and B, foroxymithine, K-26, aspergillomarasmine A and B, and ganoderic acid K. Their structures and producing organisms are summarized in Umezawa (1989).

4. References

Aoyagi, T., 1989, in: *Bioactive Metabolites from Microorganisms* (M. E. Bushell and U. Grafe, eds.), Elsevier, Amsterdam, pp. 403–418.

Aoyagi, T., Takeuchi, T., Matsuzaki, A., Kawamura, K., Kondo, S., Hamada, M., Maeda, K., and Umezawa, H., 1969, *J. Antibiot.* 22(6):283–286.

Aoyagi, T., Tobe, H., Kojima, F., Hamada, M., Takeuchi, T., and Umezawa, H., 1978, *J. Antibiot.* 31(6):636–638.

Aoyagi, T., Yoshida, S., Nakamura, Y., Shigihara, Y., Hamada, M., and Takeuchi, T., 1990, *J. Antibiot.* 43(2):143–148.

Fukuhara, K., Katsura, M., and Murao, S., 1982, *Agric. Biol. Chem.* 46(6):1707–1710.

Hagiwara, H., Miyazaki, K., Matuo, Y., Yamashita, J., and Horio, T., 1981, *Biochem. Biophys. Res. Commun.* 98:488–493.

Hanada, K., Tamai, M., Yamagishi, M., Ohmura, S., Sawada, J., and Tanaka, I., 1978, *Agric. Biol. Chem.* 42(3):523–528.

Imada, C., Maeda, M., Hara, S., Taga, N., and Simidu, U., 1986, *J. Appl. Bacteriol.* 60:469–476.

Inaoka, Y., Tamaoki, H., Takahashi, S., Enokita, R., and Okazaki, T., 1986, *J. Antibiot.* 39(10):1368–1377.

Kaise, H., Shinohara, M., Miyazaki, W., Izawa, T., Nakano, Y., Sugawara, M., Sugiura, K., and Sasaki, K., 1979, *J. Chem. Soc. Chem. Commun.* 16:726–727.

Kennedy, A. R., and Little, J. B., 1978, *Nature* **276**:825–826.

Meyn, M., Rossman, S., and Troll, W., 1977, *Proc. Natl. Acad. Sci. USA* **74**:1152–1156.

Miyano, T., Tomiyasu, M., Iizuka, H., Tomisaka, S., Takita, T., Aoyagi, T., and Umezawa, H., 1972, *J. Antibiot.* **25**(8):489–491.

Morishima, H., Takita, T., Aoyagi, T., Takeuchi, T., and Umezawa, H., 1970, *J. Antibiot.* **23**(5):263–265.

Murao, S., and Watanabe, T., 1977, *Agric. Biol. Chem.* **41**(7):1313–1314.

Murao, S., Shin, T., Katsu, Y., Nakatani, S., and Hirayama, K., 1985, *Agric. Biol. Chem.* **49**(3):895–897.

Ogura, K., Maeda, M., Nagai, M., Tanaka, T., Nomoto, K., and Murachi, T., 1985, *Agric. Biol. Chem.* **49**(3):799–805.

Ohno, H., Saheki, T., Awaya, J., Nakagawa, A., and Omura, S., 1978, *J. Antibiot.* **31**(11):1116–1123.

Saino, T., Someno, T., Ishii, S., Aoyagi, T., and Umezawa, H., 1988, *J. Antibiot.* **41**(2):220–225.

Sano, S., Ikai, K., Kuroda, H., Nakamura, T., Obayashi, A., Ezure, Y., and Enomoto, H., 1986, *J. Antibiot.* **39**(12):1674–1684.

Suda, H., Aoyagi, T., Hamada, M., Takeuchi, T., and Umezawa, H., 1972, *J. Antibiot.* **25**(4):263–265.

Suda, H., Aoyagi, T., Takeuchi, T., and Umezawa, H., 1973, *J. Antibiot.* **26**(10):621–623.

Takahashi, S., Ohishi, Y., Kato, H., Noguchi, T., Naito, H., and Aoyagi, T., 1989, *Exp. Cell Res.* **183**:399–412.

Tanaka, T., Suda, H., Naganawa, H., Hamada, M., Takeuchi, T., Aoyagi, T., and Umezawa, H., 1984, *J. Antibiot.* **37**(6):682–684.

Umezawa, H., 1989, in: *Natural Products Isolation* (G. H. Wagman and R. Cooper, eds.), Elsevier, Amsterdam, pp. 481–538.

Umezawa, H., Aoyagi, T., Morishima, H., Kunimoto, S., Matsuzaki, M., Hamada, M., and Takeuchi, T., 1970, *J. Antibiot.* **23**(8):425–427.

Umezawa, H., Aoyagi, T., Okura, A., Morishima, H., Takeuchi, T., and Okami, Y., 1973a, *J. Antibiot.* **26**(12):787–789.

Umezawa, H., Miyano, T., Murakami, T., Takita, T., Aoyagi, T., Takeuchi, T., Naganawa, H., and Morishima, H., 1973b, *J. Antibiot.* **26**(10):615–617.

Umezawa, H., Aoyagi, T., Suda, H., Hamada, M., and Takeuchi, T., 1976, *J. Antibiot.* **29**(1):97–99.

Umezawa, H., Aoyagi, T., Ohuchi, S., Okuyama, A., Suda, H., Takita, T., Hamada, M., and Takeuchi, T., 1983, *J. Antibiot.* **36**(11):1572–1575.

Umezawa, H., Aoyagi, T., Ogawa, K., Naganawa, H., Hamada, M., and Takeuchi, T., 1984a, *J. Antibiot.* **37**(4):422–425.

Umezawa, H., Aoyagi, T., Ogawa, K., Iinuma, H., Naganawa, H., Hamada, M., and Takeuchi, T., 1984b, *J. Antibiot.* **39**(9):1088–1090.

Umezawa, H., Aoyagi, T., Tanaka, T., Suda, H., Okuyama, A., Naganawa, H., Hamada, M., and Takeuchi, T., 1985, *J. Antibiot.* **38**(11):1629–1630.

Umezawa, K., Matsushima, T., and Sugimura, T., 1977, *Proc. Jpn. Acad.* **53B**:30–33.

Yoshida, S., Naganawa, H., Aoyagi, T., Takeuchi, T., Takeuchi, Y., and Kodama, Y., 1991, *J. Antibiot.* **44**(6):579–581.

8

Protease Inhibitor Synthesis by MCF-7 Breast Cancer Cells

THOMAS H. FINLAY, SUSAN S. KADNER, and SNAIT TAMIR

1. Introduction and Scope of the Chapter

It is well established that proteolytic enzymes play a significant role in the expression of the malignant phenotype including the loss of growth regulation, invasiveness, and formation of metastases (Liotta *et al.*, 1991). Tumor cell-derived proteases have multiple activities and have been shown to degrade basement membrane components, stimulate angiogenesis, and promote tumor cell proliferation and migration. Tumor cells may also be responsible for the elaboration of proteolytic enzymes by host cells such as the endothelium, stroma, or components of the immune system. Studies using an *in vitro* amnion invasion assay, shown to provide a rigorous test for tumor cell invasion *in vivo* (Yagel *et al.*, 1989), suggest the involvement of a protease cascade in the invasion process. Although there is some controversy regarding the specific proteases participating in the cascade, plasminogen activator, plasmin, stromelysin, type IV collagenase, and interstitial collagenase appear to be important (Ostrowski *et al.*, 1986; Persky *et al.*, 1986; Whitham *et al.*, 1986; Mignatti *et al.*, 1987; Strous *et al.*, 1988). Tissue-type plasminogen activator has been identified in breast cancer cytosol and its concentration may be of some prognostic significance (Duffy *et al.*, 1988). There is also a large body of evidence suggesting that metastasis is facilitated by thrombus formation (Saito *et al.*, 1980; Gasic *et al.*, 1983). Tumor cells have been shown to induce platelet aggregation through the generation of

THOMAS H. FINLAY, SUSAN S. KADNER, and SNAIT TAMIR • Department of Obstetrics and Gynecology, New York University Medical Center, New York, New York 10016.
Protease Inhibitors as Cancer Chemopreventive Agents, edited by Walter Troll and Ann R. Kennedy. Plenum Press, New York, 1993.

thrombin and a specific membrane protein responsible for thrombin generation has been isolated from several tumor cell lines (Cavanaugh *et al.*, 1988).

Extracellular proteases may play a role in tumorigenesis without being directly involved with invasion and metastasis. Insulinlike growth factors, particularly IGF-I, appear to be important local mitogenic factors involved with autocrine/paracrine regulation of breast cancer cell proliferation (Osborne *et al.*, 1990). IGF-I binds more tightly to its binding protein, BF-3, than it does to its receptor and proteolysis of BF-3 may be an obligate requirement for IGF-I release (Giudice *et al.*, 1990). One of the BF-3 cleaving proteases appears to be neutralized by α_1-antichymotrypsin (α_1-ACHY), an inhibitor of extracellular chymotrypsin-like enzymes (Stenman *et al.*, 1991). Breast cancer cells are able to synthesize both IGF-I binding factors and α_1-ACHY (Masot *et al.*, 1985; Tamir *et al.*, 1990; DeLeon *et al.*, 1990) and it is possible that interactions between these and a cell surface protease may serve to regulate IGF-I activity. Proteolytic cleavage is required to split out the soluble, 50-amino-acid form of transforming growth factor α (TGFα) from its membrane-bound precursor on the surface of transformed cells (Bringman *et al.*, 1987) and it has been suggested that this process may constitute an important regulatory step in the release of soluble growth factors from cell surface-bound precursors (Massague, 1990). The release of TGFα appears to be an efficient process in most cell types resulting in the accumulation of pro-TGFα on the cell surface. The residues, Ala-Ala-Ala-Val-Val and Leu-Leu-Ala-Val at the two sites of cleavage (E' and E" in Fig. 1), should both be susceptible to hydrolysis by a yet-to-be-identified elastase-like enzyme (Teixido *et al.*, 1990). In HL-60 cells, inhibition of the expression of myeloblastin, a serine protease having sequence homology to human neutrophil elastase including the primary substrate binding site, has been shown to block proliferation and induce differentiation (Bories *et al.*, 1989). Myeloblastin appears to be a "granzyme" identical to proteinase 3, Wegener's autoantigen, and AGP7 (Gupta *et al.*, 1990). These are proteases of unknown function released from azurophil granules in neutrophils and lymphocytes which may serve as regulators of cellular proliferation and autocrine growth factors in the hemopoietic system (Jenne and Tschopp, 1989). The physiological substrate of myeloblastin/AGP7 or possible relationship to the TGFα protease is not known; however, one would expect both proteases to be neutralized by α_1-antitrypsin (α_1-AT), the major human extracellular elastase inhibitor (see below).

TGFα, which is structurally and functionally related to EGF, can interact with the EGF receptor and elicit a similar mitogenic response in a variety of cells (Derynck, 1988). TGFs have been implicated in the autocrine growth of both human and rodent tumor cells and have been shown to reversibly confer properties generally associated with the transformed phenotype on nontransformed fibroblasts. In rat fibroblasts, transfection with human TGFα appears to contribute to neoplastic transformation, while in transgenic mice, overexpression of TGFα has been shown to result in epithelial hyperplasia and breast carcinoma

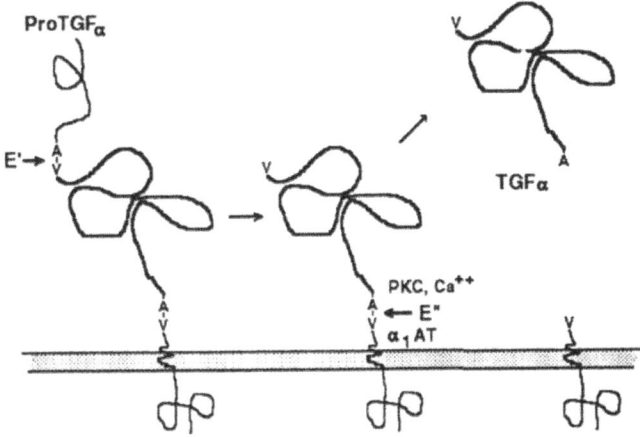

Figure 1. Two-step cleavage of pro-TGFα from the cell surface (after Massague, 1990). Each cleavage is presumed to be catalyzed by one or more endogenously synthesized elastase-like enzymes. Only the second cleavage (by E'') appears to be rate limiting for the release of free TGFα. Pro-TGFα can interact with EGF/TGFα receptors on the surface of adjacent cells, effecting cell–cell adhesion and mitogenesis (Clarke *et al.*, 1989). Cleavage may be an obligate step in a process to generate two active forms of TGFα each with different properties. Recent evidence suggests that the cleavage at E'' is stimulated independently by serum factors, Ca^{2+}, and phorbol esters (Anklesaria *et al.*, 1990; Pandiella and Massague, 1991). It is possible that the activity of these elastase-like enzymes may also be regulated by α$_1$-AT or a second extracellular elastase inhibitor, secretory leukoprotease inhibitor (Rice and Weiss, 1990).

(Rosenthal *et al.*, 1986; Sandgren *et al.*, 1990). Estrogen and TGFα have been shown to interact in the modulation of growth of human breast cancer cells and it was initially suggested that TGFα acts as an autocrine mediator of estrogen-stimulated growth in estrogen-dependent breast cancer cells (Bates *et al.*, 1988). The role of TGFα now appears to be more complicated as TGFα-mediated transformation may also require increased EGF receptor levels (DiMarco *et al.*, 1989). In MCF-7 breast cancer cells, blockade of the EGF receptor, while inhibiting TGFα-induced growth, had little effect on estrogen-stimulated growth, suggesting that TGFα is not the primary mediator of the growth effects of estrogen (Arteaga *et al.*, 1988). Similarly, transfected MCF-7 cells expressing high levels of TGFα also require estrogen for growth *in vitro* or for tumor formation in nude mice (Clarke *et al.*, 1989). How estrogens, growth factors, proteases, and protease inhibitors interact to regulate cell growth in breast cancer cells is not clear at present.

While a role for endogenously synthesized proteases in tumorigenesis is accepted, there is little information available regarding the role of endogenously synthesized protease inhibitors, despite the fact that exogenous protease inhibitors have been shown to suppress tumorigenesis in both *in vitro* and *in vivo* systems (Mignatti *et al.*, 1987; Persky *et al.*, 1986; Strous *et al.*, 1988; Saito *et al.*, 1980; Gasic *et al.*, 1983). Epidemiological studies have suggested an association of a diet containing legumes with reduced incidence of breast, colon, and prostatic cancer (Friedman, 1986; Troll *et al.*, 1984). A trivial explanation for this phenomenon is that it occurs only as a consequence of the blockage of protein adsorption (Yavelow *et al.*, 1983). Plant protease inhibitors have been shown to inhibit oncogenic transformation and the promotion of C3H/10T^1/2 cells in culture, and an intracellular protease which may be important in oncogenic transformation has been identified in this cell line, suggesting that the protease inhibitors are not acting solely as inhibitors of adsorption (Yavelow *et al.*, 1985; Billings *et al.*, 1987). Several tumor cell lines have been found to secrete protease inhibitors (Lee *et al.*, 1982; Gendler and Tokes, 1984; Ray *et al.*, 1982) as well as proteases and it is an intriguing possibility that the specificity and amount of protease inhibitors produced by a tumor cell may have an effect on its metastatic potential. In this chapter we discuss the synthesis of two protease inhibitors, α_1-AT and α_1-ACHY, by MCF-7 breast cancer cells. We also compare the regulation of the synthesis of these proteins by various cell types and speculate about their possible role in the modulation of tumorigenesis and metastasis.

2. α_1-AT and α_1-ACHY

2.1. Function and Properties

α_1-AT and α_1-ACHY are 68- and 53-kDa plasma glycoproteins belonging to the serpin (for *ser*ine *p*rotease *in*hibitor) supergene family (Travis and Salvasen, 1983). This group of proteins, which also includes antithrombin III, α_1-antiplasmin, and C1-esterase inhibitor, is responsible for the control of a wide range of physiological activities modulated by proteolytic enzymes such as blood coagulation, fibrinolysis, complement activation, implantation, and aspects of the inflammatory response. Serpins neutralize proteases through the formation of stable, inactive, 1:1 complexes which after formation are rapidly cleared from the circulation. Complex formation occurs after cleavage of a unique peptide bond in the inhibitor causes a dramatic conformational change (Stein *et al.*, 1990; Pemberton *et al.*, 1988). α_1-AT and α_1-ACHY play major roles in the host response to trauma and inflammation (Travis *et al.*, 1988). The primary role of α_1-AT, which is present at high levels in human plasma (1.5–3.5 mg/ml), appears to be the neutralization of elastases released by leukocytes at sites of inflammation. α_1-ACHY, present in plasma at somewhat lower levels (0.2–0.5 mg/ml), is thought to neutralize chymotrypsin-like proteases such as cathepsin G which are also released by leukocytes and mast cells at inflammatory sites. The protease specificity of α_1-AT and α_1-ACHY are quite different; while α_1-AT can inhibit a wide range of proteases found in plasma such as PMN elastase, chymase, thrombin, and plasmin, α_1-ACHY is effective only against chymotrypsin-like proteases such as chymase and cathepsin G (Travis and Salvasen, 1983; Schechter *et al.*, 1989). α_1-AT and α_1-ACHY have a high degree of functional and structural similarity. The amino acid sequences of the two proteins show an overall homology of 42% and their protease binding sites, although structurally different, are located in the same general region. The homology extends to the DNA level: intron locations of the two human genes on chromosome 14 are identical (Bao *et al.*, 1987). Corticosteroid binding globulin (CBG), the major glucocorticoid carrier in the circulation, is also a member of the serpin supergene family (Hammond *et al.*, 1987). CBG is cleaved by elastase at a locus analogous to the locus cleaved by elastase in α_1-AT and cleavage results in decreased glucocorticoid binding (Hammond *et al.*, 1990). Since local elastase levels depend to a large degree on local levels of α_1-AT, delivery of glucocorticoids to inflammatory sites may be regulated by a mechanism involving the interaction of elastase and α_1-AT. An essential methionine residue in α_1-AT is easily oxidized *in vivo* by oxidants released from leukocytes. Oxidation blocks inhibitory activity against elastase (Beatty *et al.*, 1982). This is probably necessary under normal physiologic conditions to transiently turn off α_1-AT activity in the immediate vicinity of an inflammatory site.

2.2. Site of Synthesis

α_1-AT and α_1-ACHY are synthesized primarily by hepatocytes and to a lesser degree by monocytes (Perlmutter *et al.*, 1985; Mornex *et al.*, 1986). MCF-7 human breast cancer cells, a cell line of epithelial origin, have been shown to synthesize and secrete α_1-ACHY and synthesis is stimulated by estrogens (Masot *et al.*, 1985). We have confirmed these observations and in addition have shown that MCF-7 cells can also synthesize α_1-AT (Tamir *et al.*, 1990). Consistent with this is a report of the synthesis of α_1-AT by a human intestinal epithelial cell line (Perlmutter *et al.*, 1989a). α_1-ACHY may also be synthesized by the brain as a recent report suggests that it is a major constituent of the plaques found in the brains of individuals with Alzheimer's disease (Abraham and Potter, 1989) where it can inhibit the activity of a cell surface chymotrypsin-like protease (Nelson and Siman, 1990). The immunohistochemical localization of α_1-AT in many tissues has been reported, although this should be viewed with caution because of possible contamination by α_1-AT from plasma (Finlay *et al.*, 1981). Transgenic mice containing multiple copies of the human α_1-AT gene have been shown to express human α_1-AT in their liver, kidney, stomach, small intestine, spleen, thymus, adrenal glands, ovaries, testes, and pancreas (Carlson *et al.*, 1988), suggesting the nonhepatic synthesis of α_1-AT to be a common phenomenon. Preliminary results from this laboratory show the presence of α_1-AT and α_1-ACHY mRNA in freshly obtained placental trophoblastic tissue

from postpartum placentas of various gestational ages and in JAR choriocar-
cinoma cells (Bergman *et al.*, 1991). Synthesis of α_1-AT and α_1-ACHY proteins
by the JAR cells was also demonstrated by SDS-PAGE of ^{35}S-methionine-
labeled proteins immunoprecipitated from metabolically labeled cells in culture
using specific antibodies to α_1-AT and α_1-ACHY. It is possible that in the
trophoblast as in other tissues, protease inhibitors play a role both in modulating
the inflammatory response and in regulating growth processes.

While the amount of α_1-AT and α_1-ACHY produced by nonhepatic cells is
small in comparison to that produced by hepatocytes, it may be important in
increasing α_1-AT levels at sites of inflammation. For example, alveolar macrophages (which represent approximately 10% of the cells of the alveolar structures) and monocytes of the lower respiratory tract are located at sites where
α_1-AT is needed to block the action of neutrophil elastase. α_1-AT and α_1-ACHY
isolated from plasma have both been shown to inactivate human chymase, a
chymotrypsin-like protease released by tissue mast cells (Schechter *et al.*, 1989).
It is possible that the protease inhibitors synthesized by epithelial cells have a
similar function. Although α_1-AT is present at high levels in plasma, because of
its size it only diffuses into tissues slowly and levels outside of the circulation are
quite low. α_1-AT levels on the epithelial surface of the lower respiratory tract are
only 10% that of the plasma (Wewers *et al.*, 1987). Whether this represents
diffusion from the plasma or endogenous synthesis is unknown.

2.3. Regulation of Synthesis

Although more is known regarding α_1-AT and α_1-ACHY synthesis in hepatocytes than in other cell types, it is probable that the cell-specific expression of
these proteins is not simply the result of a single cell-specific factor but rather the
result of a combination of factors present at varying levels in all cells. α_1-AT and
α_1-ACHY are acute-phase proteins and their levels in plasma can increase three-
to fourfold during the host response to trauma/inflammation. Expression of
α_1-AT by human hepatocytes and monocytes is regulated by the inflammatory
mediator IL-6 (Andrus *et al.*, 1988a; Perlmutter *et al.*, 1989b; Castell *et al.*,
1989) while two other cytokines, IL-1 and TNF, appear to be less effective
(Andus *et al.*, 1988b). We have found similar but not identical effects in MCF-7
cells (see below). In monocytes, expression of α_1-AT decreases during maturation while it increases in Caco 2 cells (an enteric epithelial cell line) as they
differentiate into enteric villous-type cells (Perlmutter *et al.*, 1988a). Endotoxin
has been shown to increase α_1-AT synthesis in monocytes (but not in hepatocytes) by increasing the translational efficiency of α_1-AT mRNA. Also in monocytes, α_1-AT synthesis may be regulated by elastase (perhaps by an elastase–
α_1-AT complex) (Perlmutter *et al.*, 1988b). The presence of a receptor for the
α_1-AT–elastase complex in hepatocytes suggests a similar mechanism (Fuchs *et
al.*, 1984). The existence of liver-specific *trans*-acting factors (HNF-1/LF-B1)

able to regulate transcription of α_1-AT and other proteins has been reported by a number of groups (Couritois *et al.*, 1987; Schorpp *et al.*, 1988; Frain *et al.*, 1989) but these appear to be responsible for general liver-specific protein synthesis and not for the increased protein synthesis occurring during the acute-phase reaction. In man the α_1-AT gene appears to transcribed from different promoters in the hepatocyte and monocyte (Perlino *et al.*, 1987): no information is yet available regarding transcription in other cell types. Synthesis of α_1-AT (and most likely α_1-ACHY) by the liver appears to be at least partially under endocrine control. In man, both diethylstilbestol (a synthetic estrogen) and Danazol (a synthetic androgen) increase plasma α_1-AT levels without an apparent general stimulation of liver protein synthesis (Liberman *et al.*, 1971; Gadek *et al.*, 1980). Results from this laboratory confirm similar endocrine control in the mouse (Nathoo and Finlay, unpublished observations).

3. α_1-AT and α_1-ACHY in MCF-7 Cells

3.1. MCF-7 Breast Cancer Cell Line

The MCF-7 cell line, originally derived from the pleural effusion of a patient with a malignant carcinoma of the breast, retains many of the properties of the differentiated mammary epithelial cell including estrogen sensitivity and the ability to synthesize mammary gland-associated proteins (Soule *et al.*, 1973). MCF-7 cells, when injected into athymic, nude mice, form tumors in the presence of estrogens (Russo *et al.*, 1976). It thus provides a convenient model system for the examination of hormonal control of tumorigenesis and metastasis (Shin, 1979; Huseby *et al.*, 1984; Osborne *et al.*, 1985; Niwa *et al.*, 1989). Like many other tumor cell lines, MCF-7 cells independently passaged in different laboratories, display a considerable degree of heterogeneity. Differences in antigenic phenotype (Hand *et al.*, 1983), estrogen responsiveness (Osborne *et al.*, 1987), plasminogen activator activity (Katzenellenbogen *et al.*, 1984), amplification of the N-*ras* oncogene (Graham *et al.*, 1985), and most importantly, tumorigenicity in nude mice (Osborne *et al.*, 1987) have all been reported in variant MCF-7 sublines. It has been demonstrated by a number of investigators that metastatic MCF-7 cells in culture synthesize and secrete α_1-ACHY and that its synthesis is stimulated by estradiol (Masot *et al.*, 1985; Gendler and Tokes, 1986). MCF-7 cells in culture synthesize and secrete a number of proteins in response to estrogen stimulation which may play a role in tumorigenesis and metastasis such as oncogenes, growth factors, proteases, and protease inhibitors. Stimulation of specific protein synthesis by MCF-7 cells is complex and is not completely understood and can be accomplished by estradiol (E_2) acting directly or indirectly, i.e., via the autocrine action of an E_2-stimulated growth factor. As mentioned above, MCF-7 cells synthesize and secrete both α_1-ACHY and α_1-AT and that synthesis is stimulated by E_2. It is unclear, however, whether α_1-AT and α_1-ACHY play roles in the tumorigenic/metastatic process or are only present in response to a real or anticipated inflammatory stimulus.

3.2. Synthesis of α_1-AT and α_1-ACHY by MCF-7 Cells

Because of a possible role for endogenous protease inhibitors as modulators of tumorigenesis and metastasis as well as the inflammatory response, we began a systematic study of α_1-AT and α_1-ACHY synthesis by different MCF-7 breast cancer cell sublines to see if there was a correlation between protease inhibitor synthesis and tumorigenic/metastatic potential. Preliminary experiments were designed to explore protease inhibitor synthesis by MCF-7 cells, establish a relationship between protease inhibitors and tumorigenesis or metastasis of MCF-7 cells in nude mice, and develop a model system in which the effects of protease inhibitor synthesis by MCF-7 cells growing in soft agar could be studied.

Synthesis of α_1-AT and α_1-ACHY by MCF-7 cells in confluent monolayer culture was examined under conditions designed to minimize the effects of changes in cell number (Tamir et al., 1990). Protein synthesis was monitored by immunoprecipitation followed by SDS-PAGE of ^{35}S-labeled proteins, and mRNA levels by Northern blotting with specific cDNA probes. In initial experiments using the MCF-7 cell subline originally obtained from the Michigan Cancer Research Foundation at the 203rd passage, we looked for the production of protease inhibitors in serum-free media by immunoblotting with commercial antibodies to human α_1-AT and α_1-ACHY. Serum-free media were necessary because of cross-reacting materials in fetal bovine serum (FBS). A time-dependent increase in immunoreactive α_1-AT and α_1-ACHY in spent media was seen with higher levels of both inhibitors in media from cells maintained in the presence of estradiol. However, because the MCF-7 cells did not grow well in serum-free media, results from these experiments were somewhat variable and difficult to quantitate. In subsequent experiments, cells were grown in media containing 10% FBS (charcoal-treated to remove endogenous steroids) and [^{35}S]methionine. Radiolabeled α_1-AT and α_1-ACHY were identified and quantitated by immunoprecipitation followed by SDS-PAGE. The rates of α_1-AT and α_1-ACHY synthesis were approximately equal and doubled in the presence of 10 nM E_2 (Fig. 2). Immunoblotting and immunoprecipitation yielded comparable results, confirming hormonally sensitive synthesis of both protease inhibitors. Similar results were obtained by Northern blot analysis. Incubation of spent media with [^{125}I]trypsin or [^{125}I]chymotrypsin resulted in the formation of stable complexes identical to the complexes formed between these proteases and the protease inhibitors in plasma showing the release of active protease inhibitors by MCF-7 cells in culture.

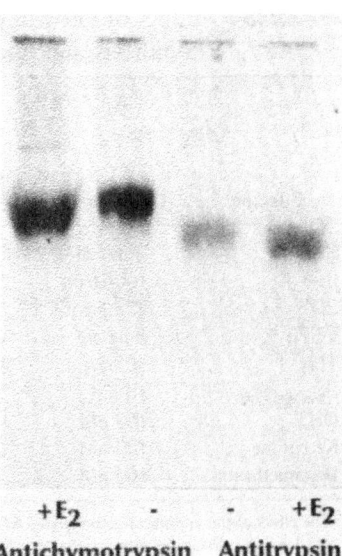

Figure 2. Production of α_1-AT and α_1-ACHY by MCF-7 cells in culture in the presence and absence of estradiol. Cells were incubated in phenol red-free media containing 10% charcoal-treated fetal bovine serum with and without 10 nM estradiol for 48 hr. At the end of the incubation period, cells were transferred to methionine-free media containing 0.15 mCi/ml ^{35}S methionine for 6 hr. ^{35}S-labeled α_1-AT and α_1-ACHY in the media were identified and quantitated by autoradiography after immunoprecipitation and SDS-PAGE (Tamir *et al.*, 1990).

$+E_2$ -   - $+E_2$

Antichymotrypsin   Antitrypsin

3.3. Kinetics of α_1-AT and α_1-ACHY Synthesis and Secretion

MCF-7 cells were subjected to pulse labeling with [^{35}S]methionine to follow the kinetics of protease inhibitor synthesis. At various intervals, α_1-AT and α_1-ACHY in the media and lysed cells were identified by autoradiography after immunoprecipitation and SDS-PAGE. Labeled α_1-AT in the media reached a maximum at 3 hr, then declined and was not apparent after 6 hr. The size of the major intracellular form of α_1-AT was approximately 44 kDa which is consistent with that reported for unglycosylated α_1-AT synthesized from MCF-7 cell RNA. A minor form of approximately 51 kDa, which is probably partly glycosylated α_1-AT, was also found intracellularly. Labeling of the 44-kDa form reached a maximum 30 min after pulse labeling and then diminished. Ninety minutes after pulse labeling, the presence of any newly synthesized α_1-AT protein in the cell cytosol was no longer detectable. Our observations of the kinetics of α_1-AT and α_1-ACHY synthesis by MCF-7 cells are consistent with those reported for monocytes and hepatocytes by others (Perlmutter *et al.*, 1985).

3.4. Stimulation of α_1-AT and α_1-ACHY Synthesis by Steroid Hormones, Inflammatory Mediators, and Growth Factors

To gain a further understanding of the mechanisms governing the synthesis and release of protease inhibitors by MCF-7 cells, we examined the effects of a diverse group of potential effectors including inflammatory mediators, growth

Table I. Effect of Growth Factors and Steroids on α_1-AT and α_1-ACHY
Synthesis and mRNA Levels in MCF-7 (203P) Cells[a]

		Fold increase over control[b]			
		α_1-AT		α_1-ACHY	
Effector	Concentration	Protein	mRNA	Protein	mRNA
IL-1	4 ng/ml	2.66 ± 0.65	8.18	3.46 ± 1.60	n.d.[c]
IL-6	100 U/ml	2.29 ± 0.11	2.74 ± 0.47	1.52 ± 0.06	2.26 ± 0.03
EGF	25 ng/ml	2.30 ± 0.46	2.29 ± 1.00	1.41 ± 0.07	1.40 ± 0.08
TGFβ	5 ng/ml	1.71 ± 0.82	1.40 ± 0.20	n.d.	n.d.
TPA	50 ng/ml	2.31 ± 0.23	4.10 ± 0.15	2.65 ± 0.33	3.66 ± 1.96
E_2	10 nM	2.16 ± 0.36	2.60 ± 0.21	2.43 ± 0.12	2.19 ± 0.16
DHT	100 nM	1.71 ± 0.32	1.14 ± 0.02	1.18 ± 0.28	1.41 ± 0.16
Keoxifene	100 nM	1.48 ± 0.18	1.65 ± 0.33	0.54 ± 0.10	0.48 ± 0.19
Dexamethasone	100 nM	n.d.	2.54 ± 0.68	n.d.	4.83 ± 0.16

[a]The effect of the various effectors on α_1-AT and α_1-ACHY synthesis was accomplished by immunoprecipitation of
^{35}S-labeled cells as described in the text. Steady-state mRNA levels were determined by Northern blot analysis of
cells grown on cells treated in an identical fashion in the absence of [^{35}S]methionine.
[b]Mean ± S.D. for 3–7 separate determinations.

factors, and steroid hormones on α_1-AT and α_1-ACHY synthesis in two MCF-7
cell sublines: the MCF-7 (203P) subline (Table I) which secretes both inhibitors
and the MCF-7 (ML) subline (Table II) which secretes predominantly α_1-ACHY
(Table III). Our primary interest was to determine whether protease inhibitor
synthesis by MCF-7 cells could be stimulated without a general increase in cell
growth. Confluent cells were maintained in charcoal–dextran-treated FBS to
which was added the test substance. After 60 hr, cells were washed and incubated 12 hr longer in media containing the test substances plus [^{35}S]methionine.
Labeled α_1-AT and α_1-ACHY were quantitated and identified as described
above. Steady-state RNA levels were determined by Northern blot analysis on
cells treated in an identical fashion except for the presence of [^{35}S]methionine.
Total RNA was isolated by the guanidinium isothiocyanate method and 20-μg
samples were electrophoresed on 1% agarose/formaldehyde gels. After transfer
to GeneScreen nylon membranes, the RNA was hybridized with ^{32}P-labeled
human α_1-AT and α_1-ACHY cDNA probes (Tamir *et al.,* 1990). After autoradiography, the first probe was washed off and the blot rehybridized with a ^{32}P-
labeled β-actin cDNA probe. Quantitation was accomplished by densitometry
after autoradiography. In preliminary experiments it had been determined that
maximum stimulation of protease inhibitor accumulation occurred after 72 hr.
Although there were some differences in α_1-AT and α_1-ACHY synthesis by
different MCF-7 sublines, IL-1, IL-6, EGF, TGFβ, E_2, dexamethasone, and TPA
were found to stimulate protein synthesis and increase mRNA levels for both
inhibitors two- to fourfold without substantially increasing the incorporation of

Table II. Effect of Growth Factors and Steroid Hormones on α_1-ACHY Synthesis and mRNA Levels in MCF-7 (ML) Cells

		Fold increase over control	
Effector	Concentration	mRNA	Protein
IL-1	4 ng/ml	2.42 ± 0.32	2.27 ± 0.21
IL-6	100 U/ml	2.53 ± 0.19	2.59 ± 0.59
EGF	25 ng/ml	1.94 ± 0.04	2.42 ± 0.29
TGFβ	5 ng/ml	2.61 ± 0.04	1.48 ± 0.17
TPA	50 ng/ml	3.86 ± 1.01	2.97 ± 0.25
E_2	10 nM	3.05 ± 0.34	4.18 ± 0.91
TPA + E_2	50 ng/ml, 10 nM	8.06 ± 0.60	n.d.
DHT	100 nM	2.09 ± 0.07	n.d.
Keoxifene	100 nM	0.60 ± 0.24	n.d.
Retinoic acid	100 nM	n.d.[b]	2.37 ± 0.48
Dexamethasone	100 nM	n.d.	3.99 ± 0.77

[a]Mean ± S.D. for 3–12 separate determinations. Changes in protein and mRNA levels were determined as described in Table I.
[b]n.d., not determined.

[³H]thymidine into DNA. In each instance, steady-state mRNA levels increased by a corresponding amount, suggesting that regulation occurred at the level of transcription although nuclear runoff experiments will have to be performed to show that this is actually the case. It is possible that the addition of any of the above growth factors could stimulate the MCF-7 cells to progress from G_0 to G_1; however, the fact that actin transcription is constant in control cells or cells treated with E_2, TPA, or EGF makes this possibility unlikely.

Table III. Estrogen Receptor Number and Protease Inhibitor Synthesis in MCF-7 Sublines

MCF-7 cell subline	Estrogen receptor[a] (fmole E_2/mg protein)	Protease inhibitor synthesis[b]	
		α_1-AT	α_1-ACHY
203P	133.6 ± 70.7	10.6 ± 4.9	26.1 ± 7.6
300P	(not done)	20.4 ± 7.9	22.1 ± 10.9
ML	36.7 ± 18.8	ND[c]	165.2 ± 109
BK	92.3 ± 4.4	ND	ND

[a]n = 10 experiments, three samples per experiment.
[b]n = 4–5. Determined by immunoprecipitation from spent media of cells grown with [³⁵S]methionine. Values are reported as ³⁵S immunoprecipitated as a percentage of total ³⁵S incorporated into protein × 10^2.
[c]ND, not detected.

It may be noteworthy that the antiestrogen keoxifene inhibited synthesis of α_1-ACHY and decreased its messenger levels in both sublines while stimulating synthesis of α_1-AT in the 203P subline. These results indicate subtle differences in the effects of antiestrogens and perhaps estrogens on the synthesis of the two proteins. Whether this occurs at the transcriptional or posttranslational level is unclear. There is precedence for this paradoxical effect of antiestrogens. Recently it has been reported that tamoxifen, a nonsteroidal estrogen structurally similar to keoxifene (Black et al., 1983), and E_2 have opposite effects on c-jun mRNA levels in avian liver and oviduct (Lau et al., 1991). Differences in the effects of E_2 and keoxifene on the synthesis of α_1-AT and α_1-ACHY could also be due to a direct effect on the conformation of the endoplasmic reticulum as it has been shown that while both E_2 and tamoxifen bind to the endoplasmic reticulum, the complexes formed are not the same (Brown and Sharp, 1990). As described below, preliminary experiments from this laboratory suggest a correlation between decreased synthesis of α_1-AT and α_1-ACHY by MCF-7 cells and tumorigenesis in nude mice. The nature of the specific proteases involved with tumorigenesis inhibited by α_1-ACHY and α_1-AT under these conditions is unknown. It is also unclear whether they are of MCF-7 cell or host origin, and, if they originate in the host, whether similar proteases are found in man.

Treatment of MCF-7 cells with TPA has yielded confusing results: long-term treatment (5 days) appears to inhibit cell proliferation concomitant with a 33% decrease in E_2 receptor number while increasing total protein synthesis twofold (Guilbaud et al., 1988). In our hands, TPA at 50 ng/ml caused an approximately threefold stimulation of the synthesis of both α_1-AT and α_1-ACHY by MCF-7 cells. Stimulation of α_1-ACHY and α_1-AT synthesis by E_2 and TPA was additive which is consistent with the observation that TPA and E_2 modulate transcription by different mechanisms. However, under some conditions E_2 can stimulate c-fos mRNA (Wilding et al., 1988) and TPA can modulate E_2 receptor synthesis (Guilbaud et al., 1988), suggesting that the effects of TPA and E_2 can be linked. Phorbol esters, such as TPA, promote tumorigenesis by potentiating the effect of subthreshold doses of carcinogens (Slaga, 1983) through the persistent stimulation of protein kinase C (Nishizuka, 1984). Stimulation of protein kinase C results in increased transcription of a number of genes responsible for tumorigenesis and metastasis such as the proto-oncogenes c-fos, c-jun, and c-myc (Greenberg and Ziff, 1984; Lau et al., 1991) and the proteases collagenase and stromelysin (Whitham et al., 1986). Phorbol ester-inducible genes have generally been shown to contain a common cis element recognized by the nuclear factor AP-1 (Angle et al., 1987). Various cells have been shown to synthesize proteases in response to exposure to TPA (plasminogen activator, stromelysin) (Montesano and Orci, 1985). The induction of protease inhibitor synthesis by TPA in epithelial cells may be a generalized response to an anticipated increase in protease levels after exposure to TPA or other inflammatory mediators such as IL-1 and IL-6.

3.5. Production of α_1-AT and α_1-ACHY by Various MCF-7 Sublines

Four different MCF-7 sublines were examined for their ability to synthesize α_1-AT and α_1-ACHY in the presence and absence of E_2 (Table III). The 300P subline is a variant of the parent MCF-7 (203P) subline which arose during the course of these studies after approximately 100 passages. Synthesis of both α_1-AT and α_1-ACHY by the 203P and 300P sublines is E_2-mediated. What may be significant is the apparent twofold greater synthesis of α_1-AT by the 300P subline. The ML subline is able to synthesize high levels of α_1-ACHY but little if any α_1-AT (occasionally low levels of α_1-AT synthesis were detected in E_2-stimulated cells). No detectable synthesis of either inhibitor was observed with the BK subline. Results consistent with the above were obtained by Northern blot analysis. Under these conditions, however, low levels of α_1-AT mRNA transcription by the ML subline and of α_1-AT and α_1-ACHY mRNA transcription in the BK subline can be detected. E_2 receptors in the MCF-7 cells (106 cells/sample) were quantitated using a standard dextran-treated charcoal method as described in the methods and materials. The 203P, ML, and BK sublines were all found to contain E_2 receptors (Table III); however, there appears to be no relationship between E_2 receptor number and protease inhibitor synthesis.

4. Perspectives and Conclusions

We have demonstrated the synthesis and secretion of fully active α_1-AT by MCF-7 human breast cancer cells in culture. The α_1-AT in conditioned media was identified immunologically by Western blotting and by complex formation with [125I]trypsin. True synthesis was established by immunoprecipitation from the media of cells grown in the presence of [35S]methionine and by the presence of α_1-AT mRNA determined by Northern blotting with an α_1-AT cDNA probe. As has been shown earlier for α_1-ACHY (Masot *et al.*, 1985), synthesis of α_1-AT is stimulated by E_2. What may be a significant observation is that different MCF-7 cell sublines vary widely in their ability to synthesize and secrete α_1-AT and α_1-ACHY. The ability to synthesize these protease inhibitors does not appear to depend on E_2 receptor number. The relevance of these observations would take on added significance if it could be demonstrated that normal and/or malignant breast tissue synthesize protease inhibitors *in vivo* and if there were differences in the amounts of protease inhibitors synthesized.

It has been estimated that of patients who develop malignant tumors, 50% can be cured by current therapeutic modalities such as drugs, surgery, or radiation (Chamber, 1986). Of the remainder, the majority will die as a result of metastases largely because the widespread initiation of metastatic colonies often occurs before the primary tumor can be detected and treated. This is particularly true for breast cancer where approximately 25% of patients with stage I tumors have already developed metastatic disease at the time of initial diagnosis (Hellman and Harris, 1987). Recent evidence suggests the existence of a highly penetrant dominant allele conferring susceptibility to breast cancer in some families (Newman *et al.*, 1988). If the tumorigenic/metastatic potential of a cancer cell is a function of the amount or ratio of amounts of the protease inhibitors and proteases, then it is possible that parenteral administration of protease inhibitors before the onset of detectable disease could be of some use in these individuals. Pharmacologic stimulation of endogenous protease inhibitor synthesis or reduction in protease levels by the tumor or the surrounding tissues might have a similar effect. At the very least, our studies should provide a new set of biochemical markers that may be of prognostic value in breast cancer.

ACKNOWLEDGMENT. Supported in part by Grant CA02071 from the National Institutes of Health.

5. References

Abraham, C. R., and Potter, H., 1989, The protease inhibitor, α1-antichymotrypsin, is a component of the brain amyloid deposits in normal aging and Alzheimer's disease, *Ann. Med.* **21**:77–81.

Andus, T., Geiger, T., Hirano, T., Kishimoto, T., and Heinrich, P. C., 1988a, Action of human interleukin 6, interleukin 1α and tumor necrosis factor on the mRNA induction of acute-phase proteins, *Eur. J. Immunol.* **18**:739–746.

Andus, T., Geiger, T., Hirano, T., Kishimoto, T., Tran-Thi, T. A., Decker, K., and Heinrich, P. C., 1988b, Regulation of synthesis and secretion of major rat acute-phase proteins by recombinant human interleukin-6 (BSF-2/IL-6) in hepatocyte primary cultures, *Eur. J. Biochem.* **173**:287–293.

Angle, P., Baumann, I., Stein, B., Delius, H., Rahmsdorf, H. J., and Herrlich, P., 1987, 12-o-tetradecanoyl-phorbol-13-acetate (TPA) induction of the human collagenase gene is mediated by an inducible enhancer element located in the 5′-flanking region, *Mol. Cell. Biol.* **7**:2256–2266.

Anklesaria, P., Texido, J., Laiho, M., Pierce, J. H., Greenberger, J. S., and Massague, J., 1990, Cell–cell adhesion mediated by binding of membrane-anchored transforming growth factor α to epidermal growth factor receptors promotes cell proliferation, *Proc. Natl. Acad. Sci. USA* **87**:3289–3293.

Arteaga, C. L., Coronado, E., and Osborne, C. K., 1988, Blockade of the epidermal growth factor receptor inhibits transforming growth α-induced but not estrogen-induced growth of hormone-dependent human breast cancer, *Mol. Endocrinol.* **2**:1064–1069.

Bao, J. J., Sifers, R. N., Kidd, V. J., Ledley, F. D., and Woo, S. L., 1987, Molecular evolution of serpins: Homologous structure of the human alpha 1-antichymotrypsin and alpha 1-antitrypsin genes, *Biochemistry* **26**:7755–7759.

Bates, S. E., Davidson, N. E., Valverius, E. M., Dickson, R. B., Kudlow, J. E., Freter, C., Tam, J. P., Lippmann, M. E., and Salamon, D. S., 1988, Expression of transforming growth factor alpha and its messenger ribonucleic acid in human breast cancer: Its regulation by estrogen and its possible functional significance, *Mol. Endocrinol.* **2**:543–545.

Beatty, K., Robertie, P., Senior, R. M., and Travis, J., 1982. Determination of oxidized alpha-1-proteinase inhibitor in serum, *J. Lab. Clin. Med.* **100**:186–192.

Bergman, D., Kadner, S. S., Chan, Y., Dowling, V., Esterman, A., Young, B. K., and Finlay, T.

H., 1991, Synthesis of α_1-antichymotrypsin and α_1-antitrypsin by human trophoblast cells, Abstract #358, Presented at the 38th Annual Meeting of the Society for Gynecologic Investigation, San Antonio, Tex.

Billings, P. C., St. Clair, W., Ryan, C. A., and Kennedy, A. R., 1987, Inhibition of radiation-induced transformation of C3H/10T1/2 cells by chymotrypsin inhibitor from potatoes, *Carcinogenesis* **8**:809–812.

Black, L. J., Jones, C. D., and Falcone, J. F., 1983, Antagonism of estrogen action with a new benzothiophene derived antiestrogen, *Life Sci.* **32**:1031–1036.

Bories, D., Raynal, M. C., Solomon, D. H., Darzynkiewicz, Z., and Cayre, Y. E., 1989, Down regulation of a serine protease, myeloblastin, causes growth arrest and differentiation of promyelocytic leukemia cells, *Cell* **59**:959–968.

Bringman, T. S., Lindquist, P. B., and Derynck, R., 1987, Different transforming growth factor-α species are derived from a glycosylated and palmitoylated transmembrane precursor, *Cell* **48**:429–440.

Brown, M., and Sharp, P. A., 1990, Human estrogen receptor forms multiple protein–DNA complexes, *J. Biol. Chem.* **265**:11238–11243.

Carlson, J. A., Rogers, B. B., Sifers, R. N., Hawkins, H. K., Finegold, M. J., and Woo, S. L. C., 1988, Multiple tissues express alpha 1-antitrypsin in transgenic mice and man, *J. Clin. Invest.* **82**:26–36.

Castell, J. V., Gomez-Lechon, M. J., David, M., Andus, T., Geiger, T., Trullenque, R., Fabra, R., and Heinrich, P. C., 1989, Interleukin-6 is the major regulator of acute phase protein synthesis in adult human hepatocytes, *FEBS Lett.* **242**:237–239.

Cavanaugh, P. G., Sloane, B. F., and Honn, K. V., 1988, The role of the coagulation system in tumor cell induced platelet aggregation and metastasis, *Hemostasis* **18**:37–46.

Chamber, B. A., 1986, Present status and future prospects for treatment of metastatic cancer, in: *Mechanisms of Cancer Metastasis: Potential Therapeutic Implications* (K. V. Honn, W. E. Powers, and B. F. Sloane, eds.), Nijhoff, The Hague, pp. 15-22.

Clarke, R., Brunner, N., Katz, D., Glanz, P., Dickson, R. B., Lippman, M. E., and Kern, F. G., 1989, The effects of a constitutive expression of transforming growth factor-α on the growth of MCF-7 human breast cancer cells *in vitro* and *in vivo*, *Mol. Endocrinol.* **3**:372–380.

Couritois, G., Morgan, J. G., Campbell, L. A., Fourel, G., and Crabtree, G. R., 1987, Interaction of a liver-specific nuclear factor with the fibrinogen and α_1-antitrypsin promoters, *Science* **238**:688–692.

DeLeon, D. D., Bakker, B., Wilson, D. M., Lamson, G., and Rosenfeld, R. G., 1990, Insulin-like growth factor binding proteins in human breast cancer cells: Relationship to hIGFBP-2 and hIGFBP-3, *J. Clin. Endocrinol. Metab.* **71**:503–532.

Derynck, R., 1988, Transforming growth factor α, *Cell* **54**:593–595.

Dickson, R. B., and Lippman, M. E., 1987, Estrogenic regulation of growth and polypeptide growth factor secretion in human breast carcinoma, *Endocr. Rev.* **8**:29–43.

DiMarco, E., Pierce, J. H., Fleming, T. P., Kraus, M. H., Molloy, C. J., Aaronson, S. A., and DiFiore, P. P., 1989, Autocrine interaction between TGFα and the EGF-receptor: Quantitative requirements for induction of the malignant phenotype, *Oncogene* **4**:831–838.

Duffy, M. J., O'Grady, P., and O'Siorain, 1988, Plasminogen activator. A new marker in breast cancer, in: *Progress in Cancer Research and Therapy 3*, Volume 35 (F. Brescani, R. J. B. King, M. E. Lippman, and D. L. Page, eds.), Raven Press, New York, pp. 300–303.

Finlay, T. H., Katz, J., Rasums, A., Seiler, S., and Levitz, M., 1981, Estrogen-stimulated uptake of α1-protease inhibitor and other plasma proteins by the mouse uterus, *Endocrinology* **108**:2129–2136.

Frain, M., Swart, G., Monaci, P., Nicosia, A., Stampfli, S., Rainer, F., and Cortese, R., 1989, The liver-specific transcription factor LF-B1 contains a highly diverged homeobox DNA binding domain, *Cell* **59**:145–157.

Friedman, M., (ed.), 1986, *Nutritional and Toxicological Significance of Enzyme Inhibitors in Foods*, Plenum Press, New York.

Fuchs, H. E., Michalopouls, G. K., and Pizzo, V. S., 1984, Hepatocyte uptake of α1-proteinase inhibitor–trypsin complexes in vitro: Evidence for a shared uptake mechanism for proteinase complexes of α1-proteinase inhibitor and antithrombin III, *J. Cell Biochem.* **25**:231–243.

Gadek, J. E., Fulmer, J. D., Gelfand, J. A., Frank, M. M., Petty, T. L., and Crystal, R. G., 1980, Danazol-induced augmentation of serum α1-antitrypsin levels in individuals with marked deficiency of this antiprotease, *J. Clin. Invest.* **66**:82–87.

Gasic, G. J., Viner, E. D., Budzynski, A. I., and Gasic, G. P., 1983, Inhibition of lung tumor colonization by leech salivary gland extracts from *Haementeria ghilianni, Cancer Res.* **43**:1633–1636.

Gendler, S. J., and Tokes, Z. A., 1984, Active proteinase inhibitors associated with human breast epithelial cells, *J. Cell Biochem.* **26**:157–167.

Gendler, J., and Tokes, Z. A., 1986, Expression of an active proteinase inhibitor by human breast epithelial cells, *Biochim. Biophys. Acta* **882**:242–253.

Giudice, L. C., Farrell, E. M., Pham, H., Lamson, G., and Rosenfeld, R. G., 1990, Insulin-like growth factor binding proteins in maternal serum throughout gestation and in the puerperium: Effects of a pregnancy-associated serum protease activity, *J. Clin. Endocrinol. Metab.* **71**:806–816.

Graham, K. A., Richardson, C. L., Minden, M. D., Trent, J. M., and Buick, R. N., 1985, Varying degrees of amplification of the N-ras oncogene in the human breast cancer cell line MCF-7, *Cancer Res.* **45**:2201–2205.

Greenberg, M. E., and Ziff, E. B., 1984, Stimulation of 3T3 cells induces transcription on the c-fos proto-oncogene, *Nature* **311**:433–438.

Guilbaud, N., Pichon, M. F., Faye, J. C., Bayard, F., and Valette, A., 1988, Modulation of estrogen receptors by phorbol diesters in human breast MCF-7 cell line, *Mol. Cell. Endocrinol.* **56**:157–163.

Gupta, S. K., Niles, J. L., McCluskey, R. J., and Arnaout, M. A., 1990, Identity of Wegener's autoantigen (p29) with proteinase 3 and myeloblastin, *Blood* **76**:2162.

Hammond, G. L., Smith, C. L., Goping, I. S., Underhill, D. A., Harley, M. J., Reventos, J., Mustos, N. A., Gunalus, G. L., and Bardin, C. W., 1987, Primary structure of human corticosteroid binding globulin, deduced from hepatic and pulmonary cDNAs, exhibits homology with serine protease inhibitors, *Proc. Natl. Acad. Sci. USA* **84**:5153–5157.

Hammond, G. L., Smith, C. L., Paterson, N. A., and Sibbald, W. J., 1990, A role for corticosteroid-binding globulin in delivery of cortisol to activated neutrophils, *J. Clin. Endocrinol. Metab.* **71**:34–39.

Hand, P. H., Nuti, M., Colcher, D., and Schlom, J., 1983, Definition of antigenic heterogeneity and modulation among human mammary carcinoma cell populations using monoclonal antibodies to tumor-associated antigens. *Cancer Res.* **43**:728–735.

Hellman, S., and Harris, J. R., 1987, The appropriate breast cancer paradigm, *Cancer Res.* **47**:339–342.

Huseby, R. A., Maloney, T. M., and McGrath, C. M., 1984, Evidence for a direct growth-stimulating effect of estradiol on human MCF-7 cells in vivo, *Cancer Res.* **44**:2654–2659.

Jenne, D. E., and Tschopp, J., 1989, Granzymes, a family of serine proteases released from granules of cytolytic T lymphocytes upon T cell receptor stimulation, *Immunol. Rev.* **103**:53–71.

Katzenellenbogen, B. S., Norman, M. J., Eckert, R. L., Peltz, S. W., and Mangel, W. F., 1984, Bioactivities, estrogen receptor interactions and plasminogen activator-inducing activities of tamoxifen and hydroxytamoxifen isomers in MCF-7 human breast cancer cells, *Cancer Res.* **44**:112–119.

Lau, C. K., Subramanian, M., Rasmussen, K., and Spelsberg, T. C., 1991, Rapid induction of the *c-jun* protooncogene in the avian oviduct by the antiestrogen tamoxifen, *Proc. Natl. Acad. Sci. USA* **88**:829-833.

Lee, D., Shochat, D., and Gold, D. V., 1982, α1-Proteinase inhibitor production by human adenocarcinomas xenotransplanted into nude mice, *J. Natl. Cancer Inst.* **69**:381-385.

Liberman, J., Mittman, C., and Kent, J. R., 1971, Screening for heterozygous α₁-antitrypsin deficiency with diethylstilbestrol and effect of oral contraceptives, *J. Am. Med. Assoc.* **217**:1198-1206.

Liotta, L. A., Steeg, P. S., and Stetler-Stevenson, W. G., 1991, Cancer metastasis and angiogenesis: An imbalance of positive and negative regulation, *Cell* **64**:327-336.

Masot, O., Buskevitch, P. P., Capony, F., Garcia, M., and Rochefort, M., 1985, Estradiol increases the production of α1-antichymotrypsin in MCF-7 and T47D breast cancer cell lines, *Mol. Cell. Endocrinol.* **42**:207-214.

Massague, J., 1990, Transforming growth factor α: A model for membrane-anchored growth factors, *J. Biol. Chem.* **265**:21393-21396.

Mignatti, P., Robbins, E., and Rifkin, D., 1987, Tumor invasion through the human amniotic membrane: Requirement for a proteinase cascade, *Cell* **47**:487-498.

Montesano, R., and Orci, L., 1985, Tumor-promoting phorbol esters induce angiogenesis in vitro, *Cell* **42**:469-477.

Mornex, J. F., Chytil-Weir, A., Martinet, Y., Courtney, M., LeCocq, J. P., and Crystal, R., 1986, Expression of the α1-antitrypsin gene in mononuclear phagocytes of normal and α1-antitrypsin-deficient individuals, *J. Clin. Invest.* **77**:1952-1961.

Nelson, R. B., and Siman, R., 1990, Clipsin, a chymotrypsin-like protease in rat brain which is irreversibly inhibited by α₁-antifchymotrypsin, *J. Biol. Chem.* **265**:3836-3843.

Newman, B., Austin, M. A., Lee, M., and Kung, M. K., 1988, Inheritance of human breast cancer: Evidence for autosomal dominant transmission in high-risk families, *Proc. Natl. Acad. Sci. USA* **85**:3044-3048.

Nishizuka, Y., 1984, The role of protein kinase C in cell surface signal transduction and tumor promotion, *Nature* **308**:693-698.

Niwa, T., Bradlow, H. L., Fishman, J., and Swaneck, G. E., 1989, Determination of estradiol 2- and 16β-hydroxylase activities in MCF-7 human breast cancer cells in culture using radiometric analysis, *J. Steroid Biochem.* **33**:311-314.

Osborne, C. K., Hobbs, K., and Clark, G. M., 1985, Effect of estrogens and antiestrogens on growth of human breast cancer cells in athymic nude mice, *Cancer Res.* **45**:584-590.

Osborne, C. K., Hobbs, K., and Trent, J. M., 1987, Biological differences among MCF-7 human breast cancer cell lines from different laboratories, *Breast Cancer Res. Treat.* **9**:111-121.

Osborne, C. K., Clemmons, D. R., and Arteaga, C. L., 1990, Regulation of breast cancer growth by insulin-like growth factors, *J. Steroid Biochem. Mol. Biol.* **37**:805-809.

Ostrowski, L. E., Ahsan, A., Suthar, B. P., Bain, D. L., Wong, C., Patel, A., and Schultz, R. M., 1986, Selective inhibition of proteolytic enzymes in an *in vivo* model for experimental metastasis, *Cancer Res.* **46**:4121-4128.

Pandiella, A., and Massague, J., 1991, Multiple signals activate cleavage of the membrane transforming growth factor-α precursor, *J. Biol. Chem.* **266**:5769-5773.

Pemberton, P. A., Stein, P. E., Pepys, M. B., Potter, J. M., and Carrell, R. W., 1988, Hormone binding globulins undergo serpin conformation change in inflammation, *Nature* **336**:257-258.

Perlino, E., Cortese, R., and Ciliberto, G., 1987, The human α1-antitrypsin gene is transcribed from two different promoters in macrophages and hepatocytes, *EMBO J.* **6**:2767-2771.

Perlmutter, D. H., Cole, F. S., Kilbridge, P., Rossing, T. H., and Colten, H. R., 1985, Expression of the α1-proteinase inhibitor gene in human monocytes and macrophages, *Proc. Natl. Acad. Sci. USA* **82**:795-799.

Perlmutter, D. H., Travis, J., and Punsal, P. I., 1988a, Distinct and additive effects of elastase and endotoxin on expression of α1-antiproteinase inhibitor in mononuclear phagocytes, *J. Biol. Chem.* **263**:16499–16503.

Perlmutter, D. H., Travis, J., and Punsal, P. I., 1988b, Elastase regulates synthesis of its inhibitor, α1-proteinase inhibitor, and exaggerates the defect in homozygous piZZ α1 PI deficiency, *J. Clin. Invest.* **81**:1774–1780.

Perlmutter, D. H., Daniels, J. D., Auerbach, H. S., De Schryver, K. K., Winter, H. S., and Alpers, D. H., 1989a, The alpha-1-antitrypsin gene is expressed in a human intestinal epithelial cell line, *J. Biol. Chem.* **264**:9485–9490.

Perlmutter, D. H., May, L. T., and Sehgal, P. B., 1989b, Interferon β2/interleukin 6 modulates synthesis of α1-antitrypsin in human mononuclear phagocytes and in human hepatoma cells, *J. Clin. Invest.* **84**:138–144.

Persky, B., Ostrowski, L. E., Pagast, P., Ahasan, A., Schultz, R. M., 1986, Inhibition of proteolytic enzymes in the in vitro model for basement membrane invasion, *Cancer Res.* **46**:4129–4134.

Ray, M. B., Gebos, K., Callea, F., and Desmet, D. V., 1982, α1-Antitrypsin immunoreactivity in gastric carcinoid, *Histopathology* **6**:289–297.

Rice, W. G., and Weiss, S. J., 1990, Regulation of proteolysis at the neutrophil–substrate interface by secretory leukoprotease inhibitor, *Science* **249**:178–181.

Rosenthal, A., Lindquist, P. B., Bringman, T. S., Goeddel, D. V., and Derynck, R., 1986, Expression in rat fibroblasts of a human transforming growth factor-α cDNA results in transformation, *Cell* **48**:301–309.

Russo, J., Brennan, M. J., and Rich, M. A., 1976, Induction of tumor growth by inoculation of a human breast cancer cell (MCF7) into ovary or pituitary grafted nude mice, *Proc. Am. Assoc. Cancer Res.* **17**:16–19.

Saito, D., Sawamura, M., Umezawa, K., Kanai, Y., Furihata, C., Matsushima, T.,and Sugimura, T., 1980, Inhibition of experimental blood-borne lung metastasis by protease inhibitors, *Cancer Res.* **40**:2539–2542.

Sandgren, E. P., Luetteke, N. C., Palmiter, R. D., Brinster, R. L., and Lee, D. C., 1990, Overexpression of TGFα in transgenic mice: Induction of epithelial hyperplasia, pancreatic metaplasia, and carcinoma of the breast, *Cell* **61**:1121–1135.

Schechter, N. M., Sprows, J. L., Schoenberger, O. L., Lazarus, G. S., Cooperman, B. S., and Rubin, H., 1989, Reaction of human skin chymotrypsin-like proteinase chymase with plasma proteinase inhibitors, *J. Biol. Chem.* **264**:21308–21315.

Schorpp, M., Kugler, W., Wagner, U., and Ryffel, G. U., 1988, Hepatocyte-specific promoter element HP1 of the xenopus albumin gene interacts with transcriptional factors of mammalian hepatocyte, *J. Mol. Biol.* **202**:307–320.

Shin, S. I., 1979, Use of nude mice for tumorigenicity testing and mass propagation, *Methods Enzymol.* **58**:370–379.

Slaga, T. J., 1983, Cellular and molecular mechanisms of tumor promotion, *Cancer Surv.* **2**:595–612.

Soule, H. D., Vasquez, J., Long, A., Albelbert, S., and Brennan, M. A., 1973, Human cell line from a pleural effusion derived from a breast carcinoma, *J. Natl. Cancer Inst.* **51**:1409–1416.

Stein, P. E., Leslie, A. G., Finch, J. T., Turnell, W. G., McLaughlin, P. J., and Carrell, R. W., 1990, Crystal structure of ovalbumin as a model for the reactive centre of serpins, *Nature* **347**:99–102.

Stenman, U. H., Leinonen, J., Alfthan, H., Rannikko, S., Tuhkanen, K., and Alfthan, O., 1991, A complex between prostrate-specific antigen and alpha 1-antichymotrypsin is the major form of prostate-specific antigen in serum of patients with prostatic cancer: Assay of the complex improves clinical sensitivity for cancer, *Cancer Res.* **51**:222–226.

Strous, G. J., van Kerkhof, P., Dekker, J., and Schwartz, A. L., 1988, Metalloendoprotease inhibitors block protein synthesis, intracellular transport, and endocytosis in hepatoma cells, *J. Biol. Chem.* **263**:18197–18204.

Tamir, S., Kadner, S. S., Katz, J., and Finlay, T. H., 1990, Regulation of antitrypsin and anti-chymotrypsin synthesis by MCF-7 breast cancer cell lines, *Endocrinology* **127**:1319–1328.

Teixido, J., Wong, S. T., Lee, D., and Massague, J., 1990, Generation of transforming growth factor-α from the cell surface by an O-glycosylation-independent multistep process, *J. Biol. Chem.* **265**:6410–6415.

Travis, J., and Salvasen, G. S., 1983, Human plasma proteinase inhibitors, *Annu. Rev. Biochem.* **52**:655–709.

Travis, J., Shieh, B. H., and Potempa, J., 1988, The functional role of acute phase plasma proteinase inhibitors, *Tokai J. Exp. Clin. Med.* **13**:313–320.

Troll, W., Frenkel, K., and Wiesner, R., 1984, Protease inhibitors as anticarcinogens, *J. Natl. Cancer Inst.* **73**(6):1245–1250.

Wewers, M. D., Casolaro, M. A., and Crystal, R. G., 1987, Comparison of α1-antitrypsin levels and antineutrophil elastase capacity of blood and lung in a patient with the α1-antitrypsin phenotype null-null before and during α1-antitrypsin augmentation therapy, *Am. Rev. Respir. Dis.* **135**:539–543.

Whitham, S. E., Murphy, G., Angel, P., and Rahmsdorf, H. J., 1986, Comparison of human stromelysin and collagenase by cloning and sequence analysis, *Biochem. J.* **240**:913–916.

Wilding, G., Lippman, M. E., and Gelman, E. P., 1988, Effects of steroid hormones and peptide growth factors on protooncogene c-fos expression in human breast cancer cells, *Cancer Res.* **48**:802–805.

Yagel, S., Khokha, R., Denhardt, D. T., Kerbel, R. S., Parhar, R. S., and Lala, P. K., 1989, Mechanisms of cellular invasiveness: A comparison of amnion invasion in vitro and metastatic behavior in vivo, *J. Natl. Cancer. Inst.* **81**:768–775.

Yavelow, J., Finlay, T. H., Kennedy, A. R., and Troll, W., 1983, Bowman–Birk soybean protease inhibitor as an anticarcinogen, *Cancer Res.* **43**:2454–2459.

Yavelow, J., Collins, M., Birk, Y., and Troll, W., 1985, Nanomolar concentrations of Bowman–Birk soybean protease inhibitor suppress X-ray induced transformation in vitro, *Proc. Natl. Acad. Sci. USA* **82**:5395–5399.

9

Analysis of Structure–Activity Relationships of the Bowman–Birk Inhibitor of Serine Proteinases
Toward a Rational Design of New Cancer Chemopreventive Agents

PETER FLECKER

1. Introduction

Proteinase inhibitors are a class of the various dietary inhibitors of mutagenesis and carcinogenesis (Hayatsu *et al.*, 1988). Schelp and Pongpaew (1988) have recently hypothesized that protection against cancer may result from an increase of endogenous proteinase inhibitors such as α_2-macroglobulin induced by diets that are low in calories and fat. The Bowman–Birk inhibitor (BBI) of serine proteinases, a double-headed polypeptide–inhibitor of trypsin and chymotrypsin, is one of the most potent cancer chemopreventive agents (Yavelow *et al.*, 1983, 1985). Recently, this property has been substantiated in an *in vivo* investigation using mice (St. Clair *et al.*, 1990) that were exposed to dimethylhydrazine, a potent chemical carcinogen. Therefore, BBI is currently being considered as an attractive candidate for studies directed toward the prevention of several forms of cancer that are widespread in Western societies. BBI is a small single-chain polypeptide of 71 amino acids with two subdomains directed toward trypsin and chymotrypsin/elastase, respectively (Fig. 1). This protein is the prototype of a

PETER FLECKER • Institute for Physiological Chemistry, University of Mainz, W-6500 Mainz, Germany.

Protease Inhibitors as Cancer Chemopreventive Agents, edited by Walter Troll and Ann R. Kennedy. Plenum Press, New York, 1993.

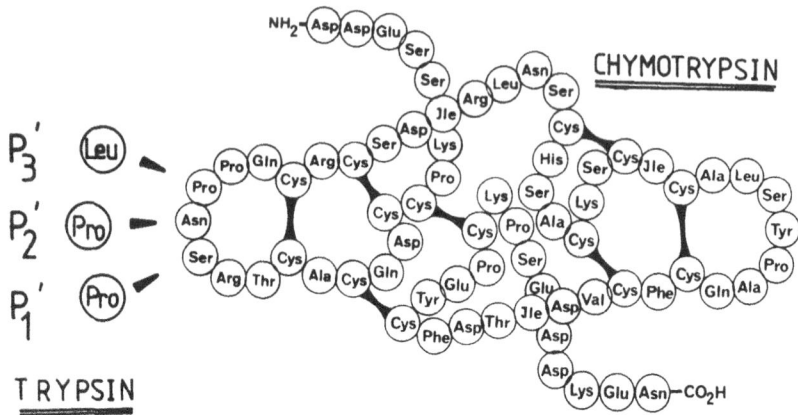

Figure 1. Covalent structure of Bowman–Birk-type proteinase inhibitors (reproduced from Flecker, 1987). The amino acid sequence of the molecule modified at positions 16 and 27 is given. The single amino acid replacements in the trypsin-reactive subdomain are shown.

family of proteinase inhibitors occurring in legumes. The three-dimensional structure of several BBI-type proteinase inhibitors in the free form (Suzuki *et al.*, 1987; Chen *et al.*, 1992) and complexed with trypsin (Tsunogae *et al.*, 1986) were published recently. The structure of BBI in solution has been determined by NMR spectroscopy (Werner and Wemmer, 1991, 1992). The inhibitory subdomains of BBI are rigidified into a polycyclic, clearly arranged and highly conserved structural framework. BBI-type proteinase inhibitors fulfill many of the criteria of an attractive model for protein engineering studies (Fersht, 1985). Presently, major efforts are devoted to the pathophysiological elucidation and pathobiochemical characterization of the role of limited proteolysis in the course of malignant transformation. However, these efforts will eventually culminate in the rational design of specific chemical agents directed toward those proteolytic enzymes that are involved in malignant transformation.

Both the pathobiochemical and pathophysiological research on the one hand and the chemical fields of protein engineering and rational drug design on the other are relatively new disciplines, being in their infancy in many essential respects.

In this account, the state of the art in protein engineering studies on BBI with reference to published material is assessed. The present status of biological research is discussed briefly to draw conclusions on its relation to the fields of protein and chemical drug design in the future.

2. *Biological Aspects*

Considerable progress in the elucidation of the cancer chemopreventive activity of BBI and other proteinase inhibitors was achieved in the last few years.

These efforts were summarized in the meeting report edited by Troll and Kennedy (1989). According to this report a considerable number of proteolytic reactions occurring in carcinogenesis are involved:

1. Several intracellular target proteins of BBI comprising proteolytic activities were isolated by conventional techniques (Billings et al., 1987) and affinity chromatography on BBI–Sepharose (Billings et al., 1988).
2. The occurrence of chymotrypsin-like proteinase at the membrane of fibroblast cells acting as cellular receptors of BBI was reported (Yavelow et al., 1987a,b).
3. Transformation of chick embryo fibroblasts by Rous sarcoma virus is blocked efficiently by a monoclonal antibody directed toward plasminogen activator (results of Dr. Quigley and his colleagues, discussed by Troll and Kennedy, 1989).
4. Proteinase inhibitors are active suppressors of oncogene expression as shown by Dr. Garte in the inhibition of transformation of fibroblasts by the H-ras oncogene. A substantial reduction of the levels of c-myc RNA was reported by Dr. Chang (discussed by Troll and Kennedy, 1989).
5. The destruction of basement membranes in the course of metastasis is also prevented by treatment with respective proteinase inhibitors (results of Dr. Goldfarb, discussed by Troll and Kennedy, 1989). Generally, proteinase inhibitors are assumed to prevent carcinogenesis in the proliferative phase of malignant transformation. The addition of these agents at some later stage is without any protective effect. However, not all proteinase inhibitors are active as chemopreventive agents of cancer.

For instance, the ras p21 oncogene product, displaying partial sequence homology to cystatins, a class of cysteine proteinase inhibitors (reviewed by Barrett et al., 1986), is an effective inhibitor of cathepsins B and L (Hiwasa et al., 1987a,b).

These enzymes may be involved in the lysosomal proteolysis of growth factor receptors in the course of their physiological downregulation on the one hand and regulation of cAMP-dependent type II A protein kinase activity on the other. According to the model of Hiwasa (1988), the inhibition of these physiological reactions might stimulate unlimited cell growth via activation of competence genes that induce biochemical tumor markers themselves as demonstrated in the role of the c-fos protein as a trans activator of collagenase gene expression (Schönthal et al., 1988).

However, no hasty generalizations can be advanced at the present. Increased proteolytic activities closely resembling model reactions with cathepsin L on a dephosphorylated 70-kDa substrate of protein kinase C were detected in the case of ras-transformed fibroblasts. These experiments in E. Racker's group point to some connection between tumor malignancy of cells and cathepsin L (Laumas et al., 1989).

In any case, both beneficial and deleterious proteolytic reactions will have to be considered in the course of work directed toward the development of cancer chemopreventive agents. Deleterious proteinases involved in malignant transformation will have to be inhibited by these agents with maximal specificity.

Any success in this direction will require a firm chemical understanding of the mechanism and the fine specificity of proteinase–inhibitor interactions in submolecular detail. This is the main intention of our work.

3. Prospects of Protein Engineering for the Design of Anticarcinogenic Agents

A complementary approach to biological studies on the mechanism of malignant transformation is chemical tinkering with some active compound on the basis of chemical intuition and perception of structural analogy. The resulting derivatives are subjected to various *in vitro* and *in vivo* testing procedures. This intuitive approach of the medicinal chemist, although tedious, has already led to the discovery of many useful compounds since the early days of chemotherapy (see Witkop, 1981, for a historical commentary). It has provided tremendous impact not only to chemotherapy, but also to the acquisition of models in biology (see Elion, 1989, for a discussion).

Today, such an approach could also be applied to proteins as BBI via site-directed modification of their natural or fully synthetic genes (Engels and Uhlmann, 1989).

Therefore, the unambiguous identification and structural elucidation of the target enzymes of this inhibitor is a major scientific challenge. The rational design of agents for chemoprevention of cancer certainly will profit from such information supplemented by data on the reactivities of these proteinases with synthetic substrates on the one hand and knowledge-based structure prediction methods (Blundell *et al.*, 1988) on the other. Nevertheless, we still might not have enough basic knowledge required for designing agents that interfere in malignant transformation, even if x-ray crystallographic data of all of the target enzymes of anticarcinogenic proteinase inhibitors were available at high resolution (Laskowski and Kato, 1980).

What are the essential structural features of the mode of action and the fine specificity of BBI? In our opinion, these questions cannot be answered on the basis of x-ray crystallographic studies alone. X-ray crystallography does not refer to transition states of enzymatic reactions. Therefore, the analysis should be supplemented with protein engineering studies (Fersht, 1985). However, how can conformational effects in a given mutation be distinguished from functional effects with scrutiny if we consider our ignorance of the protein folding code (Jaenicke, 1987)? This problem is of crucial importance for any clear-cut interpretation of results. Deleterious effects on the stability (Knowles, 1987) and refolding properties (Goldenberg *et al.*, 1989) of a protein in the course of a protein engineering study should always be considered.

How should a complete breakdown of inhibitory activity observed in a mutant proteinase inhibitor be best interpreted? Is it a consequence of a significant perturbation of the three-dimensional structure of the protein or vice versa, due to a lack of some local structural element essential for the activity of the inhibitor? The crucial importance of the selection of a model protein allowing some preliminary test for structural integrity of the mutants, which could be performed quickly with small quantities of material, was taken into account from the beginning of this project.

BBI was selected as a suitable model protein mainly on the basis of this consideration. This protein has two closely aligned trypsin- and chymotrypsin-inhibitory subdomains that are not completely independent of one another in terms of their activities (Odani and Ikenaka, 1978) and spectroscopic properties (Birk et al., 1980). Therefore, one of these domains could be used as an internal standard for the detection of conformational perturbations in the mutants.

4. A New Approach to BBI-Type Proteinase Inhibitors by Synthetic Gene Technology

The author published the first approach to a BBI-type proteinase inhibitor by recombinant DNA techniques some time ago (Flecker, 1987).

The sequence of this protein was modified in two positions in accordance with published sequence homologies in the Bowman–Birk family. A polypeptide sequence devoid of an internal methionine was generated by a $Met^{27} \rightarrow Ile^{27}$ mutation. This manipulation was a chemical prerequisite for the expression as a fusion protein and subsequent cyanogen bromide cleavage at the NH_2-terminal methionine residue.

In addition to that, a $Lys^{16} \rightarrow Arg^{16}$ mutation was introduced to investigate the details of binding of the P_1 side chain of the inhibitor to the amino acids Asp^{189} and Ser^{190} located in the primary specificity pocket of trypsin (see below).

A DNA sequence, coding for the inhibitor, was selected according to the rules for preferential codon usage of proteins expressed at high levels in E. coli. An NH_2-terminal Met codon was introduced for the subsequent cyanogen bromide cleavage. A maximum of singular restriction sites was introduced, to facilitate simple insertion of short oligonucleotide duplexes carrying the desired modifications. The complete synthetic gene coding for the BBI-type proteinase inhibitor is shown in Fig. 2. This sequence was dissected retrosynthetically at the singular SphI site into two subfragments that were assembled from short synthetic oligodeoxyribonucleotides. The synthetic effort required for the redesign of the gene by resynthesis of complete DNA stretches could be kept at a minimum this way. Interested readers are referred to the original publication for further details of the synthetic and cloning procedures (Flecker, 1987). All attempts to express the BBI-type proteinase inhibitor directly in standard systems under

```
EE                   H                         S
CC        N M        I                  N      A D
OO        L B        N                  L      U P
RR        A O        F                  A      3 N
*1        3 2        1                  3      A 1
 /
     AATTCATGGACGACGAATCTTCCAAACCATGTTGCGATCAGTGT
1    --- --- -+------- -+--- ---- +------ --+----- 45
     GTACCTGCTGCTTAGAAGGTTTGGTACAACGCTAGTCACA

     MetAspAspGluSerSerLysProCysCysAspGlnCys


T                         F
T          AMT            N          F
H          FLH            U          O
1          LUA            4          K
2          311            H          1
 /
     GCTTGCACGCGTTCCAACCCGCCGCAGTGCCGTTGCTCTGACATC
46   --- +---------+- ------ +---------+----- -- + 90
     CGAACGTGCGCAAGGTTGGGCGGCGTCACGGCAACGAGACTGTAG

     AlaCysThrArgSerAsnProProGlnCysArgCysSerAspIle


                         N              H F
                         NSS            I NH
                         LPP            N UH
                         AHH            P DA
                         311            1 31
                          //             /
     CGTCTCAACTCTTGCCACTCCGCATGCAAATCTTGTATTTGCGCT
91   - ---- --+---------+- --- ---+--- ----+----- 135
     GCAGAGTTGAGAACGGTGAGGCGTACGTTTAGAACATAAACGCGA

     ArgLeuAsnSerCysHisSerAlaCysLysSerCysIleCysAla


          S                   H
          HBNCD           H   I
          PCCRD           P   N
          ANIFE           H   D
          21111           1   2
           //
     CTGTCTTACCCGGCTCAGTGCTTCTGTGTTGACATCACCGACTTC
136  --- +---------+------ ---+------ - +-------- + 180
     GACAGAATGGGCCGAGTCACGAAGACACAACTGTAGTGGCTGAAG

     LeuSerTyrProAlaGlnCysPheCysValAspIleThrAspPhe


          T                   B        M
          A                   B        B
          Q                   V        O
          2                   2        2

     TGCTACGAACCGTGCAAACCGTCTGAAGACGACAAAGAAAACTAA
181  ---- -----+--- ------+ ------- -+------- -+-- -- 225
     ACGATGCTTGGCACGTTTGGCAGACTTCTGCTGTTTCTTTTGATT

     CysTyrGluProCysLysProSerGluAspAspLysGluAsnEnd


          H
          SAIT
          ACNA
          LCDQ
          1121
           /
     TAAG
226  ----+---- 234
```

Figure 2. The DNA sequence of the synthetic gene coding for the BBI-type proteinase inhibitor. The restriction sites are also shown.

control of the *tac* promoter or in respective secretion systems to any significant level were not successful. No proteinase inhibitory activity or any band in SDS gels at the expected molecular mass of the inhibitor was detectable. This points to a pronounced instability in *E. coli* which is probably the result of rapid digestion of this small polypeptide in the bacterial cells. This is in accord with the observations of other authors who faced similar difficulties in their attempts to express small proteinase inhibitors in *E. coli* directly.

BBI is a protein that is rigidified by many disulfide bridges. Such proteins frequently are not secreted easily, presumably because they are not easily unfolded during the transition through the membrane of the periplasmatic space of *E. coli* (Nilsson *et al.*, 1989).

So far, only a standard fusion protein strategy on a fragment of β-galactosidase has been successful. Respectable quantities of intracellular fusion protein were obtained using this approach (Fig. 3), which can be purified further by simple precipitation procedures (unpublished results in our laboratory). However, the subsequent cyanogen bromide cleavage yielded a complex mixture of proteins containing low levels of trypsin-inhibitory activity. The consideration that the major portion of the material of interest might be distributed into a complex mixture of molecules that are cross-linked via intermolecular disulfide bridges did not render further purification attempts of any value. Instead, the crude cyanogen bromide cleavage product was reduced under denaturing condi-

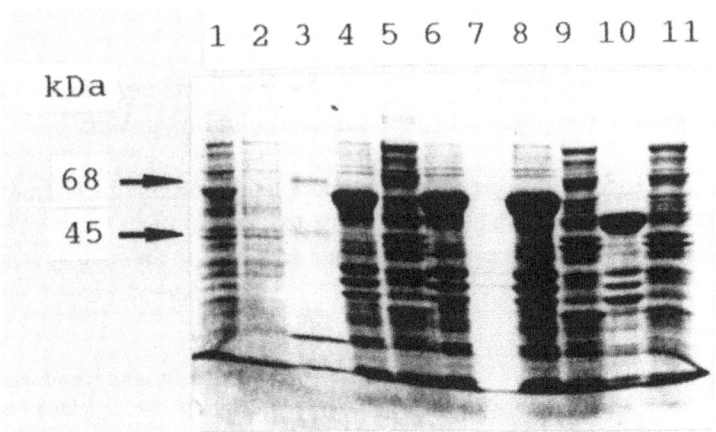

Figure 3. Expression of the parent BBI-type inhibitor as fusion protein with a fragment of β-galactosidase. (1) Total extract of *E. coli* transformed with pLZP WB1/PF17 after and (2) without induction with IPTG. (3) Molecular mass standards at 45 and 68 kDa. (4, 6, 8) Successive Na_2HPO_4 precipitations of fusion protein; (5, 7, 9) corresponding supernatants. (10) Expression of the β-galactosidase fragment in vector pLZP WB1 alone after Na_2HPO_4 precipitation; (11) corresponding supernatant. The increase of the molecular mass of fusion protein in lane 8 relative to lane 10 is apparent. (From Flecker, 1987.)

tions and subjected to subsequent renaturation (Ahmed *et al.*, 1975; Hogle and Liener, 1973). A high dilution of protein during refolding turned out to be of crucial importance to avoiding formation of intermolecular disulfide bridges and obtaining satisfactory yields of active material.

The crude expression product was reported to contain approximately 25% of fusion protein according to densitometric scanning of the gel shown in Fig. 3 (lane 8). From the relative molecular masses of the β-galactosidase fragment (54 kDa) and the inhibitor (8 kDa), a theoretical yield of 1.2 mg based on 32 mg of crude fusion protein is calculated. The 320 μg of active inhibitor obtained after affinity chromatography on trypsin–Sepharose, corresponds to an isolated yield of 27% over three steps of cyanogen bromide cleavage, refolding, and the affinity chromatographic purification. The inhibitor is highly homogeneous as judged by SDS gel electrophoretic and HPLC data (Fig. 4). The inhibitory constant of this material determined by the method of Green and Work (1953) was 2.6×10^{-10} M which is in full agreement with the value of 2.8×10^{-10} M reported by Seidl and Liener (1972) within experimental error.

Obviously, structurally different but energetically equivalent modes of interaction of P_1Lys and the respective Arg residues operate in the primary specificity of trypsin as shown in Fig. 5 (Craik *et al.*, 1985). Expression of the β-galactosidase fragment alone, cyanogen bromide cleavage, and application of the refolding protocol gave no significant trypsin-inhibitory activity. Therefore, the trypsin-inhibitory activity was due to the expressed and refolded inhibitor exclusively.

5. Trypsin–Sepharose as a Matrix with Complementary Structure Is Required for Refolding of Proteinase Inhibitor Variants

On the basis of this preparatory work, studies on site-directed mutagenesis in the trypsin-reactive subdomain were started.

The chymotrypsin-reactive subdomain was used as an internal standard for

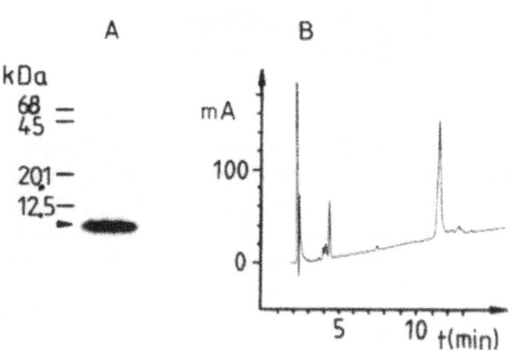

Figure 4. Analysis of the parent inhibitor after refolding and affinity chromatography on trypsin–Sepharose. (A) Gel electrophoretic analysis on a 15% SDS–gel stained with Coomassie blue. A molecular mass of the inhibitor of 8 kDa is confirmed. (B) HPLC analysis of the material after affinity chromatography. The peak eluted at $t = 11.5$ min is the only trypsin-inhibitory material found. (From Flecker, 1987.)

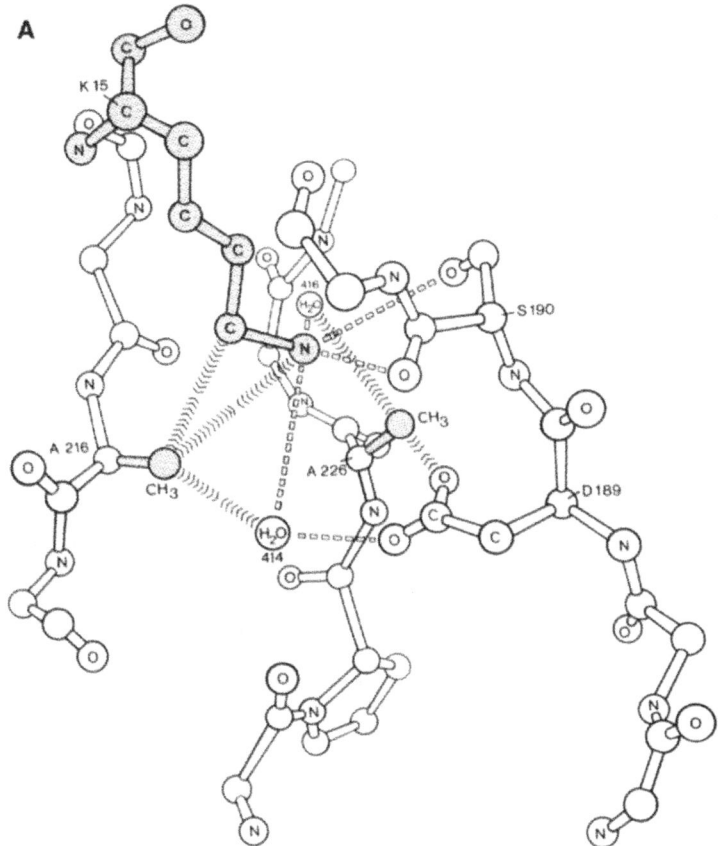

Figure 5. Comparison of binding modes of different ligands in the primary specificity pocket of trypsin. The binding of Lys[15] of pancreatic trypsin inhibitor (A) and benzamidine (B) is a model for the binding modes of the side chain of arginine. Note: a further hydrogen bond between the amino group of Lys and the Ser[190] carbonyl oxygen atom is gained in (A) and lost in (B) resulting in energetic equivalence of binding modes of Lys and Arg in the primary specificity pocket of trypsin. (Reproduced from Craik *et al.*, 1985, with permission. Copyright by the American Association for the Advancement of Science.)

the detection of structural perturbations in the course of these experiments. Here, reference will be given to the following published examples (Flecker, 1989):

$$P_1'\,Ser \rightarrow Pro$$
$$P_2'\,Asn \rightarrow Pro$$
$$P_3'\,Pro \rightarrow Leu$$

to illustrate the importance of detecting and controlling refolding problems in the course of protein engineering studies. These point mutations do not occur in the

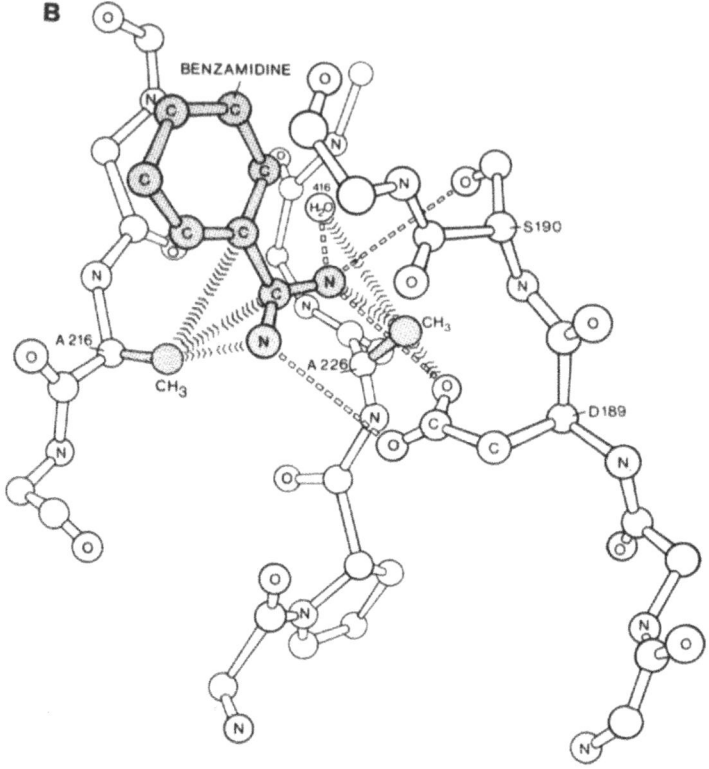

Figure 5. (Continued)

BBI family (see Ikenaka and Norioka, 1986, for a review on the amino acid sequences of BBI-type proteinase inhibitors).

These mutants were constructed in our laboratory recently, to address some questions concerning the mechanism of proteinase inhibitors (Laskowski and Kato, 1980). Their biochemical characterization and kinetic properties will be published elsewhere (Flecker, manuscripts in preparation). The expression, cyanogen bromide cleavage, and the initial refolding experiments were performed in close analogy to the parent protein.

However, the amount of trypsin-reactive material was reduced dramatically in comparison with that of the chymotrypsin-reactive subdomain (Figs. 6–8, cf. a and c). In the case of the P_2'Pro variant, no trypsin-inhibitory activity was detected at all. All attempts at improving the ratio of both subdomains toward the desired stoichiometric ratio of 1:1 by systematic variation of the refolding conditions as the addition of stabilizing Hofmeister salts (Creighton, 1980) and the presence of thioredoxin from *Corynebacterium nephridii* as a method for refolding disulfide-containing proteins (Pigiet and Schuster, 1986) were without benefit. After some time of unsuccessful experimentation, the idea arose to use trypsin as a matrix with complementary structure for the refolding and subse-

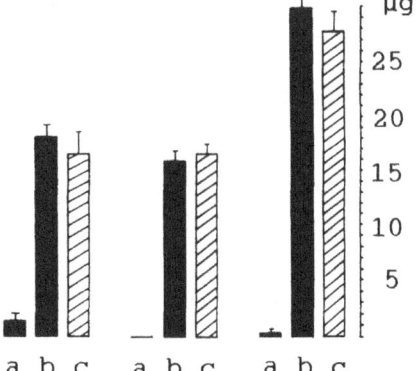

Figures 6–8. Summary of titration experiments in both proteinase inhibitory subdomains of the P_1'Pro (Fig. 6), the P_2'Pro (Fig. 7), and the P_3'Leu (Fig. 8) variants of the Bowman–Birk inhibitor. Amount of (a) trypsin-reactive material after refolding in solution without trypsin–Sepharose (Flecker, 1987); (b) trypsin-reactive material after refolding in the presence of trypsin–Sepharose (Flecker, 1989); (c) the constant amount of chymotrypsin-reactive material obtained in the absence and presence of trypsin–Sepharose. (Reproduced from Flecker, 1989.)

quent affinity purification steps of the variants. The ratio of both proteinase inhibitory subdomains was shifted to the stoichiometric ratio of 1:1 as shown by inspection of bars a–c in Figs. 6–8. Bar a refers to the amount of trypsin obtained by the refolding procedure in the absence of the matrix, b refers to the respective amount of trypsin-reactive subdomain obtained in the presence of trypsin–Sepharose, and c represents the amount of chymotrypsin-reactive subdomain which was constant within experimental error by both refolding procedures.

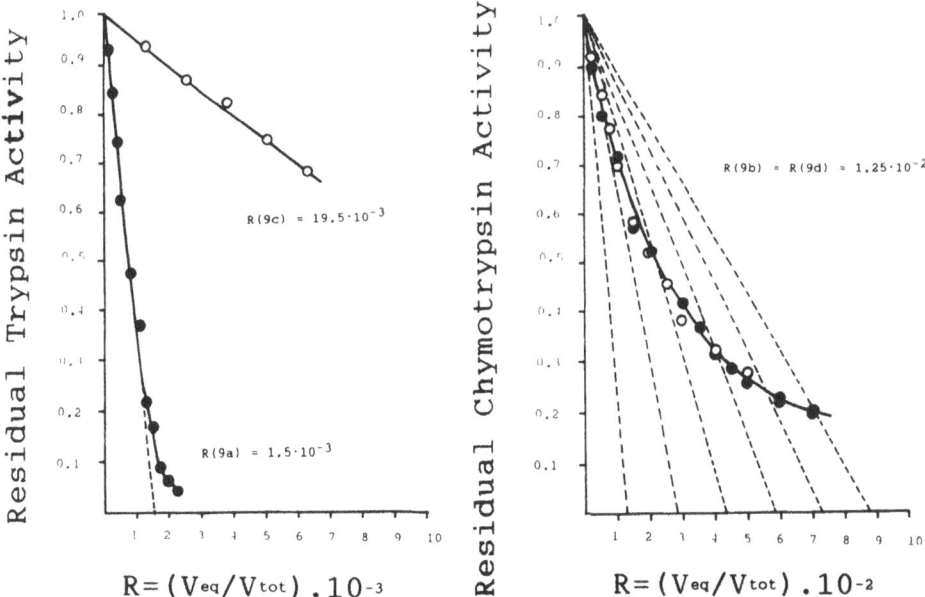

Figure 9. Titration of both subdomains of the P_1'Pro variant of the parent inhibitor. Refolding in the presence of trypsin–Sepharose (●): titration with trypsin (curve a) and chymotrypsin (curve b). Refolding in the absence of trypsin–Sepharose (○): titration with trypsin (curve c) and chymotrypsin (curve d). (Reproduced from Flecker, 1989.)

The analysis is shown in detail by comparing the titration curves of the P_1'Pro variant with trypsin after refolding in the presence (Fig. 9a,b) and absence (Fig. 9c,d) of trypsin–Sepharose. The titration curves with chymotrypsin are superimposable within experimental error. The amount of the internal standard is not affected by the matrix as expected for a point mutation in the trypsin-reactive subdomain. No trypsin- or chymotrypsin-inhibitory activities were found in the combined flow-throughs of the affinity chromatography experiment. This shows that the stoichiometric ratio of 1:1 was not the result of a simple affinity chromatographic step on trypsin–Sepharose. No chymotrypsin-inhibitory activity is detectable in the nonspecific flow-throughs of the affinity chromatographic experiments.

The possibility that minor amounts of trypsin-reactive subdomain were bound and eluted together with chymotrypsin-reactive material can be ruled out unequivocally. Excess chymotrypsin-reactive material should be detected in the nonspecific flow-throughs of the trypsin–Sepharose column in this case.

6. BBI Has Structural Similarity to the COOH-Terminal Part of the B Chain of Laminin

Recently, the author asked Dr. R. F. Doolittle to search his protein sequence bank with regard to BBI. It was hoped that further hypotheses or at least some new aspect on the cancer chemopreventive activity of BBI might emerge from this computer search which could be tested experimentally. As we presently do not have any resources to get involved in these experiments ourselves, we communicate the result to the scientific community in the hope that some other laboratory will pick up the problem.

The COOH-terminal region in the B chain of mouse laminin, which is located at the bottom of the cross-shaped structure of this molecule, was the only protein in his sequence bank that displayed any resemblance to BBI as shown in Fig. 10.

However, the structural analogies between both proteins are mainly restricted to the distribution of the cysteine residues although there is no strict match in the distribution of cysteine residues in both molecules. Nevertheless, the similarities are much greater than would be expected by chance (Dr. Doolittle, personal communication). Laminin is presently considered (see Engel, 1989, for a review) as a growth-stimulating molecule involved in the control of differentiation of various cell types. It was shown to increase the metastatic ability of tumor cells (Terranova et al., 1984). The growth-promoting activity of laminin as a large structural protein allows "more localized and regulated action in comparison to small, more diffusible growth factors" (Engel, 1989).

The increased amount of laminin on the surface of malignant cells is a well-established observation which was correlated to tumor growth and invasiveness (see Iwamoto et al., 1987, and references cited therein).

D D E S S K P C C D Q C A C   T K S N P P Q C   R C S D M R
L S S V C D P N G G Q C Q C R P N V V G R T C N R C A P G T

L N S C H S A C K S C I C A L S Y P A Q C F C V D I T D
F G F G P N G C K P C D C H L Q G S A S A F C D A I T G Q C

F C Y E P C K P S E D D K E N
H C F Q G I Y A R Q C D R C L

Figure 10. Amino acid sequence alignment of the Bowman–Birk inhibitor (upper line) and amino acids No. 829–903 in the B_1 chain of laminin of the mouse (lower line). Identical amino acids are framed.

Beyond the particular case of laminin, the occurrence of many disulfide bridges in peptide and protein growth factors has been noted in the literature. The structural motif of a "trefoil" disulfide loop in breast cancer-associated peptide (pS2), pancreatic spasmolytic polypeptide (PSP), and the spasmolysins is just one of the many examples presently being discussed in the literature (Thim, 1989). The structural analogies between the family of BBI-type proteinase inhibitors on the one hand and growth factors on the other point to the idea that BBI not only prevents proteolytic reactions, but could also interfere with the deregulation of growth factor receptors in the course of malignant transformation. Of course, this tentative proposal remains to be tested experimentally at the biochemical level.

7. Conclusions

We have published the first approach to a BBI-type proteinase inhibitor via genetic engineering (Flecker, 1987). Despite previous reports on cDNA and genomic clones coding for this protein (Hammond *et al.*, 1984), the stage was not set for production of this inhibitor via genetic techniques due to serious refolding problems faced in this molecule containing seven disulfide bridges in a single chain of 71 amino acids. Clinical tests on BBI will critically depend on the production of larger quantities of correctly refolded and highly purified protein. Preparations from natural sources are contaminated by agglutinins (Fritz, 1980). This problem should not appear with material expressed in *E. coli*.

My recent paper (Flecker, 1989) describing the refolding protocol in the presence of trypsin–Sepharose is the first description of a refolding technique for mutant proteinase inhibitors on a matrix with complementary structure.

Our initial reservations (Flecker, 1987) toward interpreting activities of mutant proteins without any control regarding conformational integrity are most clearly confirmed by the P_2'Pro variant. This material is devoid of trypsin-inhibitory activity on refolding in the absence of the matrix, but a very active inhibitor of trypsin after refolding in its presence.

Any statement that the "natural" amino acids in the $P_1'-P_3'$ stretch of the BBI family were "required for activity" would not really be accurate. Instead, deleterious effects on the refolding properties of our mutants occur, which can be bypassed by the trypsin–Sepharose technique.

Now, the platform is set for studies on the structure–activity relationship of BBI via site-directed mutagenesis. Presently, we are confined to inhibition studies on target proteinases with known three-dimensional structure such as trypsin and chymotrypsin. We have 15 variants of BBI in our hands. Some of these variants have been designed as more potent inhibitors of standard serine proteinases than the parent BBI-type proteinase inhibitor by simple chemical considerations. Of course, as long as the structure of the proteinases involved in malignant transformation and other receptors of BBI remain unknown, we may not have reached solid ground for attempting any rational design of anticarcinogenic proteinase inhibitors. Clearly, more biochemical data on the cleavage specificities of these proteinases are required.

Nevertheless, the physical and chemical principles governing specificity and catalysis are very likely the same or very similar in all serine proteinases and the interactions with their corresponding inhibitors. Therefore, preliminary studies on model proteinases with known three-dimensional structure could become an important preliminary step in the direction of designing anticarcinogenic agents with improved properties in the future. A firm identification of the structural elements of BBI that are essential for the activity of this molecule should become important in the course of designing synthetic proteinase inhibitors of lower molecule weight. Such agents are expected to have superior properties with respect to drug targeting and delivery.

Hopefully, new strategies for the chemoprevention and more gentle approaches to a chemotherapy of cancer will eventually result.

ACKNOWLEDGMENTS. I thank the National Cancer Institute of the U.S.A. for its hospitality. Travel expenses were covered by Birch & Davis Associates, Inc., which is gratefully acknowledged. I am grateful to Professor R. F. Doolittle for his friendly help in the course of a computer search. Our work is supported by the Deutsche Forschungsgemeinschaft.

8. References

Ahmed, A. K., Schaffer, S. W., and Wettlaufer, C. B., 1975, *J. Biol. Chem.* **250**:8477–8482.
Barrett, A. J., Rawlings, N. D., Davies, M. E., Machleidt, G., Salvesen, G., and Turk, V., 1986, in: *Proteinase Inhibitors* (A. J. Barrett and G. Salvesen, eds.), Elsevier, Amsterdam, pp. 515–587.

Billings, P. C., Carew, J. A., Keller-McGandy, C., Goldberg, A. L., and Kennedy, A. R., 1987, *Proc. Natl. Acad. Sci. USA* **84**:4801–4805.

Billings, P. C., St. Clair, W., Owen, A. J., and Kennedy, A. R., 1988, *Cancer Res.* **48**:1798–1802.

Birk, Y., Jibson, M. D., and Bewley, T. A., 1980, *Int. J. Peptide Protein Res.* **15**:193–199.

Blundell, T., Carney, D., Gardner, S., Hayes, F., Howlin, B., Hubbard, T., Overington, J., Singh, D. A., Sibanda, B. L., and Sutcliffe, M., 1988, *Eur. J. Biochem.* **172**:513–520.

Chen, P., Rose, J., Love, R., Wei, C. H., and Wang, B. C., 1992, *J. Biol. Chem.* **267**:1990–1994.

Craik, C. S., Largman, C., Fletcher, T., Roczniak, S., Barr, P. J., Fletterick, P., and Rutter, W. J., 1985, *Science* **228**:291–297.

Creighton, T. E., 1980, *J. Mol. Biol.* **144**:521–550.

Elion, G. B., 1989, *Science* **244**:41–47.

Engel, J., 1989, *FEBS Lett.* **251**:1–7.

Engels, J. W., and Uhlmann, E., 1989, *Agnew. Chem.* **101**:733–752.

Fersht, A., 1985, *Enzyme Structure and Mechanism*, Freeman, San Francisco.

Flecker, P., 1987, *Eur. J. Biochem.* **166**:151–156.

Flecker, P., 1989, *FEBS Lett.* **252**:153–157.

Fritz, H., 1980, *Ciba Found. Symp.* **75**:351–379.

Goldenberg, D. P., Frieden, R. W., Haack, J. A., and Morrison, T. B., 1989, *Nature* **338**:127–132.

Green, N. M. and Work, E., 1953, *Biochem. J.* **54**:347–352.

Hammond, R. W., Foard, D. E., and Larkins, B. A., 1984, *J. Biol. Chem.* **259**:9883–9890.

Hayatsu, H., Arimoto, S., and Negishi, T., 1988, *Mutat. Res.* **202**:429–446.

Hiwasa, T., 1988, *Biol. Chem. Hoppe-Seyler* **369**(Suppl.):239–241.

Hiwasa, T., Sakiyama, S., Noguchi, S., Ha, J. M., Miyazawa, T., and Yokoyama, S., 1987a, *Biochem. Biophys. Res. Commun.* **146**:731–738.

Hiwasa, T., Yokoyama, S., Ha, J. M., Noguchi, S., and Sakiyama, S., 1987b, *FEBS Lett.* **211**:23–26.

Hogle, J. M., and Liener, I. E., 1973, *Can. J. Biochem.* **51**:1014–1020.

Ikenaka, T. and Norioka, S., 1986, in: *Prokeinase Inhibitors* (A. J. Barrett and G. Salvesen, eds.) Elsevier, Amsterdam, pp. 301–474.

Ikenaka, T., and Norioka, S., 1983, in: *Proteinase Inhibitors: Medical and Biological Aspects* (N. Katunuma, H. Umezawa, and H. Holzer, eds.), Jpn. Sci. Soc. Press, Tokyo/Springer-Verlag, Berlin, pp. 45–53.

Iwamoto, Y., Robey, F. A., Graf, J., Sasaki, M., Kleinman, H. K., Yamada, Y., and Martin, G. R., 1987, *Science* **238**:1132–1134.

Jaenicke, R., 1987, *Prog. Biophys. Mol. Biol.* **49**:117–237.

Knowles, J. R., 1987, *Science* **236**:1252–1258.

Laskowski, M., Jr., and Kato, I., 1980, *Annu. Rev. Biochem.* **49**:593–626.

Laumas, S., Abdel-Ghany, M., Leister, K., Resnick, R., Kandrach, A., and Racker, E., 1989, *Proc. Natl. Acad. Sci. USA* **86**:3021–3025.

Nilsson, B., Bermann-Marks, C., Hober, S., and Anderson, S., 1989, Anniversary Congress of the University of Groningen, "Prospects in Protein Engineering," Poster Abstract No. 040.

Odani, S., and Ikenaka, T., 1978, *J. Biochem.* **83**:747–753.

Pigiet, V. P., and Schuster, B. J., 1986, *Proc. Natl. Acad. Sci. USA* **83**:7643–7647.

St. Clair, W. H., Billings, P. C., Carew, J. A., Keller-McGandy, C., Newberne, P., and Kennedy, A. R., 1990, *Cancer Res.* **50**:580–586.

Schelp, F. P., and Pongpaew, P., 1988, *Int. J. Epidemiol.* **17**:287–292.

Schönthal, A., Herrlich, P., Rahmsdorf, H. J., and Ponta, H., 1988, *Cell* **54**:325–334.

Seidl, D. S. and Liener, I. E., 1972, *J. Biol. Chem.* **247**:3533–3538.

Suzuki, A., Tsunogae, Y., Tanaka, I., Yamane, T., Ashida, T., Norioka, S., Hara, S., and Ikenaka, T., 1987, *J. Biochem.* **101**:267–274.

Terranova, V. P., Williams, J. E., Liotta, L. A., and Martin, G. R., 1984, *Science* **226**:982–985.

Thim, L., 1989, *FEBS Lett.* **250**:85–90.

Troll, W., and Kennedy, A. R., (eds.), 1989, *Cancer Res.* **49**:499–502.

Tsunogae, Y., Tanaka, I., Yamane, T., Kikkawa, J., Ashida, T., Ishikawa, C., Wanatabe, K., Nakamura, S., and Takahashi, K., 1986, *J. Biochem.* **100**:1637–1646.

Werner, M. H., and Wemmer, D. E., 1991, *Biochemistry* **30**:3356–3364.

Werner, M. H., and Wemmer, D. E., 1992, *Biochemistry* **31**:999–1010.

Witkop, B., 1981, *Naturwiss. Rundsch.* **34**(9):361–379.

Yavelow, J., Finlay, T. H., Kennedy, A. R., and Troll, W., 1983, *Cancer Res.* (Suppl.) **43**:2454s–2459s.

Yavelow, J., Collins, M., Birk, Y., Troll, W., and Kennedy, A. R., 1985, *Proc. Natl. Acad. Sci. USA* **82**:5395–5399.

Yavelow, J., Caggana, M., and Beck, K. A., 1987a, *Cancer Res.* **47**:1598–1601.

Yavelow, J., Scott, C. B., and Mayer, T. A., 1987, *Cancer Res.* **47**:1602–1607.

10

Prevention of Cancer by Vitamin B_3 (Nicotinamide and Nicotinic Acid)
A Protease Inhibitor Available in Pure Form

WALTER TROLL

1. Introduction

Protease inhibitors (PIs) occur widely throughout plant and animal systems. Their role in preventing diseases in animals includes controlling blood clotting and contributing to the prevention of cancer. A workshop organized by the National Cancer Institute on "Protease Inhibitors as Cancer Chemopreventive Agents" concluded with the following recommendations for future research: (1) research and development of sources of PIs, (2) analysis of human foods for PI content, (3) evaluation of cancer incidence data in relation to PI content and characteristics in the diet of human populations, (4) animal studies on the efficacy of PIs in cancer prevention, and (5) studies on the mechanism of action of anticarcinogenic PIs (Troll et al., 1987).

One difficulty in carrying out these studies is the availability of sufficient quantities of pure PIs that can be used in animal experiments to determine the mechanism of their chemopreventive action. The discovery that nicotinamide is an inhibitor of two characteristic proteases, chymotrypsin and trypsin, offers new opportunities to study these actions (Troll et al., 1987, 1990). Nicotinamide and nicotinic acid (NA) have been identified as vitamin B_3, the principal vitamin necessary to prevent pellagra and esophageal cancer. This essential nutrient is a precursor of the coenzyme nicotinamide adenine dinucleotide (NAD^+). NAD^+ is

WALTER TROLL • Department of Environmental Medicine, New York University Medical Center, New York, New York 10016.

Protease Inhibitors as Cancer Chemopreventive Agents, edited by Walter Troll and Ann R. Kennedy. Plenum Press, New York, 1993.

an important component for oxyradical modulation and DNA repair. Nico-tinamide is hydrolyzed by proteases to ammonia plus NA. Nicotinamide, NA, and the related aromatic amides have been shown to have striking indications of possessing anticarcinogenic properties. It has been demonstrated that they are involved in deletion of oncogenes in NIH-3T3 cells (Nishizuka, 1984), and suppression of ornithine decarboxylase (Sakamoto et al., 1987), tumor promo-tion, and oxygen radical induction (Troll et al., 1987, 1990, 1992). Since NA and nicotinamide are vitamins, they offer an opportunity for human epidem-iological studies investigating the relationship between their consumption and the occurrence of cancer.

2. Dietary PIs Suppress Cancer

The "Western" diet, which consists of a high proportion of meat and a relatively low proportion of vegetables, appears to be responsible for a higher rate of breast, colon, and prostatic cancers. In contrast, diets rich in rice, maize, and beans lower the incidence of these cancers. Since seeds contain high concen-trations of PIs, they may limit the occurrence of these cancers in humans (Wyn-der et al., 1971; Armstrong and Doll, 1975; Carroll, 1975; Phillips, 1975; Correa, 1981). The initial clue for this possibility was discovered when the synthetic PIs trypsin or chymotrypsin were applied to mouse skin and shown to interfere with tumor promotion in two-stage carcinogenesis when promoted with 12-O-tetradecanoyl-phorbol-13-acetate (TPA) (Troll et al., 1970). Fur-ther observations demonstrated that tumor development was suppressed by feed-ing PIs. ϵ-Amino-caproic acid, an inhibitor of plasminogen activator, blocks dimethylhydrazine-induced colon cancer when added to the drinking water of mice (Corasanti et al., 1982). Diets containing soybean PIs reduce the appear-ance of tumors in mouse skin treated with 4-nitroquinoline-N-oxide and TPA (Troll et al., 1979), breast tumors in Sprague–Dawley rats subjected to ionizing radiation (Troll et al., 1980), spontaneous liver cancer in C3H mice (Becker, 1981), and colon cancer in mice (Weed et al., 1985). The possible mechanisms of this anticarcinogenesis may include interference with oxyradical formation by neutrophils, suppression of oncogene expression, and interference with adeno-sine diphosphate ribosyltransferase.

3. Interference with Oxyradical Formation

Tumor promoters, including the phorbol esters teleocidin and aplysiatoxin, induce a respiratory burst in polymorphonuclear leukocytes (PMNs), which re-sults in the formation of superoxide anion radicals ($\cdot O_2^-$), hydrogen peroxide (H_2O_2), hydroxyl radicals, and singlet oxygen (Hozumi et al., 1972; Badwey and

Table I. Inhibition of Radioactive Casein Digestion
by Trypsin/Chymotrypsin

Inhibitor	Concentration of inhibitor (mM)	Inhibition (%)	
		Chymotrypsin[a]	Trypsin[a]
Nicotinamide	10	7	6
	20	22	12
	40	53	14
	60	52	40
Benzamide	10	57	24
	20	64	37
	40	76	44
	60	88	64
3-Aminobenzamide	10	34	6
	20	50	27
	40	69	31
	60	72	40

[a]Twenty nanograms chymotrypsin or trypsin per assay.

Karnovsky, 1980; Fantone and Ward, 1982; Formisano *et al*, 1983; Kinzel *et al.*, 1986; Narisawa *et al.*, 1989). Phorbol derivatives that are inactive as tumor promoters (i.e., phorbol, phorbol diacetate, and 4-*O*-methyl-TPA) fail to elicit production of $\cdot O_2^-$ and H_2O_2 by PMNs (Frenkel and Chrzan, 1987; Frenkel *et al.*, 1987). PIs have been shown to suppress the formation of oxyradicals and H_2O_2 in human neutrophils treated with tumor promoters. In an extensive study by Frenkel and co-workers (Frenkel *et al.*, 1987; and this chapter), the PIs that interfered with chymotrypsin were identified as the primary agents responsible for this effect.

Nicotinamide, benzamide, and aminobenzamide preferentially inhibit chymotrypsin (Table I) and suppress the induction of $\cdot O_2^-$ by TPA-treated neutrophils, as shown by measuring cytochrome reduction (Table II) (Troll *et al.*, 1987, 1990). Oxygen radicals, H_2O_2, and organic peroxide have been identified as being contributors to tumor promotion (Slaga *et al.*, 1981).

Table II. Suppression of $\cdot O_2$ Formation
in TPA-Treated Human Neutrophils

Concentration of inhibitor	Inhibition (%)		
	Nicotinamide	Benzamide	3-Aminobenzamide
2 mM	18	23	15
5 mM	23	34	48
10 mM	35	84	73

Wattenberg (1985) first identified the existence of chemopreventive agents that interfere with carcinogenesis by demonstrating the activation of a procarcinogen to a carcinogen by the P_{450} oxidative enzymes. He showed that oxidation contributes to the formation of active initiating carcinogens. Interestingly, all of the more recently observed chemopreventive agents, including PIs, nicotinamide, vitamin A, retinoids, and sarcophytol A, interfere with oxidation by suppressing oxyradicals and H_2O_2 induction by promoting carcinogens.

Another possible mechanism is the modification of genetic materials, which leads to oncogene activation. Promotion modified the DNA bases resulting from oxyradical production by the action of TPA on neutrophils (Frenkel and Chrzan, 1987; Frenkel et al., 1987). This may lead to the activation of oncogenes (Garte et al., 1987; Cox et al., 1991). The contribution of oncogenes to promotion was demonstrated by Balmain, who showed in mouse skin that transfection by oncogenes mimicked promotion (Quintanilla et al., 1986). Oncogene expression is suppressed by chemopreventive agents (e.g., ras oncogene transformation of NIH-3T3 cells is suppressed by PIs, retinoids, sarcophytol A, and tamoxifen). The suppression of oncogene-induced transformation serves as a useful method for measuring and identifying these anticarcinogenic agents, and may present another important mechanism of chemoprevention.

4. Suppression of Transformation-Caused Oncogene Transfection

Nicotinamide, NA, and other inhibitors of poly adenosine diphosphate ribose [poly(ADP)ribose] polymerase were shown to cause a loss of exogenously supplied H-ras genes from NIH-3T3 cells with suppression of oncogene expression. The same mechanism may be responsible for the repression of H-ras oncogene expression in many other PIs. Garte et al. (1987) demonstrated that H-ras oncogene-induced transformation can be inhibited by leupeptin, antipain, ε-aminocaproic acid, and α_1-antitrypsin. Antipain, a low-molecular-weight PI that may be used to determine the effect that time of addition has on repressing H-ras oncogenes, surprisingly was only effective when added 3 days after transfection with ras DNA. Inhibition of cell transformation occurred only when antipain was added to NIH-3T3 cells 3 to 9 days after transfection with ras, demonstrating that it interferes with the late stage of oncogene expression. A specific time-related role for the c-myc oncogene in the growth of radiation-induced rat tumors was recently demonstrated by Garte et al. (1990), who showed that myc's participation in tumor growth was associated with the late stage of promotion or progression. This and the demonstrations by Billings et al. (1986) and Chang et al. (1985) that myc-oncogene expression is suppressed by the Bowman–Birk inhibitor (BBI) in 10T½ cells suggest a general suppression of selected oncogenes by PIs. Further support resulted from the demonstration that addition of 3-aminobenzamide suppressed transformation of NIH-3T3 cells by the H-ras, v-raf, and v-mos oncogenes when it was added 3 to 9 days after transfection (Diamond *et al.*, 1989). An oncogene that is similar to H-*ras* in causing transformation of NIH-3T3 cells was demonstrated in human coronary artery plaques (Penn *et al.*, 1986). The action of NA in suppressing arteriosclerosis in humans may be due to deletion of this oncogene (Nishizuka, 1984; Troll *et al.*, 1990). The amide inhibitors also mimic the effects of other PIs in preventing differentiation of *Arbacia punctulata* to plutei, which is stimulated by transfection with the H-*ras* oncogene (Davidson *et al.*, 1986; Troll and Corcoran, 1989).

5. Suppression of Carcinogenesis

5.1. Suppression of Two-Stage Carcinogenesis by Applying PIs to Mouse Skin

Two-stage carcinogenesis in mouse skin can be considered a working model for describing the processes necessary for tumor formation. Two distinct biological processes of chemical tumorigenesis were identified in mouse skin: (1) initiation caused by a single application of a subcarcinogenic dose of a variety of carcinogens, including 7,12-dimethylbenz(*a*)anthracene (DMBA) or nitroquinoline-*N*-oxide, and (2) promotion caused by multiple applications of the tumor promoters TPA, teleocidin, aplysiatoxin, and by other inflammatory agents or hormones. Initiation is thought to be due to a somatic mutation expressed perhaps by activating the H-*ras* oncogene. A single application lasts for the lifetime of the animal. The action of tumor promoters differs from initiation in that it is biologically reversible and is influenced by environmental factors including nutrition. Tumor promoters cause induction of enzymes, including proteases and protein kinase C. The contribution of proteases to promotion was supported by the demonstration that inhibitors of trypsin [tosyl-L-lysine chloromethyl ketone (TLCK)] or chymotrypsin [tosylphenylalanine chloromethyl ketone (TPCK)] were shown to suppress promotion when painted on mouse skin. These compounds inhibit trypsin or chymotrypsin by forming a covalent adduct with histidine in the active site of the protease. When these inhibitors or the competitive substrate for trypsin, tosylarginine methyl ester (TAME), were painted on mouse skin, significant inhibition of tumor promotion was observed (Table III; Troll *et al.*, 1970). In addition to these PIs, the inhibitors naturally elaborated by streptomycetes (leupeptin, antipain, and other PIs) suppressed promotion (Hozumi *et al.*, 1972; Umezawa *et al.*, this volume). Retinoids and sarcophytol A were also initially identified as anticarcinogenes by two-stage carcinogenesis studies (Fujiki *et al.*, 1989).

5.2. Suppression of Two-Stage Carcinogenesis and Breast Cancer in Rodents by Feeding Soybean Diets

A raw soybean diet, containing a 2.21% Kunitz equivalent, suppressed two-stage carcinogenesis in mice and irradiation-induced breast cancer in rats. In

Table III. Inhibition of Tumorigenesis by Protease Inhibitors[a]

Weeks on promotion	Inhibitor treatment							
	Control		TPCK		TLCK		TAME	
	T	S	T	S	T	S	T	S
10	8	19	0	21	0	21	0	21
12	10	19	0	21	0	21	0	21
14	11	19	0	21	1	21	3	21
16	11	19	0	21	4	21	5	21
18	11	19	0	21	4	21	5	21
20	11	19	0	21	4	21	5	21
22	11	19	0	21	5	21	5	21
24	11	19	1	21	5	21	5	21
30	11	19	1	21	5	21	5	21

[a]All animals were given 10 μg of DMBA as initiator and then 5.0 μg of croton oil in acetone, applied three times weekly as promoter. The protease inhibitors TLCK, TPCK, and TAME were applied in DMSO three times weekly in 1.0-μg doses, 1 to 2 hr after applications of croton oil. All treatments were applied to ear skin of mice (the controls received DMSO alone). The average times of appearance of tumors in all three experimental groups are significantly different from the controls at $p < 0.005$. T indicates the number of tumor-bearing mice; S indicates the number of survivors.

these experiments, carcinogenesis in two animal models was studied by feeding the following PI-containing diets which showed suppression of tumor formation. Four diets were employed: (1) A raw soybean diet, containing 50% soybeans, 8% corn oil, 36% dextrose, and a 6% vitamin salt mix. (2) A casein diet, containing 32% casein, 26% corn oil, 36% dextrose, and a 6% vitamin salt mix. The higher content of corn oil in the casein diet was used to compensate for the measured fat content of soybeans, thus keeping the fat, protein and carbohydrate contents identical in these diets. (3) A heated soybean diet (200°C, 6 hr). (4) Purina rat chow. The content of trypsin inhibitor in these diets was determined by measuring the inhibition of 5 μg trypsin using benzoyl arginine-*p*-nitroanilide as the substrate (Troll *et al.*, 1979, 1980). Using purified Kunitz soybean trypsin inhibitor as a standard, the apparent concentration of trypsin inhibitor in the diets was as follows: raw soybean (2.21%; Purina rat chow, 0.78%; casein, 0.17%; and heated soybean, 0.10%).

The two-stage carcinogenesis study in ICR Swiss–Millerton mice was carried out by applying 200 μg of nitroquinoline-*N*-oxide percutaneously once to the shaved skin and followed 3 days later by applying 5 μg of TPA three times a week. The diets—raw soybean, roasted soybean, and casein—were started 2 weeks before initiation. The 20 mice on the raw soybean (high PI content) diet showed a significant delay of onset of tumor formation when compared with those on the casein or roasted soybean diet with low PI content (Fig. 1). These results are similar to those obtained when PIs were directly applied to mouse skin as previously reported (Troll *et al.*, 1970).

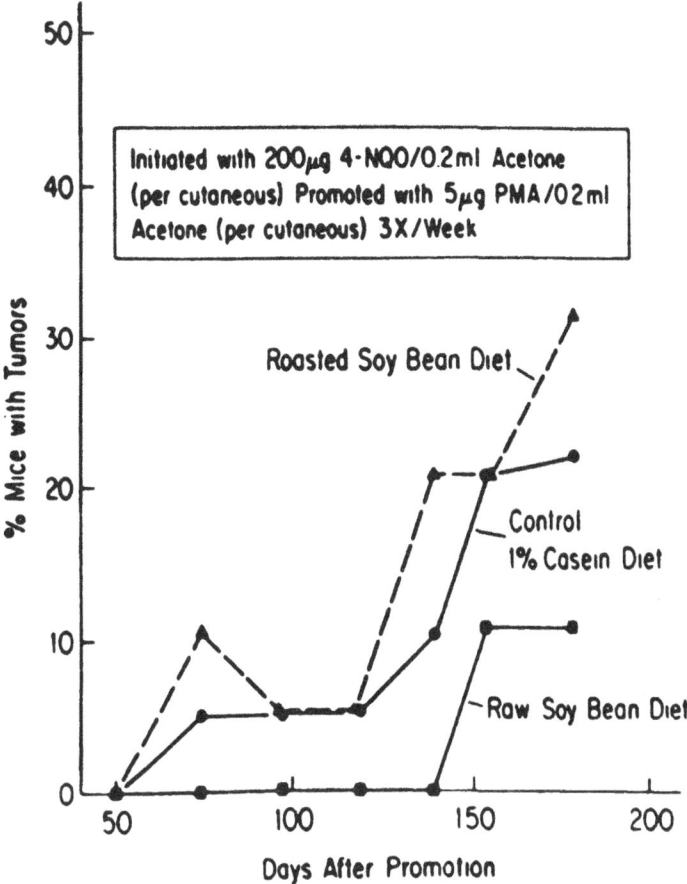

Figure 1. Number of tumors in a two-stage carcinogenesis experiment is significantly diminished when mice are fed a raw soybean diet versus mice receiving control diets (casein or roasted soybean).

These diets were also used in the experimental breast cancer studies. In these experiments the rats were irradiated with 300 R at approximately 38 R/min. The rats were 56 days old at the time of irradiation and were placed on the special diet 2 weeks before irradiation. Rats were palpated weekly and the tumors were removed when they reached a size of 2 cm.

Feeding raw soybeans and Purina rat chow had a significant effect on suppressing breast tumor formation relative to the casein-fed animals. At 10 weeks after radiation, rats on the casein diet had a significantly greater number of tumors than did rats on the soybean or Purina rat chow diet. This was true for both cancers (Fig. 2) and fibroadenomas (Fig. 3). At later time periods (35 and 52 weeks), only the soybean diet seemed to inhibit the appearance of fi-broadenomas. Moreover, only the soybean diet completely suppressed the spontaneous cancer incidence in Sprague–Dawley rats.

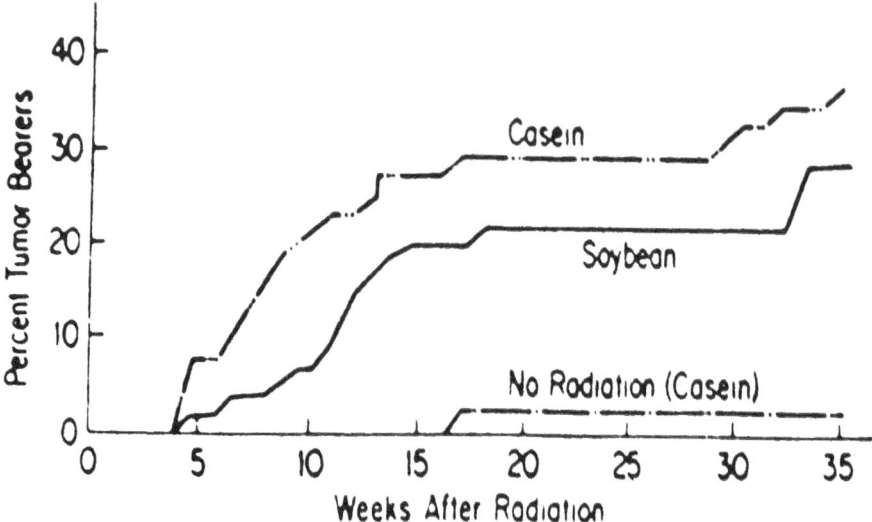

Figure 2. Effect of diets on the number of breast cancers formed in rats upon x-radiation.

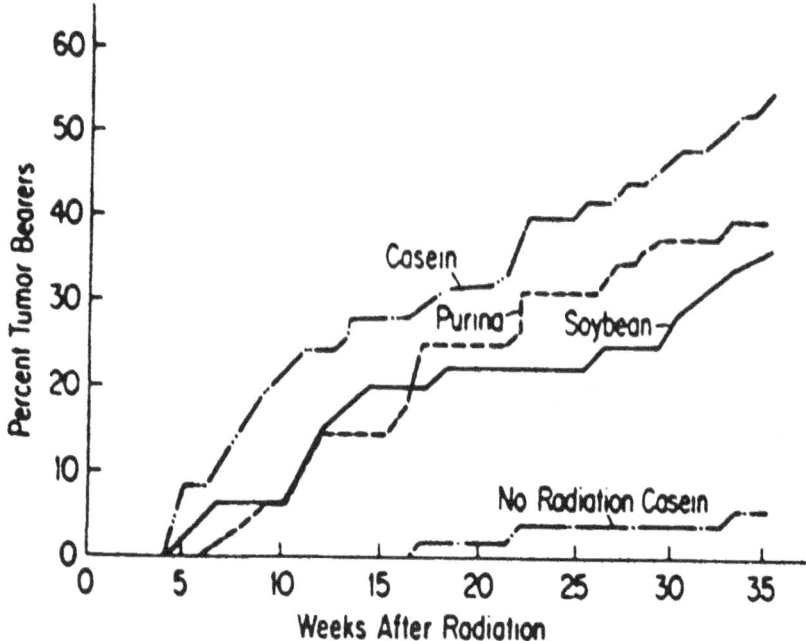

Figure 3. Effect of diets on the number of breast fibroadenomas formed in rats upon x-radiation.

Feeding soybeans or purified BBI to rodents has been shown to suppress experimental colon (Weed *et al.*, 1985) and liver (Becker, 1981) cancers. Thus, feeding diets containing PIs suppresses two-stage carcinogenesis, breast, colon, and liver cancers in rodents. These results support the view that dietary PIs may be useful in preventing human cancer.

5.3. Suppression of Tumor Promotion in Mice by Feeding NA-Supplemented Diets

Nicotinamide and benzamide had limited usefulness in preventing tumor promotion in diets of rodents because of their toxicity. NA was not toxic at high levels and demonstrated striking dose-related suppression of two-stage carcinogenesis (Troll *et al.*, 1992). In these experiments, ICR mice were initiated with 25 μg DMBA and promoted with 0.5 μg TPA three times a week. After 120 days the control mice had 22 tumors per mouse, those on a diet containing 0.1% NA had an average tumor yield of 14 per mouse, while those on a diet containing 1% NA had 8 per mouse. Diets containing 0.1% nicotinamide and benzamide showed suppression that was similar to that obtained with 0.1% NA. The tumor promoter TPA induces H_2O_2 and oxyradicals causing breakage of DNA, which results in induction of poly(ADP)ribose polymerase. Catalyzing the transfer of poly(ADP)ribose from NAD$^+$ to proteins (Berger, 1985) results in cell death and genetic damage that leads to malignant transformation. NAD$^+$ levels in human lymphocytes have been shown to be restored by feeding NA (Weitberg, 1989). In mice, NA feeding similarly may replace the NAD$^+$ lost through the H_2O_2 damage by TPA-induced neutrophils, preventing cell death and genetic damage.

6. Mechanism of Cancer Prevention by Feeding PIs

The toxicity of nicotinamide and benzamide is due to the formation of ammonia by proteases and nicotinic amidase isolated in pure form. Nicotinic deamidase, an enzyme isolated in pure form from rabbits, has many properties that are similar to serine PIs in that it acts both as an amidase and as an esterase. Similar to chymotrypsin and trypsin, it is inhibited by PIs (e.g., diisopropyl phosphate and carbobenzoxyphenylalanine chloromethyl ketone) (Gillam *et al.*, 1973). The hydrolysis of niacin has been proposed as a rate-limiting step for the formation of NAD$^+$ (Greengard *et al.*, 1969). The decreased formation of this important coenzyme may contribute to carcinogenesis and tumor promotion. PIs that suppress cancer may indirectly act by inhibiting the hydrolysis of nicotinamide. The inhibitors BBI, potato inhibitor 1, and naturally occurring chymotrypsin have been shown to suppress carcinogenesis *in vivo* and *in vitro*.

The similarity between nicotinamide and proteases was further demonstrated by showing that chymotrypsin and trypsin mimic amidase by forming ammonia from nicotinamide, benzamide, and aminobenzamide. This was done by incubating these amides with trypsin and chymotrysin at pH 7.5, and measuring ammonia formation using the fluorescence formed with fluorescamine (Udenfriend et al., 1972). The amount of ammonia formed was determined to be proportional to the enzyme concentration, which is characteristic of other amides and anilides that are used as synthetic substrates for assaying proteases. The protease-inhibitory action of these amides prevents the action of competitive substrates (Table I).

7. Concluding Remarks

A variety of cancer-preventing agents have been identified, including vitamin A, retinoids, antioxidants, and PIs. Their action in preventing cancer has been demonstrated in animal models using a variety of tumor and tissue culture systems. While epidemiological evidence in general has supported the action of these agents in preventing cancer, experiments in humans using pure compounds have not been successfully carried out. Experiments with retinoids have been planned, but the unexpected promoting action and interference with normal development in pregnancies have interfered with their execution. The lack of pure natural PIs has stopped any plans in that direction. The epidemiology of populations who consume seeds rich in PIs provides important supportive data for the putative cancer-preventing action of PIs, which are constituents of all seeds presumably to prevent their consumption by insects. However, demonstrating the action of PIs alone in preventing human cancers requires the availability of a pure PI, which can be used in a large-scale experiment in selected human populations and cancer patients where the recurrence of cancers can be monitored. Nicotinamide and NA may serve in this role. The exposure of humans to these agents can be readily measured by NAD^+ formation in erythrocytes and leukocytes. Since NA is being used to lower cholesterol and prevent arteriosclerosis, it is tempting to propose that it is the deletion of oncogenes in both systems that is responsible for this action as it is in tumor promotion.

PIs appear to interfere at three separate steps that are characteristic of tumor promotion: (1) They prevent the induction of oxyradicals by tumor promoters in neutrophils, resembling many other chemopreventive agents (e.g., retinoids) (Schuster et al., 1992; Wei and Frenkel, 1992). (2) Oxyradicals lead to the breakage of DNA, which induces poly(ADP)ribose polymerase by using NAD^+ as an intermediary and depleting it from the cells. Some PIs suppress the induction of poly(ADP)ribose, e.g., antipain, benzamide, and nicotinamide (Troll et al., 1990). (3) NAD^+ is resynthesized by NA feeding, which suppresses tumor promotion. PIs and NA are unique in their ability to suppress the early and late stages of tumor promotion. The possible role of NAD^+ levels in suppressing tumor promotion is of interest and further investigation may provide a tool for estimating the progress of cancer development.

8. References

Armstrong, B., and Doll, R., 1975, Environmental factors and cancer incidence and mortality in different countries, with special reference to dietary factors, *Int. J. Cancer* **15**:617–631.

Badwey, J. A., and Karnovsky, M. L., 1980, Active oxygen species and the functions of phagocytic leukocytes, *Annu. Rev. Biochem.* *49*:695–726.

Becker, F. F., 1981, Inhibition of spontaneous hepatocarcinogenesis in C3H/HeN mice by Edipro A, an isolated soy protein. *Carcinogenesis* **2**:1213–1214.

Berger, N. A., 1985, Symposium: Cellular response to DNA damage: The role of poly(ADP-ribose), *Radiat. Res.* **101**:4–15.

Billings, P. C., Shuin, T., Lillehaug, J., Miura, T., Roy-Burman, P., and Landolph, J. R., 1987, Enhanced expression and state of the c-myc oncogene in chemically and X-ray transformed C3H/10T¹/₂ Cl 8 mouse embryo fibroblasts, *Cancer Res.* **47**:3643–3649.

Carroll, K. K., 1975, Experimental evidence of dietary factors and hormone-dependent cancers, *Cancer Res.* **35**:3374–3383.

Chang, J. D., Billings, P. C., and Kennedy, A. R., 1985, C-myc expression is reduced in antipain-treated proliferating C3H10T¹/₂ cells, *Biochem. Biophys. Res. Commun.* **133**:830–835.

Corasanti, J. G., Hobika, G. H., and Markus, G., 1982, Interference with dimethylhydrazine induction of colon tumors in mice by ε-aminocaproic acid, *Science* **216**:1020–1021.

Correa, P., 1981, Epidemiological correlations between diet and cancer frequency, *Cancer Res.* **41**:3685–3690.

Cox, L. R., Motz, J., Troll, W., and Garte, S. J., 1991, Effects of retinoic acid on NIH3T3 cell transformation by the H-*ras* oncogene, *J. Cancer Res. Clin. Oncol.* **117**:102–108.

Davidson, D., Garte, S., and Troll, W. 1986, H-*ras* oncogene DNA affects embryonic development in the sea urchin, *Biol. Bull.* **171**:472.

Diamond, A. M., Der, C. J., and Schwartz, J. L., 1989, Alterations in transformation efficiency by the ADPRT-inhibitor 3-aminobenzamide are oncogene specific, *Carcinogenesis* **10**:383–385.

Fantone, J. C., and Ward, P. A., 1982, Role of oxygen-derived free radicals and metabolites in leukocyte-dependent inflammatory reactions, *Am. J. Pathol.* **107**:397–418.

Formisano, J., Troll, W., and Sugimura, T., 1983, Superoxide response induced by indole alkaloid tumor promoters, *Ann. N.Y. Acad. Sci.* **407**:429–431.

Frenkel, K., and Chrzan, K., 1987, Hydrogen peroxide formation and DNA base modification by tumor promoter-activated polymorphonuclear leukocytes, *Carcinogenesis* **8**:455–460.

Frenkel, K., Chrzan, K., Ryan, C., Wiesner, R., and Troll, W., 1987, Chymotrypsin-specific protease inhibitors decrease H_2O_2 formation by activated human polymorphonuclear leukocytes, *Carcinogenesis* **8**:1207–1212.

Fujiki, H., Suganuma, M., Supuri, H., Yoshizawa, S., Takagi, K., and Kobaya, M., 1989, Sarcophytols A and B inhibit tumor promotion by teleocidin in two-stage carcinogenesis in mouse skin, *J. Cancer Res. Clin. Oncol.* **115**:25–28.

Garte, S. J., Currie, D. D., and Troll, W., 1987, Inhibition of H-*ras* oncogene transformation of NIH 3T3 cells by protease inhibitors. *Cancer Res.* **47**:3159–3162.

Garte, S. J., Burns, F. J., Ashkenazi-Kimmel, T., Felber, M., and Sawey, M. J., 1990, Amplification of the c-*myc* oncogene during progression of radiation-induced rat skin tumors, *Cancer Res.* **50**:3073–3077.

Gillam, S. S., Watson, J. G., and Chaykin, S., 1973, Nicotinamide deamidase from rabbit liver. III. Inhibition and sedimentation, *Arch. Biochem. Biophys.* **157**:268–281.

Greengard, P., Petrack, B., and Kalinsky, H. J., 1969, Identification of hormonally controlled endogenous inhibitor of liver nicotinamide deamidase, *Biochim. Biophys. Acta* **184**:148–153.

Hozumi, M., Ogawa, M., Sugimura, T., Takeuchi, T., and Umezawa, H., 1972, Inhibition of tumorigenesis in mouse skin by leupeptin, a protease inhibitor from *Actinomycetes*, *Cancer Res.* **32**:1725–1729.

Kinzel, V., Fürstenberger, G., Loehrke, H., and Marks, F., 1986, Three-stage tumorigenesis in mouse skin: DNA synthesis as a prerequisite for the conversion stage induced by TPA prior to initiation, *Carcinogenesis* **7**:779–782.

Narisawa, T., Takahashi, M., Niwa, M., Fukaura, Y., and Fujiki, H., 1989, Inhibition of methylnitrosourea-induced large bowel cancer development in rats by sarcophytol A, a product from a marine soft-coral *Sarcophyton glaucum*, *Cancer Res.* **49**:3287–3289.

Nishizuka, Y., 1984, The role of protein kinase C in cell surface signal transduction and tumor promotion, *Nature* **308**:693–698.

Penn, A., Garte, S. J., Warren, L., Nesta, D., and Mindich, B., 1986, Transforming gene in human atherosclerotic plaque DNA, *Proc. Natl. Acad. Sci. USA* **83**:7951–7955.

Phillips, R. L., 1975, Role of life-style and dietary habits in risk of cancer among Seventh-Day Adventists, *Cancer Res.* **35**:3513–3522.

Quintanilla, M., Brown, K., Ramsden, M., and Balmain, A., 1986, Carcinogen-specific mutation and amplification of Ha-ras during mouse skin carcinogenesis, *Nature* **322**:78–80.

Sakamoto, M., Yanagi, S., and Kamiya, T., 1987, Inhibitory effects of niacin and its analogues on induction of ornithine decarboxylase activity by diethylnitrosamine in rat liver, *Biochem. Pharmacol.* **36**:3015–3019.

Schuster, M. G., Enriquez, P. M., Curran, P., Cooperman, B. S., and Rubin, H., 1992, Regulation of neutrophil superoxide by antichymotrypsin–chymotrypsin complexes, *J. Biol. Chem.* **267**:5056–5059.

Slaga, T. J., Klein-Szanto, A. J. P., Triplett, L. L., Yotti, L. P., and Trosko, J. E., 1981, Skin tumor promoting activity of benzoyl peroxide, a widely used free radical-generating compound, *Science* **213**:1023–1025.

Troll, W., and Corcoran, G., 1989, Nicotinamide suppresses *Arbacia punctulata* development, *Biol. Bull.* **177**:317.

Troll, W., Klassen, A., and Janoff, A., 1970, Tumorigenesis in mouse skin: Inhibition by synthetic inhibitors of proteases. *Science* **169**:1211–1213.

Troll, W., Belman, S., Wiesner, R., and Shellabarger, C. J., 1979, Protease action in carcinogenesis, in: *Biological Function of Proteinases* (H. Holzer and H. Tschesche, eds.), Springer-Verlag, Berlin, pp. 165–170.

Troll, W., Wiesner, R., Shellabarger, C. J., Holtzman, S., and Stone, J. P., 1980, Soybean diet lowers breast tumor incidence in irradiated rats, *Carcinogenesis* **1**:469–472.

Troll, W., Wiesner, R., and Frenkel, K., 1987, Anticarcinogenic action of protease inhibitors, *Adv. Cancer Res.* **49**:265–283.

Troll, W., Garte, S., and Frenkel, K., 1990, Suppression of tumor promotion by inhibitor of poly(ADP)ribose formation, in: *Antimutagenesis and Anticarcinogenesis Mechanisms II* (Y. Kuroda, D. M. Shankel, and M. D. Waters, eds.), Plenum Press, New York, pp. 225–232.

Troll, W., Belman, S., and Cohen, L. A., 1992, Nicotinic acid supplemented diets suppress tumor promotion, *Proc. Am. Assoc. Cancer Res.* **33**:131.

Udenfriend, S., Stein, S., Böhlen, P., Dairman, W., Leimgruber, W., and Weigele, M., 1972, Fluorescamine: A reagent for assay of amino acids, peptides, proteins and primary amines in the picomole range, *Science* **178**:871–872.

Wattenberg, L. W. 1985, Chemoprevention of cancer, *Cancer Res.* **45**:1–8.

Weed, H. G., McGandy, R. B., and Kennedy, A. R., 1985, Protection against dimethylhydrazine-induced adenomatous tumors of the mouse colon by the dietary addition of an extract of soybeans containing the Bowman–Birk protease inhibitor, *Carcinogenesis* **6**:1239–1241.

Wei, H., and Frenkel, K., 1992, Suppression of tumor promoter-induced oxidative events and DNA damage *in vivo* by sarcophytol A: A possible mechanism of anti-promotion, *Cancer Res.* **5:**2298–2303.

Weitberg, A. B., 1989, Effect of nicotinic acid supplementation *in vivo* on oxygen radical-induced genetic damage in human lymphocytes, *Mutat. Res.* **216:**197–201.

Wynder, E., Mabuchi, K., and Whitmore, W., 1971, Epidemiology of cancer of the prostate, *Cancer* **28:**344–360.

11

Approaches to Studying the Target Enzymes of Anticarcinogenic Protease Inhibitors

PAUL C. BILLINGS

1. Introduction

Epidemiological studies suggest that dietary factors play an important role in the etiology of cancer at many different sites (Correa, 1981; Doll and Peto, 1981). For example, high levels of legumes in the diet have been associated with lower overall cancer rates and are inversely correlated with the incidence of breast, colon, pancreatic, and prostate cancer (Mills *et al.*, 1988; Phillips, 1975). Legumes are known to contain high concentrations of protease inhibitors (Birk, 1975). Several laboratories have reported that protease inhibitors are effective suppressors of radiation- and chemical carcinogen-induced transformation *in vitro* and *in vivo* (reviewed by Kennedy and Billings, 1987; Troll *et al.*, 1984). For example, the soybean-derived Bowman–Birk protease inhibitor (BBI) (Birk, 1985) has been shown to suppress DMH-induced colon and liver carcinogenesis in mice (Billings *et al.*, 1990b; St. Clair *et al.*, 1990; Weed *et al.*, 1985) and DMBA-induced cheek pouch carcinogenesis in hamsters (Messadi *et al.*, 1986). In addition, BBI as well as several other protease inhibitors will suppress chemical- and radiation-induced transformation of mouse embryo fibroblast cells *in vitro* (Baturay and Kennedy, 1986; Yavelow *et al.*, 1985). Protease inhibitors have also been shown to inhibit the transformation of NIH 3T3 cells brought

---

PAUL C. BILLINGS • Department of Radiation Oncology, University of Pennsylvania School of Medicine, Philadelphia, Pennsylvania 19104.

Protease Inhibitors as Cancer Chemopreventive Agents, edited by Walter Troll and Ann R. Kennedy. Plenum Press, New York, 1993.

about by transfection of an activated *ras* gene (Garte *et al.*, 1987). Although the mechanisms by which protease inhibitors suppress carcinogenesis are not fully understood, we believe that these compounds exert their anticarcinogenic effects by inhibiting one or more enzymatic activities involved in the induction and/or expression of the transformed phenotype (Billings *et al.*, 1987a, 1988, 1990a). Consequently, in addition to being potent anticarcinogenic agents, protease inhibitors should be useful biochemical tools for identifying cellular enzymes involved in carcinogenesis.

In order to understand the mechanisms by which protease inhibitors suppress carcinogenesis, I feel that it is necessary to define and characterize the "target" proteins with which these compounds interact. We have employed two approaches to identify those cellular enzymes which specifically interact with the anticarcinogenic protease inhibitors. The first approach has utilized a series of defined substrates to identify enzymatic activities which are inhibited by protease inhibitors possessing anticarcinogenic activity. More recently, we have employed affinity chromatography as a tool to identify cellular enzymes which specifically interact with the anticarcinogenic protease inhibitors. For our initial studies, C3H/10T1/2 mouse embryo fibroblast cells (Resnikoff *et al.*, 1973) have been used as the source of material. This cell line has been extensively used by many investigators to study the induction of carcinogenesis by a wide variety of physical and chemical carcinogens and also the suppression of the carcinogenic process by several agents including protease inhibitors (reviewed by Kennedy and Billings, 1987).

2. Results and Discussion

2.1. Defined Substrates as Tools to Identify Proteolytic Activities Which Are Inhibited by the Anticarcinogenic Protease Inhibitors

We have screened C3H/10T1/2 cell homogenates with a variety of defined substrates to identify specific proteolytic activities which are inhibited by protease inhibitors possessing anticarcinogenic activity. Utilizing the thrombin substrate Boc-Val-Pro-Arg-MCA, we have identified an endoproteolytic activity in these cells which is inhibited by BBI, chymostatin, and TPCK, protease inhibitors which have been shown to be highly effective in suppressing radiation-induced carcinogenesis (Billings *et al.*, 1987a,b). Using conventional biochemical techniques, we have purified this peptidase to near homogeneity. The enzyme elutes as a single peak from a DEAE ion exchange column and a G-200 gel filtration column with an apparent molecular mass of approximately 70 kDa; the purified protein also runs as a single 70-kDa band on a reducing SDS-polyacrylamide gel (Billings *et al.*, 1987a). Diisopropyl fluorophosphate inhibits its activity and covalently binds to this protein, indicating that the enzyme is a

Table I. Characteristics of Boc-Val-Pro-Arg-MCA
Hydrolyzing Activity in C3H/10T1/2 Cells[a]

Molecular mass	70 kDa
Subcellular location	Cytosol
pH optimum	7
Type of enzyme	Serine protease

[a]For experimental details see Billings *et al.* (1987a) and Kennedy and Billings (1987).

serine protease. Subcellular fractionation of C3H/10T1/2 cell homogenates has localized this activity to the cytosolic (100,000g supernatant) subcellular fraction (Table I). At the present time we do not know the function of this protease. However, this enzyme has features in common with other proteases described in the literature which are involved in protein processing; hence, this enzyme may well play such a role in C3H/10T1/2 cells.

We have performed additional experiments to examine the role that this protease plays in carcinogenesis. We have investigated the effect of the substrate Boc-Val-Pro-Arg-MCA, as well as other peptide substrates on radiation transformation *in vitro*. For these studies, C3H/10T1/2 cells were seeded into dishes and then irradiated with 6 Gy of x rays. Twenty-four hours later, the medium was changed and specific groups of irradiated cells were treated with enzyme substrate for the duration of the experiment. Treatment with the protease substrate led to a reduction in the number of transformed foci resulting from radiation treatment (Table II; for details see Billings *et al.*, 1990a). Since only one proteolytic activity has been detected in these cells which cleaves this substrate (Billings *et al.*, 1987a), we believe that this substrate is suppressing carcinogenesis in a manner analogous to the anticarcinogenic protease inhibitors. Presumably, this substrate is inhibiting the endogenous activity of the 70-kDa protease by acting as a competitive substrate for this enzyme.

Table II. Effect of Protease Substrate
on Radiation Transformation[a]

Treatment	Plating efficiency (%)	Total foci[b] total dishes
Control	47	3/34
6 Gy × rays	3	41/67
6 Gy × rays + Boc-Val-Pro-Arg-MCA[a]	4	17/64

[a]C3H/10T1/2 cells were treated with substrate (16 μM) 24 hr postirradiation for the
duration of the experiment. For experimental details see Billings *et al.* (1990a).
[b]Total number of type II and type III foci observed.

2.2. The Use of Affinity Chromatography to Identify Proteins Which Specifically Interact with Anticarcinogenic Protease Inhibitors

Although the use of defined substrates allows one to potentially identify enzymatic activities which are inhibited by the anticarcinogenic protease inhibitors, it is inherently limited because it is an indirect approach and does not directly address the broader and more important question of which cellular enzymes specifically interact with the anticarcinogenic protease inhibitors. A more direct approach toward identifying those enzymes which specifically interact with protease inhibitors which suppress carcinogenesis is affinity chromatography. This technique is highly selective and will potentially allow us to identify all enzymatic activities present in C3H/10T1/2 cells which specifically interact with these inhibitors. We have utilized a BBI-affinity resin to identify proteins in C3H/10T1/2 cells which specifically interact with this inhibitor (Billings *et al.*, 1988).

An affinity resin was prepared by covalently attaching the BBI to CNBr-activated Sepharose. [The preparation and testing of the BBI-affinity matrix is described in detail in Billings *et al.* (1988).] In our initial experiments we determined which proteins present in C3H/10T1/2 cell homogenates will specifically bind to the affinity matrix. For these studies, cellular proteins were metabolically labelled with [^{35}S]-Met. The cells were disrupted and the cell homogenate was subsequently passed over the BBI-affinity resin. The column was washed extensively with binding buffer [50 mM phosphate (pH 7), 1 mM MgCl$_2$, 40 mM NaCl]; bound proteins were eluted from the BBI-affinity resin with 1 and 100 mM HCl. Equal aliquots from each fraction eluting from the column were analyzed in a liquid scintillation counter for the presence of ^{35}S-labeled protein. Those fractions containing the highest levels of labeled protein were analyzed by SDS-PAGE. While some material eluted from the affinity resin with 1 mM HCl, the majority of bound material eluted with the 100 mM HCl wash (Fig. 1). The most abundant proteins binding to the column had molecular masses of ca. 45 and 60 kDa. Preincubation of the cell homogenates with free BBI reduced the binding of these proteins to the BBI-affinity column, indicating that these proteins are specifically binding to the affinity resin.

We detected protease activity in the fractions binding to the column by using a nonspecific substrate (Billings *et al.*, 1988). While these results indicated that functional enzyme activity was binding to the BBI-affinity column, they did not provide definitive information about which of these proteins had protease activity. To directly address this question, additional experiments were performed. C3H/10T1/2 cell proteins were metabolically labeled with [^{35}S]-Met and passed over the BBI-affinity column. In order to avoid irreversible denaturation of the proteins bound to the affinity resin, the proteins were eluted from the column with urea (Fig. 2). The material eluting from the column was analyzed for protease activity on polyacrylamide gels containing gelatin as substrate (Heussen

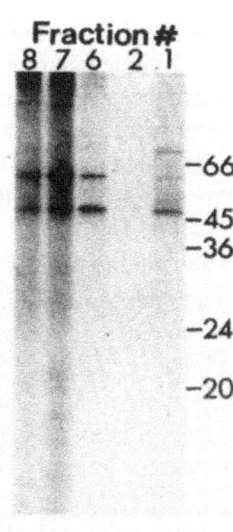

Figure 1. Analysis of cellular proteins binding to the BBI-affinity column. C3H/10T1/2 cell proteins were metabolically labeled with [^{35}S]-Met, the cells were homogenized and applied to the affinity column. The column was washed with 50 column volumes of binding buffer [50 mM phosphate buffer (pH 7), 40 mM NaCl, 1 mM MgCl$_2$]; bound proteins were eluted with 1 and 100 mM HCl. Fractions from the affinity column were counted in a liquid scintillation counter. For analysis, selected fractions containing ^{34}S-labeled protein were run on 12% SDS-polyacrylamide gels (Laemmli, 1970), the gel was stained and autoradiographed. Lanes 1–2, material eluting with the 1 mM HCl wash; lanes 6–8, material eluting with the 100 mM HCl wash. Numbers on right, molecular mass markers in kilodaltons.

and Dowdle, 1980). Under these conditions, a single band of protease activity was observed which eluted with the urea wash. Autoradiography of the zymogram revealed two labeled proteins (Fig. 2). These results indicated that functional protease activity was binding to the affinity resin. This proteolytic activity had a mass of approximately 45 kDa. Recent results indicate that this enzyme is a cytosolic serine protease.

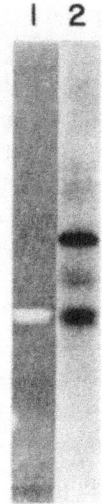

Figure 2. Elution of protease activity from the BBI-affinity column. ^{35}S-labeled C3H/10T1/2 cell proteins were passed over the BBI-affinity resin, the column was washed with 25 column volumes of binding buffer; bound proteins were eluted with 5 M urea. Twelve percent polyacrylamide gels containing 0.1% gelatin were cast (Heussen and Dowdle, 1980). Samples were applied to the gel in standard SDS-gel loading buffer containing 0.1% SDS but lacking β-mercaptoethanol and were not boiled prior to loading. The gels were run at a constant voltage of 80 V for 12 hr and then soaked in 200 ml of 2% Triton X-100 in distilled water on a gyratory shaker for 1 hr at 20°C. Next, the gels were soaked in 100 mM Tris (pH 8.0), 5 mM CaCl$_2$ for 12 hr at 37°C and then stained in amido black. Lane 1, material eluting with urea was analyzed on a gelatin-containing zymogram (note the band of protease activity); lane 2, autoradiograph of gel shown in lane 1.

In order to elucidate the mechanisms by which protease inhibitors suppress the carcinogenic process, we believe it is necessary to identify the proteins with which these compounds interact. In this report, we have summarized some of the experiments we have carried out to identify cellular enzymes in C3H/10T1/2 cells which specifically interact with BBI. Using a thrombin substrate (Boc-Val-Pro-Arg-MCA), we have identified a cytosolic, 70-kDa serine protease which is inhibited by BBI as well as several other anticarcinogenic protease inhibitors. Although the identity of this enzyme is unknown, it has features in common with other endoproteases that have been described in the literature which are involved in protein processing. Using affinity chromatography, we have identified two cellular proteins in C3H/10T1/2 cells which specifically interact with BBI (Billings et al., 1988). One of these proteins is a protease as indicated by its ability to cleave gelatin. Recent results indicate that this enzyme is a cytosolic serine protease. Currently, we are purifying this protease for protein sequencing and molecular cloning.

We have recently demonstrated that carboxypeptidase inhibitor 1 will suppress radiation-induced transformation of C3H/10T1/2 cells in vitro (Billings et al., 1989). Carboxypeptidase inhibitor 1 is known to inhibit metallo-exopeptidases but has not been shown to inhibit endoproteases (Hass and Ryan, 1981). Many peptide hormones and growth factors require posttranslational modification via proteolytic cleavage to be converted into their mature, active forms (Douglass et al., 1984; Fisher and Scheller, 1988). The conversion of a normal cell into a transformed one may well require specific growth factors and hormones. Inhibition of one, or several, of these processing enzymes by a protease inhibitor could greatly reduce the levels of mature growth factor or peptide hormone present in the cell and thus inhibit the conversion of a normal cell into a tumor cell. Our findings that inhibitors of both endoproteases and exoproteases have the ability to suppress carcinogenesis suggest that at least two types of proteolytic activities are involved in tumor cell development. One of these activities could be an endoproteolytic activity, such as the 70-kDa protease described above, which is inhibited by TPCK, chymostatin, and BBI, compounds known to inhibit endoproteases and possess anticarcinogenic activity. A second exopeptidase activity may also play an essential role in carcinogenesis; such an activity could be inhibited by carboxypeptidase inhibitor. Indeed, it is known that both endo- and exoproteolytic activities are involved in protein processing (Fisher and Scheller, 1988).

Besides being potentially useful as human cancer chemopreventive agents, protease inhibitors are powerful tools for identifying cellular enzymes involved in tumor cell development. In order to elucidate the mechanisms by which protease inhibitors suppress carcinogenesis, it will be necessary to identify and fully characterize the cellular enzymes with which the anticarcinogenic protease inhibitors interact.

ACKNOWLEDGMENTS. I thank Ms. Christine Keller-McGandy and Ms. Ann R. Morrow for technical assistance and Dr. Ann R. Kennedy for helpful discussion. This work was supported by NIH Grant CA45734.

3. References

Baturay, N. Z., and Kennedy, A. R., 1986, Pyrene acts as a cocarcinogen with the carcinogens benzo(a)pyrene, β-propiolactone and radiation in the induction of malignant transformation of cultured mouse fibroblasts; soybean extract containing the Bowman–Birk inhibitor acts as an anticarcinogen, *Cell Biol. Toxicol.* **2**:21–32.

Billings, P. C., Carew, J. A., Keller-McGandy, C. E., Goldberg, A. L., and Kennedy, A. R., 1987a, A serine protease activity in C3H/10T1/2 cells that is inhibited by anticarcinogenic protease inhibitors, *Proc. Natl. Acad. Sci. USA* **84**:4801–4805.

Billings, P. C., St. Clair, W., Ryan, C. A., and Kennedy, A. R., 1987b, Inhibition of radiation-induced transformation of C3H/10T1/2 cells by chymotrypsin inhibitor 1 from potatoes, *Carcinogenesis* **8**:809–812.

Billings, P. C., St. Clair, W., Owen, A. J., and Kennedy, A. R., 1988, Potential intracellular target proteins of the anticarcinogenic Bowman Birk protease inhibitor identified by affinity chromatography, *Cancer Res.* **48**:1798–1802.

Billings, P. C., Morrow, A. R., Ryan, C. A., and Kennedy, A. R., 1989, Inhibition of radiation-induced transformation of C3H/10T1/2 cells with carboxypeptidase inhibitor from potatoes, *Carcinogenesis* **10**:687–691.

Billings, P. C., Habres, J. M., and Kennedy, A. R., 1990a, Inhibition of radiation-induced transformation of C3H/10T1/2 cells by specific protease substrates, *Carcinogenesis* **11**:329–332.

Billings, P. C., Newberne, P. M., and Kennedy, A. R., 1990b, Protease inhibitor suppression of colon and anal gland carcinogenesis induced by dimethylhydrazine, *Carcinogenesis* **11**:1083–1086.

Birk, Y., 1975, Proteinase inhibitors from plant sources, *Methods Enzymol.* **45**:695–751.

Birk, Y., 1985, The Bowman Birk inhibitor, *Int. J. Peptide Protein Res.* **25**:113–131.

Correa, P., 1981, Epidemiologic correlations between diet and cancer frequency, *Cancer Res.* **41**:3685–3690.

Doll, R., and Peto, R., 1981, The causes of cancer: Quantitative estimates of avoidable risks of cancer in the United States today, *J. Natl. Cancer Inst.* **66**:1193–1308.

Douglass, J., Civelli, O., and Herbert, E., 1984, Polyprotein gene expression: Generation of diversity of neuroendocrine peptides, *Annu. Rev. Biochem.* **53**:665–714.

Fisher, J. M., and Scheller, R. H., 1988, Prohormone processing and the secretory pathway, *J. Biol. Chem.* **263**:16515–16518.

Garte, S. J., Currie, D. D., and Troll, W., 1987, Inhibition of oncogene transformation of NIH3T3 cells by protease inhibitors, *Cancer Res.* **47**:3159–3162.

Hass, G. M., and Ryan, C. A., 1981, Carboxypeptidase inhibitor from potatoes, *Methods Enzymol.* **80**:778–791.

Heussen, C., and Dowdle, E. B., 1980, Electrophoretic analysis of plasminogen activators in polyacrylamide gels containing sodium dodecyl sulfate and copolymerized substrates, *Anal. Biochem.* **102**:196–202.

Kennedy, A. R., and Billings, P. C., 1987, Anticarcinogenic actions of protease inhibitors, Proceedings of the 2nd International Congress on "Anticarcinogenesis and Radiation Protection" (P. Cerutti, O. F. Nygaard, and M. G. Simic, eds.), Plenum Press, New York, pp. 285–295.

Laemmli, U. K., 1970, Cleavage of structural proteins during the assembly of bacteriophage T4, *Nature* **227**:680–685.

Messadi, D. A., Billings, P. C., Shklar, G., and Kennedy, A. R., 1986, Inhibition of oral carcinogenesis by a protease inhibitor, *J. Natl. Cancer Inst.* **76**:447–452.

Mills, P. K., Beeson, W. L., Abbey, D. E., Fraser, G. E., and Phillips, R. L., 1988, Dietary habits and past medical history as related to fatal pancreas cancer risk among Adventists, *Cancer* **61**:2578–2585.

Phillips, R. L., 1975, Role of lifestyle and dietary habits in risk of cancer among Seventh Day Adventists, *Cancer Res.* **35**:3513–3522.

Reznikoff, C. A., Brankow, D. W., and Heidelberger, C., 1973, Establishment and characterization of a cloned line of C3H/10T1/2 mouse embryo cells sensitive to postconfluence inhibition of cell division, *Cancer Res.* **33**:3231–3238.

St. Clair, W. H., Billings, P. C., Carew, J. A., Keller-McGandy, C., Newberne, P., and Kennedy, A. R., 1990, Suppression of dimethylhydrazine-induced carcinogenesis in mice by dietary addition of the Bowman–Birk protease inhibitor, *Cancer Res.* **50**:580–586.

Troll, W., Frankel, K., and Weisner, R., 1984, Protease inhibitors as anticarcinogens, *J. Natl. Cancer Inst.* **73**:1245–1250.

Weed, H., McGandy, R. B., and Kennedy, A. R., 1985, Protection against dimethylhydrazine-induced adenomatous tumors of the mouse colon by the dietary addition of an extract of soybeans containing the Bowman–Birk protease inhibitor, *Carcinogenesis* **6**:1239–1241.

Yavelow, J., Collins, M., Birk, Y., Troll, W., and Kennedy, A. R., 1985, Nanomolar concentrations of Bowman Birk soybean protease inhibitor suppress x-ray induced transformation *in vitro*, *Proc. Natl. Acad. Sci USA* **82**:5395–5399.

12

Anticarcinogenic Activities of Naturally Occurring Cysteine Proteinase Inhibitors

RITA COLELLA, ANN F. CHAMBERS, and DAVID T. DENHARDT

1. Introduction

Proteases and their respective inhibitors are found in almost every biological system where proteolysis occurs. Examples of such systems include the processing of proteins during protein synthesis, activation of prohormones and proenzymes to their active forms, cellular protein turnover, digestion of endocytosed material, blood coagulation, angiogenesis, inflammation and wound healing, differentiation and tissue remodeling, invasion and metastasis, and possibly tumorigenesis. In both primary and secondary tumors, vascularization of the tumor tissue (angiogenesis) facilitates the growth and spread of the tumor, and this process also involves proteases and their inhibitors. Normal physiological processes require that the activities of the proteolytic enzymes be controlled so as to prevent excessive, unwanted damage to the tissues involved. Proteolytic activity can be regulated by modulating the synthesis or degradation of the enzyme or necessary cofactors, or via interactions with activators or inhibitors of activity.

Investigations of proteinase inhibitors have been designed to define their

RITA COLELLA and DAVID T. DENHARDT • Department of Biological Sciences, Rutgers University, Piscataway, New Jersey 08855. *Present address of R.C.:* Department of Anatomical Sciences and Neurobiology, University of Louisville School of Medicine, Louisville, Kentucky 40292. *ANN F. CHAMBERS* • The London Regional Cancer Centre, University of Western Ontario, London, Ontario, Canada N6A 4L6.

Protease Inhibitors as Cancer Chemopreventive Agents, edited by Walter Troll and Ann R. Kennedy. Plenum Press, New York, 1993.

biological roles and to investigate their potential use in commercial and therapeutic applications. Examples of the latter include the use of proteinase inhibitors to reduce virus infectivity (Korant et al., 1986; Bjorck et al., 1990), to control protein degradation occurring in pathological conditions such as the muscular dystrophies and joint destruction, to engineer plant species resistant to herbivores (Ryan, 1989), and to inhibit tumorigenesis or metastasis (Schelp and Pongpaew, 1988; Schultz et al., 1988; Troll, 1989).

A metastasizing cell must separate from the primary tumor, enter into, and subsequently escape from, the vascular or lymphatic system, and establish itself at a secondary site in the organism. This process requires that the invading cell release proteolytic enzymes in order to penetrate basement membranes and degrade the extracellular matrix. The important role of matrix metalloproteinases and their inhibitors, especially the TIMPs, in tumor development and invasion have been reviewed recently elsewhere (Khokha and Denhardt, 1989; Liotta et al., 1991). The focus here is on the control of cysteine proteinases by naturally occurring inhibitors.

2. Cysteine Proteinases

Production of two cysteine proteinases, cathepsins B and L, is augmented in many transformed cell lines and in some cases correlates with tumor cell invasion (e.g., Sloane et al., 1982, 1987, 1990; Denhardt et al., 1987; Qian et al., 1989). (Although other mammalian cysteine proteinases are known, to our knowledge none of them have been implicated in carcinogenesis.) Typically, cathepsins B and L are lysosomal enzymes involved in intracellular protein degradation; they are glycosylated and sorted to the lysosomal compartment via a mannose-6-phosphate receptor (Kirschke and Barrett, 1987; Goldberg, 1987). Mouse fibroblast procathepsin L [also known as major excreted protein (MEP)] (Denhardt et al., 1986; Portnoy et al., 1986; Mason et al., 1986b; Troen et al., 1987) has an unusually low affinity for the receptor, allowing substantial amounts to be secreted by cells whenever its endogenous synthesis is increased, for example in transformed cells (Dong et al., 1989). This low affinity of MEP/procathepsin L has been attributed either to its possession of only one phosphorylated oligosaccharide (Dong and Sahagian, 1990) or to protein determinants within the molecule that impair its interaction with the receptor (Lazzarino and Gabel, 1990). Changes in the number, affinity, or distribution of the mannose-6-phosphate receptors (at least two types of which are known) in response to transformation or other stimuli can also influence the sorting of lysosomal proteins (Achkar et al., 1990; Prence et al., 1990).

Several groups have studied the contribution cathepsins B and L make to human cancers. At acid to neutral pH, these two proteinases are effective at degrading the components of the basement membrane/extracellular matrix (collagen, laminin, fibronectin, proteoglycans, elastin) either directly or indirectly, for example by activating a prometalloproteinase (Kirschke *et al.*, 1982; Mason *et al.*, 1986a; Maciewicz *et al.*, 1987; Baricos *et al.*, 1988; Lah *et al.*, 1989a). Evidence implicating cathepsin L in basement membrane degradation and penetration has been reported (Baricos *et al.*, 1988; Yagel *et al.*, 1989). Cathepsin L mRNA levels are elevated in many types of cancers, especially those of the kidney, testis, colon, and lung (Chauhan *et al.*, 1991). The production of MEP/cathepsin L from a series of *ras*-transformed cell lines correlated with their metastatic potential (Denhardt *et al.*, 1987). Yamaguchi *et al.* (1990) have characterized both a cathepsin L-like activity, which differed in certain ways from the liver enzyme, and an intrinsic inhibitor secreted by a human pancreatic cell line.

Sheahan *et al.* (1989) observed increased specific activities of both "B-like and L-like" cathepsins in human colorectal carcinoma tissue relative to normal mucosa, particularly at the stage of bowel wall invasion. The increase in cathepsin B gene expression was even more striking at the mRNA level (Murnane *et al.*, 1991). Enhanced synthesis of cathepsin B has been demonstrated in metastatic B16 mouse melanoma cells (Sloane *et al.*, 1982; Qian *et al.*, 1989) as well as in mouse and human carcinoma explants, from which it is released into the medium (Mort and Recklies, 1986). Cathepsin B activity and mRNA expression correlate with the metastasizing potential of the B16 cells (Moin *et al.*, 1989) even though inhibitors of cathepsin B do not block invasion of the human amnion (Rohrlich *et al.*, 1986; Mignatti *et al.*, 1986). A cathepsin B-like enzyme associated with the plasma membrane in certain metastatic tumors has been described (Sloane *et al.*, 1986; Rozhin *et al.*, 1987; Erdel *et al.*, 1991). Both cathepsin L and B mRNA levels were found to be increased in metastatic, *ras*-transformed NIH 3T3 cells, in proportion to levels of *ras* expression (Chambers *et al.*, 1992).

Cathepsins B and L are inhibited by members of a superfamily of endogenous inhibitors commonly known as the cystatins. Since cystatin is also the name first given to a specific proteinase inhibitor found in egg white, we will refer collectively to members of the cystatin superfamily as CPIs (cysteine proteinase inhibitors). Their high affinity for the cysteine proteinases suggests that their primary function is the suppression of cysteine proteinase activities released from intracellular compartments or from invading organisms. Since many transformed cells produce increased amounts of one or both cathepsins, it becomes important to understand how they might be regulated by endogenous CPIs during tumorigenesis. Questions that can be raised include whether CPI expression is coordinately regulated with that of a cysteine proteinase, and whether any CPI is defective in malignant cells. Here we review the members of the cystatin superfamily, discuss their occurrence and activities in cancer cells, and speculate on the possible roles of these proteins in metastasis.

Table 1. Representative Members of the Cystatin Superfamily,
the Source from Which They Were Isolated, and Their Original Name

	Source	Name	Reference
1. Stefins			
a. No Cys	Polymorphonuclear	Stefin	Brzin *et al.* (1983)
Stefin A	leukocytes		
	Human liver	Cystatin A	Green *et al.* (1984)
	Human epithelium	Acidic CPI[a]	Järvinen and Rinne (1982)
	Rat epidermis	α-thiol proteinase in-hibitor	Takio *et al.* (1984)
b. 1 or 2 Cys	Human spleen	Neutral CPI	Järvinen and Rinne (1982)
Stefin B	Human liver	Cystatin B	Green *et al.* (1984)
	Rat liver	β-thiol proteinase in-hibitor	Takio *et al.* (1983)
2. Cystatins			
Cystatin C	Cerebrospinal fluid	Gamma trace	Grubb and Lofberg (1982)
		Human cystatin	Brzin *et al.* (1984)
		Post gamma globulin	Bollengier (1987)
Chicken cystatin	Egg white		Anastasi *et al.* (1983)
	Muscle	Muscle CPI	Wood *et al.* (1985)
Cystatin S	Human saliva	Cystatin SA	Isemura *et al.* (1984)
		Cystatin SN	Isemura *et al.* (1986)
	Rat saliva	Rat cystatin S	Shaw *et al.* (1988)
3. Kininogens			
HMW	Rat, human plasma	α₁-TPI	Ohkuba *et al.* (1988)
LMW	Rat, human plamsa	α₂-TPI	Ohkuba *et al.* (1984)
T-kininogen	Rat plasma	α-TPI	Moreau *et al.* (1986)
4. α₂-HS glycoprotein			Elzanowski *et al.* (1988),
Human His-rich			Koide (1988)
glycoprotein			

[a]HMW, high molecular weight; LMW, low molecular weight; CPI, cysteine proteinase inhibitor; TPI, thiol proteinase inhibitor.

3. The Cystatin Superfamily

Inhibitors of the cysteine proteinases have been described in virtually all tissues and biological fluids. They occur as low ($M_r \sim$ of 10,000–13,000) and high ($M_r \sim$ 60,000–80,000) molecular weight proteins. Based on their structural and chemical properties, they are classified into one superfamily composed of four families. Table I lists some of the characterized family members together with synonyms found in the literature.

Type 1: Stefins. Members of this family have approximately 100 amino acids and an M_r of about 11,000. They are not glycosylated, lack disulfide bonds, and in general are found intracellularly. The stefins can be further divided into two subfamilies depending on the presence or absence of cysteine residues.

FAMILY 1: The Stefins

```
                          MIPGGLSEAKPATPEIQEIVDKVKPQLEEKTNETY--GKLEAVQYKTQVVAG...
                          MDPGTTGIVGGVSEAKPATPEIQEVADKVKRQLEEKTNEKY--EKFKVVEYKSQVVAG...
                          MMCGAPSATQPATAETQHIADQVRSQLEEKYNKKF--PVFKAVSFKSQVVAG...
                          MMCGAPSATMPATTETQEIADKVKSQLEEKANQKF--DVFKAISFRRQVVAG...

              ...TNYYIKVRAGDNKYMHLKVFKSLPGQNEDLVLTGYQVDKNKDDELTGF
              ...QILFMKVDVGNGRFLHMKVLRGLSGDD-DLKLLDYQTNKTKNDELTDF
              ...TNYFIKVHVGDEDFVHLRVFQSLPHENKPLTLSNYQTNKAKHDELTYF
              ...TNFFIKVDVGEEKCVHLRVFEPLPHENKPLTLSSYQTDKEKHDELTYF
```

FAMILY 2: The Cystatins

```
    MAGARGCVVLLAAALMLVGAVLGSEDRSRLLGAPVPVDENDEGLQRALQFAMAEYNRASNDKYSSRVVRVISAKRQLVSG...
    MAGPLRAPLLLLAILAVALAVSPAACSSPGKPPRLVGGPMDASVEEEGVRRALDFAVGEYNKASNDMYHSRALQVVRARKQIVAG...
    MAQHLSTLLLLATLAVALAWSPKEEDRIIPGGIYDADLNDEWVQRALHFAISEYNKATEDEYYRRPLQVLRAREQTFGG...

        ...IKYILQVEIGRTTCPKSSGDLQS--CEFHDEPEMAKYTTCTFVVYSIPWLNQIKLLESKCQ
        ...VNYFLDVELGRTTCTKTQPNLDN--CPFHDQPHLKRKAFCSFQIYAVPWQGTMTLSKSTCQDA
        ...VNYFFDVEVGRTICTKSQPNLDT--CAFHEQPELQKKQLCSFEIYEVPWEDRMSLVDSRCQEA
```

FAMILY 3: Human Kininogen

```
                          QESQSEEIDCNDKDLFKAVDAALKKYNSQNQSNNQFVLYRITEATKTVGSD...
                          AEGPVVTAQYDCLGCVHPISTQSPDLEPILRHGIQYFNNNTQHSSLFMLNEVKRAQRQVVAG...
                          GKDFVQPPTKICVGCPRDIPTNSPELEETLTHTITKLNAENNATFYFKIDNVKKARVQVVAG...

        ...TFYSFKYEIKEGDCPVQSGKTWQ-DCEYKAAKAATGECTATVGKRSSTKFSVATQT-CQITP..
        ...LNFRITYSIVQTNCSKENFLFLTPDCKSLWNGD-TGECTDNAYIDIQLRIASFSQN-CDIYP..
        ...KKYFIDFVARETTCSKESNEELTESCETKKLGQ-SLDCNAEVYVVPWEKKIYPTVN-CQPLGM KININ - LIGHT CHAIN
```

Figure 1. Amino acid sequence of CPIs. The conserved G residue (shaded), the sequence QVVAG (shaded), and the presence of the disulfide bonds are indicated. The signal sequences for members of the cystatin family, deduced from their cDNA, are boxed. Each sequence is continued in order (after the QVVAG sequence or its equivalent) in the second block of sequences shown in each family. The sequences from top to bottom are: human stefin A (Machleidt *et al.*, 1983), rat stefin A (Takio *et al.*, 1984), human stefin B (Ritonja *et al.*, 1985), rat stefin B (Takio *et al.*, 1983); chicken cystatin (Colella *et al.*, 1989), human cystatin C (Abrahamson *et al.*, 1987), human cystatin S (Saitoh *et al.*, 1987); and the three cystatin-like domains that make up the heavy chain of human kininogen (Ohkubo *et al.*, 1984). The positions of the kinin fragment and the light chain of human kininogen in relation to the kininogen molecule are shown.

There is 30% sequence similarity between the stefins and the type 2 cystatins (described below) centered around a conserved QVVAG sequence. The stefins lack a sequence in the COOH-terminus found in the other families (Fig. 1).

Type 2: Cystatins. The members of the second family have approximately 115 amino acids and an M_r of roughly 13,000. They also lack carbohydrates but differ from the stefins in having two disulfide bonds per molecule near the COOH-terminus. The nucleotide sequences of four members of this family [cystatin C (Abrahamson *et al.*, 1987), cystatins S and SN (Saitoh *et al.*, 1987), and chicken egg white cystatin (Colella *et al.*, 1989)] revealed three exons and a sequence encoding a signal peptide, consistent with the predominantly extracellular location of this class of inhibitors. Chicken cystatin and cystatin C are widely expressed at the mRNA level (Saitoh *et al.*, 1987; Colella *et al.*, 1989; Abrahamson *et al.*, 1990).

Cystatin C, which has long been implicated in aspects of the inflammatory response (see Järvinen *et al.*, 1987, for review), is a potent modulator of neutrophil migration (Leung-Tack *et al.*, 1990b). Abnormalities in cystatin C structure, expression, or metabolism have been reported in cerebral amyloidosis (Ghiso *et al.*, 1986; Olafsson *et al.*, 1990) and multiple sclerosis (Bollengier, 1987). It is produced in increased amounts, possibly altered in structure, by alveolar macrophages from smokers (Warfel *et al.*, 1991). Decreased CPI activities have also been reported in animal models of muscular dystrophy (Spanier and Bird, 1982; Gopalan *et al.*, 1986).

Type 3: Kininogens. Both high- and low-molecular-weight kininogens are glycosylated plasma proteins with the same NH_2-terminal heavy chain, which contains the CPI activity, and the bradykinin moiety; they differ in the COOH-terminal light chain due to differential processing of the primary transcript (Kitamura *et al.*, 1985). Both species can modulate thrombin-induced platelet aggregation/activation (Puri *et al.*, 1991; Meloni and Schmaier, 1991). Digestion with kallikrein produces three fragments: an NH_2-terminal heavy-chain portion with CPI activity, the bradykinin moiety with vasodilatory activity, and a COOH-terminal fragment of no known function (these last two originate from the light chain).

The NH_2-terminal portion (see Fig. 1) is composed of three tandemly repeated cystatin-like domains encoded by nine exons. Sequence comparisons of the nine exons indicate that this region is characterized by a thrice-repeated pattern of one sequence domain (Kitamura *et al.*, 1985). It has been shown that the organization of the genes for four members of the cystatin family [human cystatin C (Ghiso *et al.*, 1988), chicken egg white cystatin (Colella and Bird, 1993), and human salivary cystatins S and SN (Saitoh *et al.*, 1988)] is similar to each one of the threefold repeats of the kininogen gene. Of the three cystatin domains of the kininogen molecule, two have conserved CPI activity, and one can also inhibit calpain (Salvesen *et al.*, 1986; Barrett, 1987; Bradford *et al.*, 1990). These CPIs may control inflammation by inhibiting cysteine proteinases released from damaged tissue. Inability to produce kininogens is not fatal but does lead to vascular problems (Stormorken *et al.*, 1990).

Type 4: Human histidine-rich glycoprotein (Koide, 1988) and α_2-HS glycoprotein (Elzanowski *et al.*, 1988) are two functionally unrelated negative acute-phase reactants of plasma that have two cystatin-like domains but do not appear to be effective CPIs. Plasma of patients with localized breast carcinomas and malignant melanomas contain higher levels of the histidine-rich glycoprotein in comparison with normal controls (Mannucci *et al.*, 1990).

Based on sequence comparisons and conservation of the disulfide loops, an evolutionary scheme for the cystatin superfamily has been deduced (Barrett *et al.*, 1986; Kellermann *et al.*, 1989; Rawlings and Barrett, 1990). The stefins appear to represent the superfamily archetype, which gave rise to the cystatin gene as the result of COOH-terminal divergence, possibly the acquisition of a carboxyl extension. Duplication of an early cystatin gene produced an intermediate form (the progenitor of the type 4 family members) that duplicated one of its disulfide loops to give rise to the kininogens.

4. Mode of Inhibition

The CPIs are tightly binding, reversible inhibitors of papain-like cysteine proteinases with K_i values of 10^{-8} to 10^{-12} and 1:1 stoichiometry. To different extents, various members of this family inhibit cathepsins B, H, L, S, N, dipeptidyl peptidase I, calpain, and the plant cysteine proteinases papain, chymopapain, actinidin, papaya proteinase III, and ficin but not bromelain. CPIs do not inhibit serine, metallo-, or aspartic proteinases. The x-ray crystal structure of chicken egg white cystatin has been determined (Bode et al., 1988). A computer-generated docking model based on this structure proposes that three parts of the inhibitor are in close contact with the active cleft of papain: the NH_2-terminus containing a conserved Gly residue, the first hairpin containing the conserved QXVXG sequence, and a second hairpin loop at the COOH-terminus containing a conserved Trp residue. This "tripartite wedge" structure of the inhibitor fits firmly into a cleft in the enzyme, accounting for the high affinity between the two molecules (Machleidt et al., 1989). Further details and confirmation of the essential aspects of this model, which differs fundamentally from that deduced for the serine proteinase inhibitors, have been obtained from studies on the x-ray crystal structure of recombinant human stefin B in a complex with carboxymethylated papain (Stubbs et al., 1990).

When considering the inhibition of cysteine proteinases by their inhibitors in vivo, a number of points need to be kept in mind. One is whether the CPI can function in the microenvironment where the degradation of basement membrane/extracellular matrix components is occurring. Cells are able to acidify localized microenvironments in regions of adherence and can activate cathepsins extracellularly (Silver et al., 1988; Maciewicz et al., 1989). Effective inhibition of cathepsin B or L by a CPI in this situation would require that adequate amounts of the inhibitor be able to access the microenvironment and function there. As for pH, chicken cystatin's interaction with the plant enzyme ficin is independent of pH over the range 4.0–9.0 (Sen and Whitaker, 1973).

Also relevant is the susceptibility of the CPI to inactivation. For example, cystatin C and kininogen can be inactivated by cathepsin D, thus giving this aspartic proteinase a role in regulating the activity of the cysteine proteinases (Lenarcic et al., 1991). The NH_2-terminus of cystatin is readily cleaved, resulting in truncated forms with increased K_i values perhaps due to the loss of the conserved Gly residue (Isemura et al., 1986; Machleidt et al., 1989). This interacting meshwork of proteinases and their inhibitors that impact on the invasiveness of the cell is clearly complex; obviously, there are many ways in which the cell's metastatic potential can be enhanced.

5. Cystatins and Metastasis

The breakdown of the basement membrane/extracellular matrix that occurs during metastasis is probably accomplished by the combined action of the lysosomal cathepsins, either cell-surface associated or secreted, and activated neutral metalloproteinases or serine proteinases. Among the cysteine proteinases, cathepsins B and L have been strongly implicated in contributing to the malignant phenotype in some cases, and hence it becomes important to understand how CPIs may serve to control their activity. A diagramatic representation of the possible action of cysteine proteinases and their inhibitors is shown in Fig. 2. There are indications in the literature, noted below, hinting that alterations in the structure or expression of a CPI may be a contributing factor in cancer.

Using immunofluorescence techniques, Järvinen *et al.* (1987) studied the distribution of stefin A (the first CPI demonstrated in cancer cells) and stefin B inhibitor activity in normal and malignant epithelium. In normal epithelium, stefins A and B were located in differentiated cells in the upper layers of the epithelium and absent in undifferentiated basal cells; they can therefore be considered markers of squamous cell differentiation. Stefins A and B were not found in malignant epithelium, consistent with the generalization that malignant transformation of undifferentiated cells is accompanied by the inability to differentiate normally.

Hawley-Nelson *et al.* (1988) also observed differential expression of stefin A mRNA in differentiating mouse epidermal cells; but in contrast to the protein localization results of Järvinen *et al.* (1987) discussed above, they found high steady-state levels of stefin A mRNA in cultured undifferentiated epidermal cells, levels which decreased when these cells were induced to differentiate. *In situ* hybridization analysis of stefin A mRNA in mouse skin confirmed its presence in the less differentiated basal cells. It is possible that the immunofluorescence localization of the protein may reflect the accumulation of stefin A synthesized in less differentiated cells or that the stefin A mRNA is translated only when the cells are induced to differentiate. *In situ* hybridization analysis and immunodetection of stefin A in the same tissue needs to be done to resolve this. On the basis of the observation that stefin A mRNA expression was reduced in many chemically induced murine skin carcinomas in comparison with normal epithelium, Hawley-Nelson *et al.* (1988) suggested that there was a defect in stefin A regulation in malignant cells. If the regulation of stefin A mRNA and protein synthesis is compromised in tumor cells, this would be another factor contributing to the increased cysteine proteinase production seen in tumor cells.

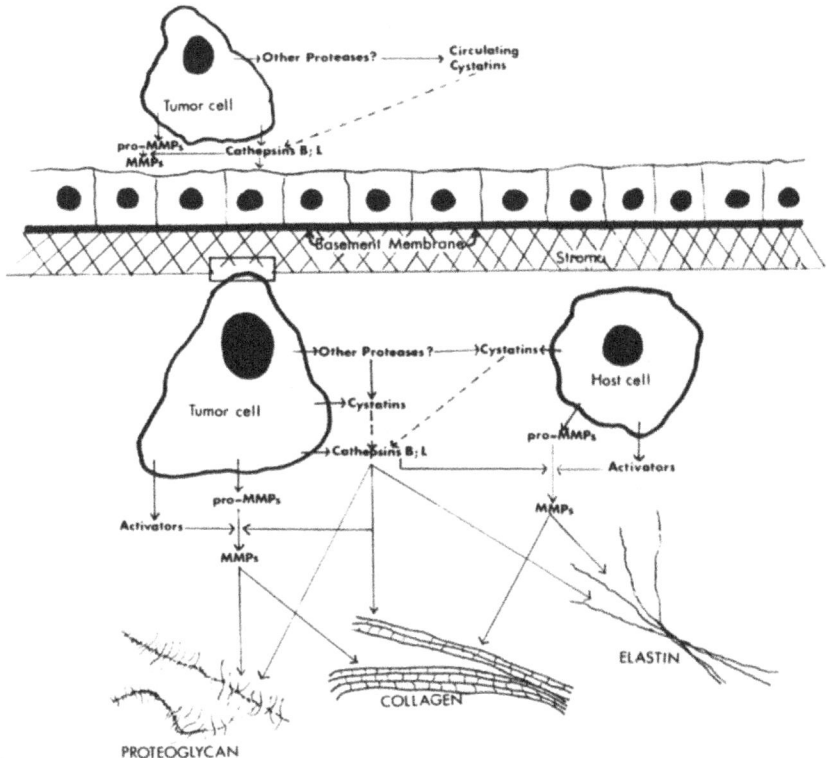

Figure 2. Schematic diagram of the possible roles of cysteine proteinases and their inhibitors during metastasis. The reactions shown are occurring in the boxed area where a tumor cell is penetrating the stroma and has established an isolated microenvironment in which acid conditions are transiently established. Cysteine proteinases can activate latent matrix metalloproteinases (MMPs) which then degrade the components of the extracellular matrix surrounding the invading cell. Cysteine proteinases can also degrade the matrix components. Both steps are regulated by secreted cysteine proteinase inhibitors (CPIs) and circulating CPIs such as the blood kininogens. Inhibition is designated by dashed lines.

Other investigators have detected CPIs in a number of carcinomas and melanomas. Rinne (1980) discovered a CPI immunologically similar to epidermal stefin A in epidermoid carcinoma, both in the primary tumor and in its metastasis. Tsushima *et al.* (1985) demonstrated the presence of a CPI with a M_r of ~ 10,000 in human melanoma tissue. This protein had characteristics and an inhibitory spectrum similar to members of the superfamily except for its smaller size. Tsushima and Hopsu-Havu (1987) showed that an extract from human squamous cell carcinomas contained stefins A, B, α-CPI (a kininogen), and a 43-kDa papain inhibitor. The 43-kDa papain inhibitor was originally isolated from psoriatic skin (Järvinen *et al.*, 1984). When human melanoma tissue was transplanted into nude mice, CPI activity increased during the tumor growth. This was due to two types of CPIs, a kininogen and stefins A and B identified by immunodiffusion studies (Tsushima *et al.*, 1988). Nishida *et al.* (1984) reported that an established human malignant melanoma line released substantial amounts of a CPI of $M_r \sim 10,300$ that differed from normal human thiol protease inhibitors. Breast cancers containing squamous cell metaplasia were shown to contain stefins A and B both inside the cancer cell and in the surrounding connective tissue (Kolář *et al.*, 1989); there appeared to be more stefin A in the fibrous stroma surrounding the less invasive cells. Two cell lines derived from breast cancers, MCF-7 and ZR-75-1, were also shown to stain positively for stefins A and B, and inhibitor production was regulated by estrogen. Cystatin C was not detected in these tumors.

There is one report of a defective stefin in a metastatic tumor (Lah *et al.*, 1989b). Stefin A isolated from a human spindle cell sarcoma had a tenfold higher K_i for liver cathepsin B relative to stefin A from normal human liver. The K_i for stefin B was similar in both tissues. The increase in K_i was characterized by both an increase in the rate of dissociation and a decrease in the rate of association. This was also true for the interaction of the sarcoma-derived stefin A with cathepsins L and H. It was suggested that stefin A isolated from the sarcoma had a different conformation than "normal" stefin A because the fluorescence spectra of the two proteins differed.

The increased cysteine proteinase activity often correlated with metastatic capacity can result from increased production of (active) enzyme or reduced inhibitor activity. For example, in a subpopulation of B16 amelanotic melanoma cells exhibiting increased cathepsin B activity, cathepsin B mRNA levels were similar to control nonmetastatic cells. The increased activity appeared to be due to a decrease in CPI activity (Rozhin *et al.*, 1990). Chambers *et al.* (1992) have observed that, in comparison with nonmetastatic NIH 3T3 cells, metastatic *ras*-transformed cells had increased levels of cathepsin L and B mRNA, as well as increased cysteine proteinase activity, in both cell extracts and conditioned media. Accompanying this increased proteinase activity was a decrease in apparent CPI activity (Chambers *et al.*, 1992). A summary of some of these findings is shown in Fig. 3. Possibly increased total proteinase activity in areas of focal degradation may degrade CPIs present; alternatively, expression of CPI genes might be downregulated in some cells in a coordinate fashion with the upregulation of cysteine proteinase genes. This latter scenario has also been suggested for metalloproteinases in these cells by Tuck *et al.* (1991), who found increased gelatinolytic activity accompanied by decreased mRNA for TIMP, relative to control cells. No matter how regulated, the effect of these changes would be increased net proteolytic degradative capacity of the tumor cells.

Very little is known concerning the role of members of the cystatin family in tumor invasion. Since they are located extracellularly, they presumably regulate cysteine proteinase activities in interstitial fluids. Rohrlich *et al.* (1986) isolated

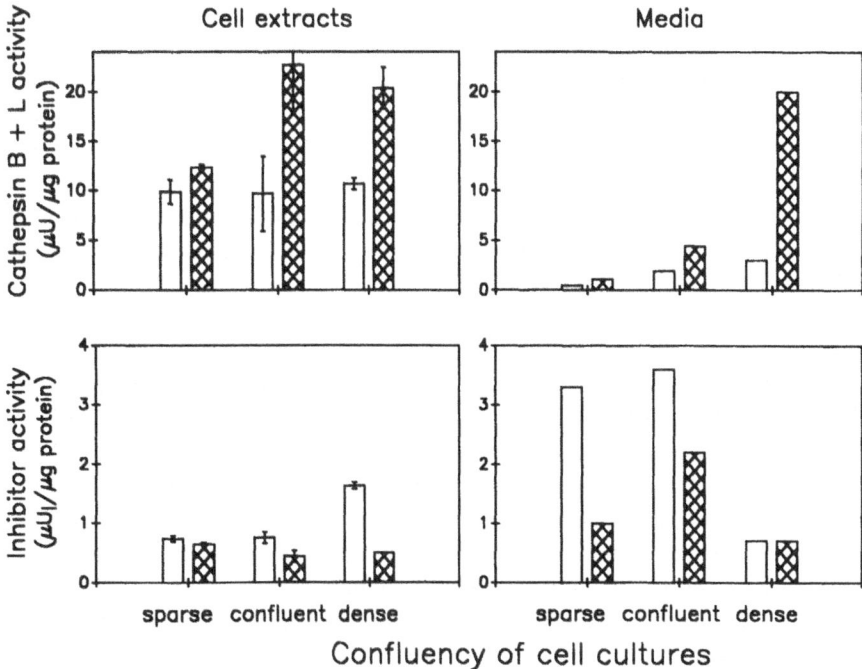

Figure 3. Net cysteine proteinase activity and cysteine proteinase inhibitor activity in NIH 3T3 cells (open bars) and in a metastatic ras-transformed derivative, PAP2 (cross-hatched bars) (Hill *et al.*, 1988). Cysteine proteinase activity in cell extracts and in conditioned media were measured using Z-Phe-Arg-NMec. CPI activity was determined from the ability of a heat-inactivated preparation to inhibit papain. Repeated experiments with sparse, confluent, and dense cell cultures consistently revealed increased proteolytic activity and unchanged or diminished inhibitor levels in the metastatic, *ras*-transformed cells (Chambers *et al.*, 1992).

human cystatin, stefin A, and other unidentified CPIs from human amniotic fluid and found that they, in contrast to inhibitors of metalloproteinases, were unable to block invasion of the human amnion by B16 melanoma cells, known to produce a cathepsin B-like activity. Likewise, Persky *et al.* (1986) did not detect inhibition of invasion when metastatic B16-F10 mouse melanoma cells were incubated in the presence of leupeptin. Mignatti *et al.* (1986) also found that CPIs were ineffective, even when preadsorbed to the membrane, at blocking invasion of the amnion by B16/BL6 cells whereas inhibitors of collagenase and plasmin were effective. Negative results such as these do not of course rule out the participation of a cysteine proteinase that is inaccessible to the inhibitor.

Using the human amnion model, Yagel *et al.* (1989) investigated the ability of several inhibitors to abrogate invasion of the basement membrane by mouse mammary carcinoma cells. Two synthetic inhibitors of cathepsin L, the peptidyl diazomethyl ketone Z-Phe-Phe-CHN$_2$ and the fluoromethylketone, Z-Phe-Ala-

CH_2F, and two natural CPIs isolated from muscle were studied. Both synthetic inhibitors suppressed invasion by 25-50%. The CPIs isolated from normal and dystrophic mouse muscle were almost as effective as the synthetic inhibitors in reducing the extent of invasion. These latter two inhibitors differed in their inhibitory spectrum. Whereas the inhibitor isolated from normal muscle inhibited both cathepsins B and L, the inhibitor isolated from dystrophic muscle did not inhibit cathepsin B (Gopalan et al., 1986). This is indirect evidence that cathepsin L may play a more important role in tumor invasion than cathepsin B in this cell line.

The members of the third cystatin superfamily, the kininogens, seem to function as acute-phase reactants (in that they are produced by host cells) during tumor cell invasion, as they do during an inflammatory response. Itoh et al. (1987) purified a CPI from the plasma of mice bearing sarcoma 180 tumors. Isolation of the inhibitor, which was more abundant in the plasma of tumor-bearing mice relative to normal mice, showed it to have a M_r of ~ 67,000. It inhibited papain, rat liver cathepsins B and L, but not cathepsin H. The inhibitor is a low-molecular-weight kininogen since it possesses amino acid sequence homology to known low-molecular-weight kininogens and releases bradykinin when incubated with kallikrein (Sueyoshi et al., 1990). The kininogen was secreted by cultured host liver cells but not by cultured sarcoma cells, suggesting that the increased plasma level of the kininogens was a host response for counteracting tumor growth.

A number of questions need to be addressed concerning the physiological significance of the members of the cystatin superfamily in cancer and in the defense mechanisms used by the host to combat transformed cells. These concern the regulation of expression of the CPIs and their chemical and biological properties, including their ability to function in focal areas of proteolysis. Hiwasa et al. (1988) have made the intriguing observation that the ras p21 proteins (which from amino acids 24 to 59 show some 60% sequence similarity to cystatin) are effective inhibitors of cathepsin L, but not cathepsin B, and can impair cleavage of the epidermal growth factor receptor in crude extracts; they speculate that ras p21 might act to inhibit receptor breakdown during endocytosis of activated receptors, thereby possibly stimulating cell proliferation. Interestingly, addition of chicken cystatin to the medium of normal mouse 3T3 fibroblasts increased the rate of cell proliferation (Sun, 1989), and repeated treatment of NIH 3T3 cells with cystatin or synthetic CPIs increased the saturation density and induced foci (Hiwasa et al. 1990).

As is so often the case, there is a Janus-like aspect to this story. We have taken the view that cysteine proteinases contributed positively to the malignant properties of the cell, and consequently inferred that the CPIs were beneficial because they inhibited proteinase activity. Alternatively, however, one could consider the impact of the CPI itself on the host's response to the tumor. For example, a CPI, e.g., cystatin C, could inhibit proteolytic attack on the cancer cell by suppressing the host's inflammatory reactions (Nishida *et al.*, 1986; Järvinen *et al.*, 1987; Leung-Tack *et al.*, 1990a). If this were the dominant effect, then excess production of cystatin C could enhance the oncogenicity of the cell!

ACKNOWLEDGMENTS. Preparation of this review was supported by funds from the National Institutes of Health (AG07972), the National Cancer Institute of Canada, and the Bureau of Biological Research, Rutgers University. AFC is a Career Scientist of the Ontario Cancer Treatment and Research Foundation.

6. References

Abrahamson, M., Grubb, A., Olafsson, I., and Lundwall, A., 1987, Molecular cloning and sequence analysis of cDNA coding for the precursor of the human cysteine proteinase inhibitor cystatin C, *FEBS Lett.* **216**:229–233.

Abrahamson, M., Olafsson, I., Palsdottier, A., Ulvsbäck, M. Lundwall, Å., Jensson, O., and Grubb, A., 1990, Structure and expression of the human cystatin gene, *Biochem. J.* **268**:287–294.

Achkar, C., Gong, Q., Frankfater, A., and Bajkowski, A. S., 1990, Differences in targeting and secretion of cathepsins B and L by BALB/3T3 fibroblasts and Moloney murine sarcoma virus-transformed BALB/3T3 fibroblasts, *J. Biol. Chem.* **265**:13650–13654.

Anastasi, A., Brown, M. A., Kembhavi, A. A., Nicklin, M. J. H., Sayer, C. A., Sunter, D. C., and Barrett, A. J., 1983, Cystatin, a protein inhibitor of cysteine proteinases, *Biochem. J.* **211**:129–138.

Baricos, W. H., Zhou, Y., Mason, R. W., and Barrett, A. J., 1988, Human kidney cathepsins B and L: Characterization and potential role in degradation of glomerular basement membrane, *Biochem. J.* **252**:301–304.

Barrett, A., 1987, The cystatins: A new class of peptidase inhibitors, *Trends Biol. Sci.* **12**:193–196.

Barrett, A. J., Fritz, H., Grubb, A., Isemura, S., Järvinen, M., Katunuma, N., Machleidt, W., Müller-Esterl, W., Sasaki, M., and Turk, V., 1986, Nomenclature and classification of the proteins homologous with the cysteine-proteinase inhibitor chicken cystatin, *Biochem. J.* **236**:312.

Bjorck, L., Grubb, A., and Kjellen, L., 1990, Cystatin C, a human proteinase inhibitor, blocks replication of herpes simplex virus, *J. Virol.* **64**:941–943.

Bode, W., Engh, R., Musil, D., Thiele, U., Huber, R., Karshikow, A., Brzin, J., Kos, J., and Turk, V., 1988, The 2.0 Å x-ray crystal structure of chicken egg white cystatin and its possible mode of interaction with cysteine proteinases, *EMBO J.* **7**:2593–2599.

Bollengier, F., 1987, Cystatin C, alias post-γ-globulin: A marker for multiple sclerosis? *J. Clin. Chem. Clin. Biochem.* **25**:589–593.

Bradford, H. N., Schmaier, A. H., and Colman, R. W., 1990, Kinetics of inhibition of platelet calpain II by human kininogens, *Biochem. J.* **270**:83–90.

Brzin, J., Kopitar, M., Turk, V., and Machleidt, W., 1983, Isolation and characterization of stefin, a cytosolic inhibitor of cysteine proteinases from human polymorphonuclear granulocytes, *Hoppe-Seylers Z. Physiol. Chem.* **364**:1475–1480.

Brzin, J., Popovic, T., Turk, V., Borchart, U., and Machleidt, W., 1984, Human cystatin, a new protein inhibitor of cysteine proteinases, *Biochem. Biophys. Res. Commun.* **118**:103–109.

Chambers, A. F., Colella, R., Denhardt, D. T., and Wilson, S. M., 1992, Increased expression of cathepsins L and B, and decreased activity of their inhibitors, in metastatic, *ras*-transformed NIH 3T3 cells, *Mole. Carcinogen* **5**:238–245.

Chauhan, S. S., Goldstein, L. J., and Gottesman, M. M., 1991, Expression of cathepsin L in human tumors, *Cancer Res.* **51**:1478–1481.

Colella, R., and Bird, J. W. C., 1993, Isolation and characterization of the chicken cystatin-encoding gene: mapping transcription start and polyadenylation sites, *Gene,* in press.

Colella, R., Sakaguchi, Y., Nagase, H., and Bird, J. W. C., 1989, Chicken egg white cystatin: Molecular cloning, nucleotide sequence, and tissue distribution, *J. Biol. Chem.* **264**:17164–17169.

Denhardt, D. T., Hamilton, R. T., Parfett, C. L. J., Edwards, D. R., St. Pierre, R., Waterhouse, P., and Nilsen-Hamilton, M., 1986, Close relationship of the major excreted protein of transformed murine fibroblasts to thiol-dependent cathepsins, *Cancer Res.* **46**:4590–4593.

Denhardt, D. T., Greenberg, A. H., Egan, S. E., Hamilton, R. T., and Wright, J. A., 1987, Cysteine proteinase cathepsin L expression correlates closely with the metastatic potential of H-ras-transformed murine fibroblasts, *Oncogene* **2**:55–59.

Dong, J., and Sahagian, G. G., 1990, Basis for low affinity binding of a lysosomal cysteine protease to the cation-independent mannose-6-phosphate receptor, *J. Biol. Chem.* **265**:4210–4217.

Dong, J., Prence, E. M., and Sahagian, G. G., 1989, Mechanism for selective secretion of a lysosomal protease by transformed mouse fibroblasts, *J. Biol. Chem.* **264**:7377–7383.

Elzanowski, A., Barker, W. C., Hunt, L. T., and Seibel-Ross, E., 1988, Cystatin domains in alpha-2-HS-glycoprotein and fetuin, *FEBS Lett.* **277**:167–170.

Erdel, M., Trefz, G., Spiess, E., Habermaas, S., Spring, H., Lah, T., and Ebert, W., 1991, Localization of cathepsin B in two human lung cancer cell lines, *J. Histochem. Cytochem.* **38**:1313–1321.

Ghiso, J., Jensson, O., and Frangione, B., 1986, Amyloid fibrils in hereditary cerebral hemorrhage with amyloidosis of Icelandic type is a variant of γ-trace basic protein (cystatin C), *Proc. Natl. Acad. Sci. USA* **83**:2974–2978.

Ghiso, J., Cowan, N., and Frangione, B., 1988, Isolation of a sequence encoding human cystatin C. Conservation of exon–intron structure between members of the cysteine proteinase inhibitors superfamily, *Biol. Chem. Hoppe-Seyler* **369**(S):205–208.

Goldberg, D. E., 1987, Biogenesis of lysosomal enzymes: Oligosaccharide chains, in: *Lysosomes: Their Role in Protein Breakdown* (H. Glauman and F. J. Ballard, eds.), Academic Press, New York, pp. 163–191.

Gopalan, P., Dufresne, M. J., and Warner, A. H., 1986, Evidence for a defective thiol protease inhibitor in skeletal muscle of mice with hereditary muscular dystrophy, *Biochem. Cell Biol.* **64**:1010–1019.

Green, G. D. J., Kembhavi, A. A., Davies, M. E., and Barrett, A. J., 1984, Cystatin-like cysteine proteinase inhibitors from human liver, *Biochem. J.* **218**:939–946.

Grubb, A., and Lofberg, H., 1982, Human γ-trace, a basic microprotein: Amino acid sequence and presence in the adenohypophysis, *Proc. Natl. Acad. Sci. USA* **79**:3024–3027.

Hawley-Nelson, P., Roop, D. R., Cheng, C. K., Krieg, T. M., and Yuspa, S. H., 1988, Molecular cloning of mouse epidermal cystatin A and detection of regulated expression in differentiation and tumorigenesis, *Mol. Carcinogenesis* **1**:202–211.

Hill, S. A., Wilson, S., and Chambers, A. F., 1988, Clonal heterogeneity, experimental metastatic ability, and p21 expression in H-ras-transformed NIH 3T3 cells, *J. Natl. Caner Inst.* **80**:484–490.

Hiwasa, T., Sakiyama, S., Yokoyama, S., Ha, J.-M., Fujita, J., Noguchi, S., Bando, Y., Kominami, E., and Katunuma, N., 1988, Inhibition of cathepsin L-induced degradation of epidermal growth factor receptors by c-Ha-ras gene products, *Biochem. Biophys. Res. Commun.* **151**:78–85.

Hiwasa, T., Sawada, T., and Sakiyama, S., 1990, Cysteine proteinase inhibitors and *ras* gene products share the same biological activities including transforming activity toward NIH3T3 mouse fibroblasts and the differentiation-inducing activity toward PC12 rat pheochromocytoma cells, *Carcinogenesis* **11**:75–80.

Isemura, S., Saitoh, E., and Sanada, K., 1984, Isolation and amino acid sequence of SAP-I an acidic protein of human whole saliva, and sequence homology with human γ-trace, *J. Biochem.* **96:**489–498.

Isemura, S., Saitoh, E., and Sanada, K., 1986, Characterization of a new cysteine proteinase inhibitor of human saliva, cystatin SN, which is immunologically related to cystatin S, *FEBS Lett.* **198:**145–149.

Itoh, N., Yokota, S., Takagishi, U., Hatta, A., and Okamoto, H., 1987, Thiol proteinase inhibitor in the ascitic fluid of sarcoma 180 tumor-bearing mice, *Cancer Res.* **47:**5560–5565.

Järvinen, M., and Rinne, A., 1992, Human spleen cysteine proteinase inhibitor. Purification, fractionation into isoelectric variants and some properties of the variants, *Biochim. Biophys. Acta* **708:**210–217.

Järvinen, M., Rinne, A., and Hopsu-Havu, V. K., 1984, Partial purification and some properties of a new papain inhibitor from psoriatic scales, *J. Invest. Dermatol.* **82:**471–476.

Järvinen, M., Rinne, A., and Hopsu-Havu, V. K., 1987, Human cystatins in normal and diseased tissues—A review, *Acta Histochem.* **82:**5–18.

Kellermann, J., Haupt, H., Auerswald, E.-A., and Müller-Ester, W., 1989, The arrangement of disulfide loops in human α_2-HS glycoprotein, *J. Biol. Chem.* **264:**14121–14128.

Khokha, R., and Denhardt, D. T., 1989, Matrix metalloproteinases and tissue inhibitor of metalloproteinases: A review of their role in tumorigenesis and tissue invasion, *Invasion Metastasis* **9:**391–405.

Kirschke, H., and Barrett, A. J., 1987, Chemistry of lysosomal proteases, in: *Lysosomes: Their role in Protein Breakdown* (H. Glauman and F. J. Ballard, eds.), Academic Press, New York, pp. 163–191.

Kirschke, H., Kembhavi, A. A., Bohley, P., and Barrett, A. J., 1982, Action of rat liver cathepsin L on collagen and other substrates, *Biochem. J.* **201:**367–372.

Kitamura, N., Kitagawa, H., Fukushima, D., Takagaki, Y., Miyata, T., and Nakanishi, S., 1985, Structural organization of the human kininogen gene and a model for its evolution, *J. Biol. Chem.* **260:**8610–8617.

Koide, T., 1988, Human histidine-rich glycoprotein gene: Evidence for evolutionary relatedness to cystatin supergene family, *Thromb. Res. Suppl.* 8:91–97.

Kolář, Z., Järvinen, M., and Negrini, R., 1989, Demonstration of proteinase inhibitors cystatin A, B and C in breast cancer and in cell lines MCF-7 and ZR-75-1, *Neoplasma* **36:**185–189.

Korant, B. D., Towatari, T., Ivanoff, L., Petteway, S., Jr., Brzin, J., Lenarcie, B., and Turk, V., 1986, Viral therapy: Prospects for protease inhibitors, *J. Cell Biochem.* **32:**91–95.

Lah, T. T., Buck, M. B., Honn, K. V., Crissman, J. D., Rao, N. C., Liotta, L. A., and Sloane, B. F., 1989a, Degradation of laminin by human tumor cathepsin B, *Clin. Exp. Metastasis* **7:**461–468.

Lah, T. T., Clifford, J. L., Helmer, K. M., Day, N. A., Moin, K., Honn, K. V., Crissman, J. D., and Sloane, B. F., 1989b, Inhibitory properties of low molecular mass cysteine proteinase inhibitor from human sarcoma, *Biochim. Biophys. Acta* **993:**63–73.

Lazzarino, D., and Gabel, C. A., 1990, Protein determinants impair recognition of procathepsin L phosphorylated oligosaccharides by the cation-independent mannose 6-phosphate receptor, *J. Biol. Chem.* **265:**11864–11871.

Lenarcic, B., Krasovec, M., Ritonja, A., Olafsson, I., and Turk, V., 1991, Inactivation of human cystatin C and kininogen by human cathepsin D, *FEBS Lett.* **280:**211–215.

Leung-Tack, J., Tavera, C., Gensac, M. C., Martinez, J., and Colle, A., 1990a, Modulation of phagocytosis-associated respiratory burst by human cystatin C: Role of the N-terminal tetrapeptide lys-pro-pro-arg, *Exp. Cell Res.* **188:**16–22.

Leung-Tack, J., Tavera, C., Martinez, J., and Colle, A., 1990b, Neutrophil chemotactic activity is modulated by human cystatin C, an inhibitor of cysteine proteinases, *Inflammation* **14:**247–258.

Liotta, L. A., Steeg, P. S., and Stetler-Stevenson, W. G., 1991, Cancer metastasis and angiogenesis: An imbalance of positive and negative regulation, *Cell* **64:**327–336.

Machleidt, W., Borchart, U., Fritz, H., Brzin, J., Ritonja, A., and Turk, V., 1983, Primary structure of stefin, a cytosolic protein inhibitor of cysteine proteinases from human polymorphonuclear granulocytes, *Hoppe-Seyler Z. Physiol. Chem.* **364**:1481–1486.

Machleidt, W., Thiele, U., Laber, B., Assfalg-Machleidt, I., Esterl, A., Wiegand, G., Kos, J., Turk, V., and Bode, W., 1989, Mechanisms of inhibition of papain by chicken egg white cystatin. Inhibition constants of N-terminally truncated forms and cyanogen bromide fragments of the inhibitor, *FEBS Lett.* **243**:234–238.

Maciewicz, R. A., Etherington, D. J., Kos, J., and Turk, V., 1987, Collagenolytic cathepsins of rabbit spleen: A kinetic analysis of collagen degradation and inhibition by chicken cystatin, *Collagen Relat. Res.* **7**:295–304.

Maciewicz, R. A., Wardale, R. J., Etherington, D. J., and Paraskeva, C., 1989, Immunodetection of cathepsins B and L present in and secreted from human pre-malignant and malignant colorectal tumor cells lines, *Int. J. Cancer* **43**:478–486.

Mannucci, P. M., Cugno, M., Bottasso, B., Marongiu, F., Maniezzo, M., Vaglini, M., and Cascinelli, N., 1990, Changes in fibrinolysis in patients with localized tumors, *Eur. J. Cancer* **26**:83–87.

Mason, R. W., Johnson, D. A., Barrett, A. J., and Chapman, H. A. 1986a, Elastinolytic activity of human cathepsin L, *Biochem. J.* **233**:925–927.

Mason, R. W., Walker, J. E., and Northrop, F. D., 1986b, The N-terminal amino acid sequences of the heavy and light chains of human cathepsin L. Relationship to a cDNA clone for a major cysteine proteinase from a mouse macrophage cell line, *Biochem. J.* **240**:373–377.

Meloni, F. J., and Schmaier, A. H. 1991, Low molecular weight kininogen binds to platelets to modulate thrombin-induced platelet activation, *J. Biol. Chem.* **266**:6786–6794.

Mignatti, P., Robbins, E., and Rifkin, D. B., 1986, Tumor invasion through the human amniotic membrane: Requirement for a proteinase cascade, *Cell* **47**:487–498.

Moin, K., Rozhin, J., McKernan, T. B., Sanders, V. J., Fong, D., Honn, K. V., and Sloane, B. F., 1989, Enhanced levels of cathepsin B mRNA in murine tumors, *FEBS Lett.* **244**:61–64.

Moreau, T., Gutman, N., Moujahed, A. E., Esnard, F., and Gauthier, F., 1986, Relationship between the cysteine-proteinase-inhibitory function of rat T kininogen and the release of immunoreactive kinin upon trypsin treatment, *Eur. J. Biochem.* **159**:341–346.

Mort, J. S., and Recklies, A. D., 1986, Interrelationship of active and latent secreted human cathepsin B precursors, *Biochem. J.* **223**:57–63.

Murnane, M. J., Sheahan, K., Ozdemirli, M., and Shuja, S., 1991, Stage-specific increases in cathepsin B mRNA content in human colorectal carcinoma, *Cancer Res.* **51**:1137–1142.

Nishida, Y., Sumi, H., and Mihara, H., 1984, A thiol protease inhibitor released from cultured human malignant melanoma cells, *Cancer Res.* **44**:3324–3329.

Nishida, Y., Tsushima, H., Toki, N., Sumi, H., and Mihara, H., 1986, Thiol protease inhibitors released from human malignant melanoma, in: *Cysteine Proteinase and Their Inhibitors* (V. Turk, ed.), Gruyter, Berlin, pp. 751–760.

Ohkubo, I., Kurachi, K., Takasawa, T., Shiokawa, H., and Sasaki, M., 1984, Isolation of a human cDNA for α_2-thiol proteinase inhibitor and its identity with low molecular weight kininogen, *Biochemistry* **23**:5691–5697.

Ohkubo, I., Namikawa, C., Higashiyama, S., Sasaki, M., Minowa, O., Mizuno, Y., and Shiokawa, H., 1988, Purification and characterization of α_1-thiol proteinase inhibitor and its identity with kinin- and fragment 1.2-free high molecular weight kininogen, *Int. J. Biochem.* **20**:243–258.

Olafsson, I., Gudmundsson, G., Abrahamson, M., Gensson, O., and Grubb, A., 1990, The amino terminal portion of cerebrospinal fluid cystatin C in hereditary cystatin C amyloid angiopathy is not truncated: Direct sequence analysis from agarose gel electrophoresis, *Scand. J. Clin. Invest.* **50**:85–93.

Persky, B., Ostrowski, L. E., Pagast, P., Ahsan, A., and Schultz, R. M., 1986, Inhibition of proteolytic enzymes in the *in vitro* amnion model for basement membrane invasion, *Cancer Res.* **46**:4129–4134.

Portnoy, D. A., Erickson, A. H., Kochan, J., Ravetch, J. V., and Unkeless, J. C., 1986, Cloning and characterization of a mouse cysteine proteinase, *J. Biol. Chem.* **261**:14697–14703.

Prence, E. M., Dong, J., and Sahagian, G. G., 1990, Modulation of the transport of a lysosomal enzyme by PDGF, *J. Cell Biol.* **110**:319–326.

Puri, R. N., Zhou, F., Hu, C. J., Colman, R. F., and Colman, R. W., 1991, High molecular weight kininogen inhibits thrombin-induced platelet aggregation and cleavage of aggregin by inhibiting binding of thrombin to platelets, *Blood* **77**:500–507.

Qian, F., Bajkowski, A. S., Steiner, D. F., Chan, S. J., and Frankfater, A., 1989, Expression of five cathepsins in murine melanomas of varying metastatic potential and normal tissues, *Cancer Res.*, **49**:4870–4875.

Rawlings, N. D., and Barrett, A. J., 1990, Evolution of proteins of the cystatin superfamily, *J. Mol. Evol.* **30**:60–71.

Rinne, A., 1980, Epidermal SH-protease inhibitor in human neoplasms and their metastases, *Pathol. Res. Pract.* **170**:172–179.

Ritonja, A., Machleidt, W., and Barrett, A. J., 1985, Amino acid sequence of the intracellular cysteine proteinase inhibitor cystatin B from human liver, *Biochem. Biophys. Res. Commun.* **131**:1187–1192.

Rohrlich, S. T., Seigfried, Z., Mignatti, P., Machleidt, W., Levy, H., and Rifkin, D. B., 1986, Characterization of low molecular mass cysteine proteinase inhibitors from human amniotic fluid, in: *Cysteine Proteinases and Their Inhibitors* (V. Turk, ed.), Gruyter, Berlin, pp. 455–471.

Rozhin, J., Robinson, D., Steven, M. A., Lah, T. T., Honn, K. V., Ryan, R. E., and Sloane, B. F., 1987, Properties of a plasma membrane-associated cathepsin B-like cysteine proteinase in metastatic B16 melanoma variants, *Cancer Res.* **47**:6620–6628.

Rozhin, J., Gomez, A. P., Ziegler, G. H., Nelson, K. K., Chang, Y. S., Fong, D., Onoda, J. M., Honn, K. V., and Sloane, B. F., 1990, Cathepsin B to cysteine proteinase inhibitor balance in metastatic cell subpopulations isolated from murine tumors, *Cancer Res.* **50**:6278–6284.

Ryan, C. A., 1989, Proteinase inhibitor gene families: Strategies for transformation to improve plant defenses against herbivores, *BioEssays* **10**:20–24.

Saitoh, E., Kim, H.-S., Smithies, O., and Maeda, N., 1987, Human cysteine-proteinase inhibitors: Nucleotide sequence analysis of three members of the cystatin gene family, *Gene* **61**:329–338.

Saitoh, E., Isemura, S., Sanada, K., Kim, H.-S., Smithies, O., and Maeda, N., 1988, Cystatin superfamily: Evidence that family II cystatin genes are evolutionarily related to family III cystatin genes, *Biol. Chem. Hoppe-Seyler* **39**:191–197.

Salvesen, G., Parkes, C., Abrahamson, M., Grubb, A., and Barrett, A. J., 1986, Human low-M$_r$ kininogen contains three copies of a cystatin sequence that are divergent in structure and in inhibitory activity for cysteine proteinases, *Biochem. J.* **234**:429–434.

Schelp, F. P., and Pongpaew, P., 1988, Protection against cancer through nutritionally-induced increase of endogenous proteinase inhibitors—A hypothesis, *Int. J. Epidemiol.* **17**:287–292.

Schultz, R. M., Silberman, S., Persky, B., Bajkowski, A. S., and Carmichael, D. F., 1988, Inhibition by human recombinant tissue inhibitor of metalloproteinases of human amnion invasion and lung colonization by murine B16-F10 melanoma cells, *Cancer Res.* **48**:5539–5545.

Sen, L. C., and Whitaker, J. R., 1973, Some properties of a ficin–papain inhibitor from avian egg white, *Arch. Biochem. Biophys.* **158**:623–632.

Shaw, P. A., Cox, J. L., Barka, T., and Naito, Y., 1988, Cloning and sequencing of a cDNA encoding a rat salivary cysteine proteinase inhibitor inducible by β-adrenergic agonists, *J. Biol. Chem.* **263**:18133–18137.

Sheahan, K., Shuja, S., and Murnane, M. J., 1989, Cysteine protease activities and tumor development in human colorectal carcinoma, *Cancer Res.* **49**:3809–3814.

Silver, I. A., Murrills, R. J., and Etherington, D. J., 1988, Microelectrode studies on the acid microenvironment beneath adherent macrophages and osteoclasts, *Exp. Cell Res.* **175**:266–276.

Sloane, B. F., Honn, K. V., Sadler, J. G., Turner, W. A., Kimpson, J. J., and Tayor, J. D., 1982,

Cathepsin B activity in B16 melanoma cells: A possible marker for metastatic potential, *Cancer Res.* **42**:980–986.

Sloane, B. F., Rozhin, J., Johnson, K., Taylor, H., Crissman, J. D., and Honn, K. V., 1986, Cathepsin B: Association with plasma membrane in metastatic tumors, *Proc. Natl. Acad. Sci. USA* **83**:2483–2487.

Sloane, B. F., Rozhin, J., Hatfield, J. S., Crissman, J. D., and Honn, K. V., 1987, Plasma membrane-associated cysteine proteinases in human and animal tumors, *Exp. Cell Biol.* **55**:209–224.

Sloane, B. F., Moin, K., Krepela, E., and Rozhin, J., 1990, Cathepsin B and its endogenous inhibitors: Their role in tumor malignancy, *Cancer Metastasis Rev.* **9**:333–352.

Spanier, A. M., and Bird, J. W. C., 1982, Endogenous cathepsin B inhibitor activity in normal and myopathic red and white skeletal muscle, *Muscle Nerve* **5**:313–320.

Stormorken, H., Briseid, K., Hellum, B., Hoem, N. O., Johansen, H. T., and Ly, B., 1990, A new case of total kininogen deficiency, *Thromb. Res.* **60**:457–467.

Stubbs, M. T., Laber, B., Bode, W., Huber, R., Jerala, R., Lenarcic, B., and Turk, V., 1990, The refined 2.4 Å X-ray crystal structure of recombinant human stefin B in complex with the cysteine proteinase papain: A novel type of proteinase inhibitor interaction, *EMBO J.* **9**:1939–1947.

Sueyoshi, T., Uwani, M., Itoh, N., Okamoto, H., Muta, T., Tokunaga, F., Takada, K., and Iwanaga, S., 1990, Cysteine proteinase inhibitor in the ascitic fluid of sarcoma 180 tumor-bearing mice is a low molecular weight kininogen, *J. Biol. Chem.* **265**:10030–10035.

Sun, Q., 1989, Growth stimulation of 3T3 fibroblasts by cystatin, *Exp. Cell Res.* **180**:150–160.

Takio, K., Kominami, E., Wakamatsu, N., Katunuma, N., and Titani, K., 1983, Amino acid sequence of rat liver thiol proteinase inhibitor, *Biochem. Biophys. Res. Commun.* **115**:902–908.

Takio, K., Kominami, K., Bando, Y., Katunuma, N., and Titani, K., 1984, Amino acid sequence of rat epidermal thiol proteinase inhibitor, *Biochem. Biophys. Res. Commun.* **121**:149–154.

Troen, B. R., Gal, S., and Gottesman, M. M., 1987, Sequence and expression of the cDNA for MEP (major excreted protein), a transformation-regulated secreted cathepsin, *Biochem. J.* **246**:731–735.

Troll, W., 1989, Protease inhibitors interfere with the necessary factors of carcinogenesis, *Environ. Health Perspect.* **81**:59–62.

Tsushima, H., and Hopsu-Havu, V. K., 1987, Cysteine proteinase inhibitors in human squamous cell carcinoma, *Acta Histochem.* **85**:23–28.

Tsushima, H., Sumi, H., Hamanaka, K., Toki, N., Sato, H., and Mihara, H., 1985, Cysteine protease inhibitors isolated from human malignant melanoma tissue, *J. Lab. Clin. Med.* **106**:712–717.

Tsushima, H., Sumi, H., Mihara, H., Joronen, I., and Hopsu-Havu, V. K., 1988, Cysteine proteinase inhibitors in human melanoma transplanted into nude mice, *Biol. Chem. Hoppe-Seyler* **369**(S):243–250.

Tuck, A. B., Wilson, S. M., Khokha, R., and Chambers, A. F., 1991, Different patterns of gene expression in *ras*-resistant and *ras*-sensitive cells, *J. Natl. Cancer Inst.* **83**:485–491.

Warfel, A. H., Cardozo, C., Yoo, O. H., and Zucker-Franklin, D., 1991, Cystatin C and cathepsin B production by alveolar macrophages from smokers and nonsmokers, *J. Leukocyte Biol.* **49**:41–47.

Wood, L., Yorke, G., Roisen, F., and Bird, J. W. C., 1985, A low molecular weight cysteine proteinase inhibitor from chicken skeletal muscle, in: *Intracellular Protein Catabolism* (J. Bond, E. Khairallah, and J. W. C. Bird, eds.), Liss, New York, pp. 81–90.

Yagel, S., Warner, A. H., Nellans, H. N., Lala, P. K., Waghorne, C., and Denhardt, D. T., 1989, Suppression by cathepsin L inhibitors of the invasion of amnion membranes by murine cancer cells, *Cancer Res.* **49**:3553–3557.

Yamaguchi, N., Chung, S. M., Shiroeda, O., Koyama, K., and Imanishi, J., 1990, Characterization of a cathepsin L-like enzyme secreted from human pancreatic cancer cell line HPC-YP, *Cancer Res.* **50**:658–663.

13

Cell Membrane Enzymes Containing Chymotrypsin-like Activity

JONATHAN YAVELOW, LORRAINE T. SCHEPIS, JOSEPH NICKELS, JR., and GEORGE RITCHIE

1. Introduction

The study of protease inhibitors and carcinogenesis has aided in the identification of proteolytic enzymes in the regulation of cell growth, invasion, and metastasis. Since the early 1970s the value of protease inhibitors in the suppression of tumorigenesis has been demonstrated in a variety of tumors (Troll *et al.*, 1970; Hozumi *et al.*, 1972; Weed *et al.*, 1985). The proteases, namely, plasminogen activator, plasmin, collagenase (Mignatti *et al.*, 1986), and cathepsin D (Sloane *et al.*, 1986), are primarily appreciated for their role in invasion and metastasis. However, Corasanti *et al.* (1982) have demonstrated that ε-aminocaproic acid suppresses dimethylhydrazine-induced colon tumors in mice, implicating a possible role for plasminogen activator in the mechanism of carcinogenesis. The control of intracellular protein turnover (Waxman *et al.*, 1985; Hershko, 1988), the maturation of polypeptide precursors (Bathurst *et al.*, 1987), the regulation of neutrophil activation (King *et al.*, 1987), and the control of sister chromatid exchange (Kennedy *et al.*, 1984) are several examples where proteases have been directly or indirectly implicated in cellular regulation.

In addition to affecting carcinogenesis *in vivo*, protease inhibitors have been shown to suppress *in vitro* cell transformation induced by a variety of carcino-

JONATHAN YAVELOW • Department of Biology, Rider College, Lawrenceville, New Jersey 08648.   *LORRAINE T. SCHEPIS* • Department of Molecular Biology, Princeton University, Princeton, New Jersey 08530.   *JOSEPH NICKELS, JR.* • Department of Microbiology and Molecular Genetics, Rutgers University, New Brunswick, New Jersey 08903.   *GEORGE RITCHIE* • Department of Physics, Rider College, Lawrenceville, New Jersey 08648.
Protease Inhibitors as Cancer Chemopreventive Agents, edited by Walter Troll and Ann R. Kennedy. Plenum Press, New York, 1993.

gens. The C3H/10T1/2 cell line has proven sensitive to radiation (Kennedy, 1984)-, chemical (Kuroki and Drevon, 1979)-, and oncogene-mediated cell transformation (Taparowsky *et al.*, 1987). All of these transformation experiments have proven to be sensitive to protease inhibitors (Yavelow *et al.*, 1985; Kuroki and Drevon, 1979; Billings *et al.*, 1987b; Baturay and Kennedy, 1986). Protease inhibitors of various specificities suppress *in vitro* transformation (for review see Kennedy, 1984) and have led to the identification of several target proteases involved in the mechanism of cell transformation (Billings *et al.*, 1987a; Yavelow *et al.*, 1987a).

The Bowman–Birk soybean proteinase inhibitor (BBI) has been shown to be an effective anticarcinogen *in vitro* (Yavelow *et al.*, 1983, 1985) and *in vivo* (Weed *et al.*, 1985). Human epidemiological studies have also suggested that legume-rich diets afford protection against breast and colon cancer (Correa, 1981). Thus, BBI may represent a nutritionally relevant anticarcinogen (Yavelow, 1986). In an effort to unravel the mechanism of anticarcinogenic action of BBI, we have mapped its anticarcinogenic domain to its chymotrypsin inhibitory activity and demonstrated its potency in nanomolar levels (Yavelow *et al.*, 1985). Recently we identified a membrane protease which is inhibited by BBI and chymostatin and hydrolyzes chymotrypsin substrates (Yavelow *et al.*, 1987a). Furthermore, using fluorescence microscopy we have identified receptor-mediated endocytosis of BBI (Yavelow *et al.*, 1987b). These studies suggest there may be a plasma membrane chymotrypsin-like protease involved in the mechanism of cell transformation which may also act as a receptor for protease inhibitors.

The particular focus of this chapter will be on cell membrane enzymes containing chymotrypsin-like enzyme activity. These proteases hypothetically act to trigger amplification cascades that irreversibly activate various cellular phenomena including transformation. This chapter will review: (1) studies with various protease inhibitors showing that chymotrypsin inhibitors effectively suppress transformation; (2) studies identifying membrane chymotrypsin-like proteases; (3) potential substrates for these chymotrypsin-like enzymes; (4) fluorescence anisotropy as a tool for studying the anticarcinogenic action of chymostatin.

2. *Effect of Chymotrypsin Inhibitors on in Vitro Cell Transformation*

We have observed that soybean BBI double-headed trypsin–chymotrypsin protease inhibitors, but not trypsin inhibitors, are capable of suppressing *in vitro* cell transformation induced by radiation (Yavelow *et al.*, 1985). Other studies with enzymatically modified BBI have shown that the chymotrypsin inhibitory domain of BBI is responsible for suppression of *in vitro* cell transformation. These results complemented by experiments showing that chymostatin also inhibits *in vitro* cell transformation of C3H/10T1/2 cells (Kuroki and Drevon,

1979; Kennedy, 1985) led us to study chymotrypsin-like proteases and their potential role in mediating cell transformation. Our observation that serum-containing media, which also contain protease inhibitors, can support *in vitro* cell transformation, whereas chymostatin and BBI suppress transformation suggests that these later protease inhibitors have a specific affinity for certain cellular components.

Certain data from these experiments have been compiled in Table I. Except for the study of Kuroki and Drevon (1979), all transformation experiments were performed in Dr. Ann Kennedy's laboratory. In the summarized experiments, protease inhibitors were added immediately after transformation and continued throughout the entire 6-week assay period. BBI consistently suppresses appearance of foci when the data are expressed as No. of foci/No. of dishes or No. of

Table I. Chymotrypsin Inhibitor Suppression of Cell Transformation

Carcinogen	Protease inhibitor (μg/ml)	No. of foci / No. of dishes	No. of dishes with foci / Total no. of dishes	Reference
X rays	Control	20/41 = 0.49	19/41 = 0.46	Yavelow et al.
	BBI (100)	8/45 = 0.18	6/45 = 0.13	(1983)
	Control	53/79 = 0.67	20/79 = 0.25	Yavelow et al.
	BBI (2.5)	10/38 = 0.26	8/38 = 0.21	(1985)
	BBI' (2.5)	2/19 = 0.11	2/19 = 0.11	
	Control	27/39 = 0.69	19/39 = 0.49	
	CPI (2.5)	1/20 = 0.05	1/20 = 0.05	
	BBI (2.5)	22/77 = 0.29	19/77 = 0.25	
	BBI(−T) (2.5)	2/20 = 0.10	2/20 = 0.10	
	BBI(−TC) (2.5)	9/20 = 0.45	7/20 = 0.35	
	Control	10/37 = 0.27	10/37 = 0.27	
	BBI (0.1)	1/39 = 0.03	1/39 = 0.03	
	Control	31/40 = 0.78	23/40 = 0.58	Billings et al.
	CI-1 (10)	4/38 = 0.11	3/38 = 0.08	(1987b)
Benzo(a)pyrene	Control	20/18 = 1.1	N.A.	Baturay and
	Crude BBI (300)	3/17 = 0.18	N.A.	Kennedy
Propiolactone	Control	33/18 = 1.8	N.A.	(1986)
	Crude BBI (300)	5/16 = 0.3	N.A.	
^{60}Co	Control	135/16 = 8.4	N.A.	
	Crude BBI (300)	11/18 = 0.6	N.A.	
Methylcholan-threne	Control	20/22 = 0.91	10/22 = 0.45	Kuroki and
	Chymostatin (50)	1/22 = 0.05	1/22 = 0.05	Drevon (1979)
X rays	Control	98/133 = 0.74	67/133 = 0.50	Kennedy
	Chymostatin (10)	1/47 = 0.02	1/47 = 0.02	(1985)
	Chymostatin (1.0)	11/89 = 0.12	11/89 = 0.12	
	Chymostatin (0.1)	6/64 = 0.09	6/64 = 0.09	

dishes containing foci/total No. of dishes. For x-ray-induced (600 rad) transformation, approximately 50% of the dishes contain foci in controls and there is approximately 0.5–0.7 focus/dish. BBI decreases this number to approximately 0.2 focus/dish or 0.2 dish containing foci/total No. of dishes. BBI' produces a decrease to 0.1 focus/dish or 0.1 dish containing foci/total No. of dishes. BBI' represents a slightly more negatively charged form of BBI. The precise difference between BBI and BBI' is currently being investigated. CPI (the trypsin and chymotrypsin inhibitor from chick peas) suppresses transformation to 0.005 focus/dish and the BBI(−T) (modified BBI such that it is a chymotrypsin inhibitor only) suppresses transformation to 0.1 focus/dish. The BBI(−TC) (modified BBI devoid of protease inhibitory activity) fails to suppress transformation with 0.45 focus/dish. Also included is an experiment where only 0.27 focus/dish was achieved in the positive control; 0.1 μg/ml BBI suppressed transformation to 0.03 focus/dish in this experiment. Precise quantitation, thus, remains difficult in C3H/10T1/2 cell transformation assays; however, in numerous independent experiments using a variety of carcinogens [e.g., benzo(a)pyrene, propiolactone, γ rays and x rays], chymotrypsin inhibitors consistently suppress the appearance of foci from 60–90% of the control. Chymotrypsin inhibitor I from potatoes (CI-1) and chick pea inhibitor (CPI) represent two other double-headed chymotrypsin inhibitors of the Bowman–Birk family which suppress cell transformation. Chymostatin is the most potent protease inhibitor where 10^{-12} M results in a statistically significant reduction of transformation (Kennedy, 1985). At 0.1 μg/ml (10^{-7} M), chymostatin yields 0.09 focus/dish or No. of dishes containing foci/total No. of dishes. Our working hypothesis is that the different chymotrypsin inhibitors have similar intracellular biochemical targets.

3. Properties of Cell Membrane Enzymes Containing Chymotrypsin-like Activity

During the past few years we have pursued the cellular target of BBI and chymostatin. We have observed low levels of chymotrypsin-like enzymes in normal and transformed C3H/10T1/2 cells. This low level of enzyme has presented problems in terms of enzyme isolation and characterization; however, it is consistent with its role in regulating specific cellular processes. The enzyme hydrolyzes specific chymotrypsin substrate (Suc-Ala-Ala-Pro-Phe p-nitroanilide or aminomethyl coumarin) as well as FITC-casein. From normal C3H/10T1/2 cells it is only extractable with detergents and is therefore an integral membrane protease. Sucrose density gradient centrifugation localizes the enzyme to the same fraction as 5′-nucleotidase (a plasma membrane marker). The partially purified enzyme (after DEAE-cellulose chromatography) hydrolyzes only specific chymotrypsin synthetic substrates, has a pH optimum of about 7.0, is stimulated by Ca^{2+} and inhibited by EDTA, BBI, chymostatin, and diisopropyl fluorophosphate (Yavelow *et al.*, 1987a; Yavelow, Schepis, and Nickels, unpublished results). For these reasons we may have a Ca^{2+}-activated chymotrypsin-like serine protease in the membranes of C3H/10T1/2 cells. The low enzyme activity could be due to the regulatory function of the protease or inappropriate assay conditions or endogenous protease–protease inhibitor complexes.

4. Potential Cellular Substrates for Membrane Chymotrypsin-like Enzymes

A model for three· different activities potentially associated with plasma membrane chymotrypsin-like proteases is diagrammed in Fig. 1. Chymostatin-sensitive protease has been detected in crude membrane preparations of Rous sarcoma virus-transformed chick embryo fibroblasts (O'Donnell-Tormey and Quigley, 1983). This enzyme may mediate the release of cell-associated plasminogen activator to an extracellular form (O'Donnell-Tormey and Quigley, 1981). It has also been reported that plasminogen activator slowly degrades fibronectin in the absence of plasminogen (Quigley *et al.*, 1987). Thus, cell attachment and subsequently cell shape may change as a result of the release of cell-associated plasminogen activator.

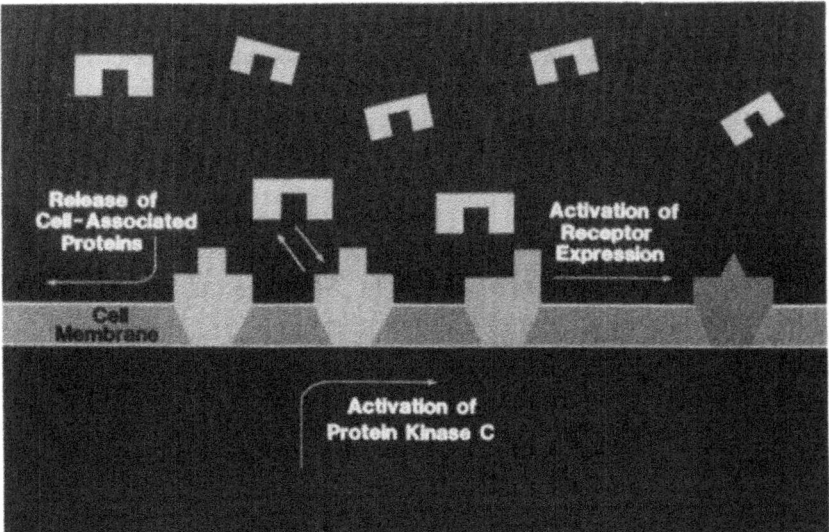

Figure 1. Representation of three possible actions catalyzed by membrane-bound proteases. White floating shapes represent protease inhibitors and light gray shapes represent the target plasma membrane protease. Release of cell-associated proteins, activation of receptor expression, and activation of protein kinase C represent three potential functions of the membrane protease.

Another instance where membrane-associated chymotrypsin-like proteases seem to be involved is in the internalization of the insulin receptor. Internalization of insulin receptors via receptor-mediated endocytosis has been blocked by the chymotrypsin substrate acetyl tyrosine ethylester (Joshen and Berhanu, 1987), suggesting that the insulin receptor's internalization may require a chymotrypsin-like protease trigger. If, in fact, the chymotrypsin-like protease can clip the cytoplasmic domain of the insulin receptor, then it would trigger endocytosis but not recycling. The irreversibility of a proteolytic clip could result in "targeting" that specific receptor for degradation—not recycling.

In addition to the direct effect of proteases on receptors, there is a poorly understood phenomenon of "receptor expression." The protease inhibitors do not directly interact with receptors; rather, they are thought to affect the access of receptor to ligand. For example, antipain and leupeptin indirectly inhibit platelet fibrinogen receptor binding to fibrinogen and subsequent serotonin release (Baldessaire *et al.*, 1985). Proteases, in other words, may affect the geometry of receptors within the membrane, thus regulating "receptor expression."

Two membrane-bound enzymes are also substrates for proteases: protein kinase C and NADPH oxidase. The neutrophil NADPH oxidase necessary for superoxide generation in activated neutrophils is activated by a protease (Yavelow *et al.*, 1982; King *et al.*, 1987). King *et al.* isolated a monoclonal antibody against neutrophil membranes which blocked neutrophil activation and superoxide generation. This antibody was also an inhibitor of chymotrypsin. The superoxide-generating oxidase is elevated in activity in phagocytosing neutrophils, although it may also be present in lower levels in other cell types. In the case of protein kinase C, the calcium- and phospholipid-dependent membrane-bound form is converted by a neutral protease to a soluble enzyme fragment which is independent of these cofactors. The relative levels of membrane-associated versus soluble kinase will obviously have enormous effects on cell growth regulation.

5. Fluorescence Anisotropy as a Tool for Studying the Anticarcinogenic Action of Chymostatin

Recently we have characterized the fluorescence of chymostatin and have observed, using the anisotropy of fluorescence polarization, the binding of chymostatin to chymotrypsin. The fluorescence anisotropy enables us to monitor protease–protease inhibitor binding directly rather than via kinetics analysis. Chymostatin exhibits a sizable fluorescence emission (410 nm) under near-UV (315 nm) excitation. Using pulsed-laser excitation we have found that chymostatin has two characteristic fluorescence lifetimes: a dominant lifetime of 4.2 nsec and a 0.4-nsec component. Fluorescence measurements for chymostatin in the presence of varying amounts of chymotrypsin revealed a plateau-type maxi-

mum in the anisotropy when the molar concentration of chymotrypsin and chymostatin were equal. Interestingly, the relatively small anisotropy value for completely bound chymostatin ($r = 0.065$) compared with the value measured for
chymotrypsin alone ($r = 0.13$) indicates that the inhibitor exhibits considerable
rotational freedom when bound to chymotrypsin. The opportunity for studying
chymostatin and its interaction with membranes using fluorescence polarization
provides additional opportunities to test the role of membrane chymotrypsin-like
proteases and transformation.

6. Conclusions

In vitro cell transformation of C3H/10T1/2 cells can be suppressed by
protease inhibitors. Chymotrypsin inhibitors are particularly effective in suppressing transformation in this system. Plasma membrane chymotrypsin-like
proteases have been detected and partially characterized and may represent a key
target for the anticarcinogenic protease inhibitors. They are present at an extremely low level and presumably represent proteases playing a regulatory role in
normal cell growth regulation. Fluorescence anisotropy of chymostatin in both
free and protease-bound forms has proven to be a successful means of observing
protease–protease inhibitor binding in the absence of substrate. This technique
will complement our kinetics analysis as we continue to study chymotrypsin
inhibitors as they interact with cell membrane proteases.

ACKNOWLEDGMENTS. This work was supported by Grant CA 47762 from the
NIH and Grant 687-046 from the New Jersey Commission for Cancer Research.

7. References

Baldessaire, J. J., Bakshian, S., Knipp, M. A., and Fisher, G. J., 1985, Inhibition of fibrinogen
receptor expression and serotonin release by leupeptin and antipain, *J. Biol. Chem.* **260**:10531–
10535.

Bathurst, J. C., Brennan, S. O., Carrell, R. W., Cousens, L. S., Brake, A. J., and Barr, P. J., 1987,
Yeast KEX 2 protease has the properties of a human proalbumin converting enzyme, *Science*
235:348–350.

Baturay, N., and Kennedy, A. R., 1986, Pyrene acts as a cocarcinogen with the carcinogens ben-
zo(a)pyrene, beta propiolactone and radiation in the induction of malignant transformation in
cultured mouse fibroblasts; soybean extract containing Bowman–Birk inhibitor acts as an anticarcinogen, *Cell Biol. Toxicol.* **2**:21–32.

Billings, P. C., Carew, J. A., Keller-McGandy, C. E., Goldberg, A. L., and Kennedy, A. R., 1987a,
A new protease activity in C3H/10T1/2 cells which is inhibited by anticarcinogenic protease
inhibitors, *Proc. Natl. Acad. Sci USA* **84**:4801–4805.

Billings, P. C., St. Clair, W., Ryan, C. A., and Kennedy, A. R., 1987b, Inhibition of radiation-
induced transformation of C3H/10T1/2 cells by chymotrypsin inhibitor 1 from potatoes, *Carcinogenesis* **8**:809–812.

Corasanti, J. G., Hobika, G. H., and Markus, G., 1982, Interference with dimethylhydrazine induction of colon tumors in mice by ε-aminocaproic acid, *Science* **216**:1020–1021.

Correa, P., 1981, Epidemiological correlations between diet and cancer frequency, *Cancer Res.* **41**:3685–3690.

Hershko, A., 1988, Ubiquitin-mediated protein degradation, *J. Biol. Chem.* **263**:15237–15240.

Hozumi, M., Ogawa, M., Sugimura, T., Takeuchi, T., and Umezawa, H., 1972, Inhibition of tumorigenesis in mouse skin by leupeptin, a protease inhibitor from Actinomycetes, *Cancer Res.* **32**:1725.

Joshen, A. L., and Berhanu, P., 1986, Chymotrypsin substrate analogues inhibit endocytosis of insulin and insulin receptors in adipocytes, *J. Cell Biol.* **103**:1807–1816.

Kennedy, A. R., 1984, Promotion and other interactions between agents in the induction of transformation *in vitro* in fibroblasts, in: *Mechanisms of Tumor Promotion*, Volume III (T. J. Slaga, ed.), CRC Press, Boca Raton, Fla., pp. 13–55.

Kennedy, A. R., 1985, The conditions for the modification of radiation transformation *in vitro* by a tumor promoter and protease inhibitors, *Carcinogenesis* **6**:1441–1445.

Kennedy, A. R., Radner, B. S., and Nagasawa, H., 1984, Protease inhibitors reduce the frequency of spontaneous chromosome abnormalities in cells from patients with Bloom's syndrome, *Proc. Natl. Acad. Sci. USA* **81**:1827–1830.

King, C. H., Goralnik, C. H., Kleinhenz, P. J., Marino, J. A., Sedor, J. R., and Mahmoud, A. A. F., 1987, Monoclonal antibody characterization of a chymotrypsin-like molecule on neutrophil membrane associated with cellular activation, *J. Clin. Invest.* **79**:1091–1098.

Kuroki, T., and Drevon, C., 1979, Inhibition of chemical transformation in C3H/10T1/2 cells by protease inhibitors, *Cancer Res.* **39**:2755–2761.

Mignatti, P., Robbins, E., and Rifkin, D. B., 1986, Tumor invasion through the human amniotic membrane: Requirement for a proteinase cascade, *Cell* **47**:487–498.

O'Donnell-Tormey, J., and Quigley, J. P., 1981, Inhibition of plasminogen activator release from transformed chicken fibroblasts by a protease inhibitor, *Cell* **27**:85–95.

O'Donnell-Tormey, J., and Quigley, J. P., 1983, Detection and partial characterization of a chymostatin-sensitive endopeptidase in transformed fibroblasts, *Proc. Natl. Acad. Sci USA* **80**:344–348.

Quigley, J. P., Gold, L. I., Schwimmer, R., and Sullivan, L. M., 1987, Limited cleavage of cellular fibronectin by plasminogen activator purified from transformed cells, *Proc. Natl. Acad. Sci. USA* **84**:2776–2780.

Sloane, B. P., Rozhin, J., Johnson, K., Taylor, H., Grisman, J. D., and Honn, K. V., 1986, Cathepsin B: Association with plasma membrane in metastatic tumors, *Proc. Natl. Acad. Sci. USA* **83**:2483–2487.

Taparowsky, E. J., Heaney, M. C., and Parsons, J. T., 1987, Oncogene mediated multistep transformation of C3H/10T1/2 cells, *Cancer Res.* **47**:4125–4129.

Troll, W., Klassen, A., and Janoff, A., 1970, Tumorigenesis in mouse skin: Inhibition by synthetic inhibitors of proteases, *Science* **169**:1211–1212.

Waxman, L., Fagan, J. M., Tanaka, K., and Goldberg, A. L., 1985, A soluble ATP-dependent system for protein degradation from murine erythroleukemia cells, *J. Biol. Chem.* **260**:11994–12000.

Weed, H., McGandy, R. B., and Kennedy, A. R., 1985, Protection against dimethylhydrazine induced adenomatous tumors of the mouse colon by the dietary addition of an extract of soybeans containing the Bowman–Birk protease inhibitor, *Carcinogenesis* **6**:1239–1241.

Yavelow, J., 1986, Role of legume-derived anticarcinogens, *N.J. Med.* **83**:233–234.

Yavelow, J., Gidlund, M., and Troll, W., 1982, Protease inhibitors from processed legumes effectively inhibit superoxide generation in response to TPA, *Carcinogenesis* **3**:135–138.

Yavelow, J., Finlay, T. H., Kennedy, A. R., and Troll, W., 1983, Bowman–Birk soybean protease inhibitor as an anticarcinogen, *Cancer Res. (Suppl.)* **43**:2454s–2459s.

Yavelow, J., Collins, M., Birk, Y., Troll, W., and Kennedy, A. R., 1985, Nanomolar concentrations of Bowman–Birk soybean protease suppress x-ray induced transformation *in vitro, Proc. Natl. Acad. Sci. USA* **82:**5395–5399.

Yavelow, J., Caggana, M., and Beck, K. A., 1987a, Proteases occurring in the cell membrane: A possible cell receptor for the Bowman–Birk type of protease inhibitors, *Cancer Res.* **47:**1598–1601.

Yavelow, J., Scott, C. B., and Mayer, T. C., 1987b, Fluorescent visualization of binding and internalization of the anticarcinogenic Bowman–Birk type protease inhibitors in transformed fibroblasts, *Cancer Res.* **47:**1602–1607.

14

The Role of Reactive Oxygen Species in Biological Damage and the Effect of Some Chemopreventive Agents

KRYSTYNA FRENKEL

1. Formation of Reactive Oxygen Species

Reactive oxygen species (ROS) can be generated by a variety of sources. The best known source is ionizing radiation which causes formation of hydroxyl radicals ($\cdot$OH), and in the presence of O_2, also superoxide anion radicals ($\cdot O_2^-$) and hydrogen peroxide (H_2O_2) (Scholes, 1983). Cellular sources cause the formation of qualitatively the same ROS but in different proportions. These ROS arise by the enzymatically mediated reduction of molecular oxygen utilizing one to four electrons donated by various cellular reducing agents (Aust *et al.*, 1985; Halliwell and Gutteridge, 1986; Vuillaume, 1987; Byczkowski and Gessner, 1988). These enzymatic processes include electron transport and redox cycling of

Abbreviations used in this chapter: BBI, Bowman–Birk inhibitor; B(a)P, benzo(a)pyrene; B(e)P, benzo(e)pyrene; COI, chicken ovoinhibitor; DMBA, 7,12-dimethylbenz(a)anthracene; dTG, thymidine glycol; GSH, glutathione; HMdU, 5-hydroxymethyl-2'-deoxyuridine; H_2O_2, hydrogen peroxide; LBI, lima bean inhibitor; Mez, mezerein; NADPH, reduced nicotinamide adenine dinucleotide phosphate; $\cdot O_2^-$, superoxide anion radicals; $\cdot$OH, hydroxyl radicals; PAHs, polycyclic aromatic hydrocarbons; PCI-2, chymotrypsin-inhibitory fragment of PtI-2; PIs, protease inhibitors; PMNs, polymorphonuclear leukocytes; PtI-1, potato inhibitor 1; PtI-2, potato inhibitor 2; ROS, reactive oxygen species; RPA, 12-O-retinoylphorbol-13-acetate; Sarp A, sarcophytol A; SBTI, soybean (Kunitz) trypsin inhibitor; SOD, superoxide dismutase; TOOI, turkey ovomucoid ovoinhibitor; TPA, 12-O-tetradecanoylphorbol-13-acetate; 8-OHdG, 8-hydroxyl-2'-deoxyguanosine; 3MC, 3-methylcholanthrene.

KRYSTYNA FRENKEL • Departments of Environmental Medicine and Pathology, New York University Medical Center, New York, New York 10016.

Protease Inhibitors as Cancer Chemopreventive Agents, edited by Walter Troll and Ann R. Kennedy. Plenum Press, New York, 1993.

endogenous quinones such as menadione (vitamin K), of chemotherapeutic quinone antibiotics such as adriamycin, daunorubicin, streptonegrin, and bleomycin, or of active agents such as paraquat. ROS can also be produced during oxidative metabolism of xenobiotics, such as polycyclic aromatic hydrocarbons (PAHs), nitroaromatics, and amines (Frenkel et al., 1988a; Leadon et al., 1988; Washburn and Di Giulio, 1988; O'Brien, 1988, Ochi and Kaneko, 1989; Wei and Frenkel, 1992b). Phagocytic cells are a very prolific source of the ROS that are generated during the respiratory burst. I will describe this last process in greater detail a little later.

ROS participate in a number of normal cellular processes, and play a positive role as bactericidal and tumoricidal agents (Vuillaume, 1987). In order to prevent the harmful side effects of ROS, organisms have elaborated a number of antioxidant defenses. These consist of the reducing agents glutathione (GSH), cysteine, and urate, as well as a number of enzymes, such as superoxide dismutase (SOD), catalase, various peroxidases including GSH peroxidase and GSH-S-transferases. In addition, there are enzymes that recognize and repair oxidative DNA damage (Teebor et al., 1988; Wallace, 1988; Breimer, 1990). The extent of these antioxidant defenses is already indicative of the potentially harmful capabilities of ROS. When ROS are formed in excessive amounts, they can overwhelm the defense mechanisms, and this can result in a variety of diseases. Conversely, some diseases cause the formation of large amounts of ROS, which then potentiate the harmful effects of the illness. The diseases that induce or are the result of a prooxidant state include rheumatoid arthritis, systemic lupus erythematosus, emphysema, adult respiratory distress syndrome, sickle-cell anemia, and a variety of malignancies such as colon, breast, and skin cancers (Dunham, 1972; McCord, 1974; Fantone and Ward, 1982; D'Onofrio et al., 1984; Biemond et al., 1986; Chester et al., 1986; Rice-Evans et al., 1986; Schacter, 1986; Vuillaume, 1987). The following are some of the harmful ROS-induced effects: connective tissue breakdown, pulmonary injury, degradation of synovial fluid, lipid peroxidation, cell lysis, vascular permeability, as well as damage to DNA (Simon et al., 1981; Fantone and Ward, 1982; Freeman and Crapo, 1982; Vercellotti et al., 1985; Burkhardt et al., 1986; Fletcher et al., 1986; Frenkel and Chrzan, 1987a; Vuillaume, 1987; Frenkel, 1989; Wei and Frenkel, 1991, 1992b). All of these processes can occur during inflammation.

Inflammation is a result of the action of phagocytic cells when upon activation they respond with a respiratory burst during which substantial amounts of ROS are generated (Badwey and Karnovsky, 1980; Klebanoff, 1980; Fantone and Ward, 1982; Freeman and Crapo, 1982). I will concentrate on the properties of one type of phagocytic cells—polymorphonuclear leukocytes (PMNs). PMNs are cells that take part in the inflammatory and immune responses, and whose normal function is to recognize, phagocytize, and destroy foreign objects such as bacteria and other opsonized particles. When these cells are activated by inappropriate stimuli, such as some lectins, allergens, and tumor promoters, large amounts of generated ROS are free to interact with the neighboring cells and impart their damaging effects on the cellular macromolecules, including DNA (Fantone and Ward, 1982; Shasby et al., 1983; Vercellotti et al., 1985; Frenkel and Chrzan, 1987a; Shacter et al., 1988; Zvillich et al., 1988; Frenkel, 1992). Regardless of the type of stimuli used, the elicited burst is characterized by a rapid consumption of oxygen followed by the almost concomitant production of $\cdot O_2^-$. These radicals can dismutate to H_2O_2 both spontaneously and enzymatically. H_2O_2 is the immediate precursor of the actual bacteriocidal species that include $\cdot OH$, hypochlorite ions, and singlet oxygen. H_2O_2 is the only one of the ROS generated that is capable of crossing through the cellular membranes with an ease almost equal to that of water (Fantone and Ward, 1982; de Mello-Filho and Meneghini, 1985; Halliwell and Gutteridge, 1986). Other ROS either need the presence of anion channels ($\cdot O_2^-$) or are too reactive to travel far ($\cdot OH$, hypochlorite).

It has been known for some time that ROS generated by phagocytic cells induce formation of DNA strand breaks in co-incubated cells (Birnboim, 1983; Dutton and Bowden, 1985). Formation of those strand breaks could be prevented by catalase, which points to H_2O_2 as the oxygen species responsible for this type of DNA damage. Since H_2O_2 by itself cannot interact with DNA (Cadet and Teoule, 1978), another species derived from it must be the ultimate damaging agent. It was shown that sister chromatid exchanges induced by H_2O_2 can be prevented by using o-phenanthroline (Meneghini, 1988), a lipophilic iron chelator, that is capable of crossing cellular membranes. This finding proves that it is a transition metal ion-induced decomposition product of H_2O_2 which is responsible for DNA breaks. Therefore, the most likely candidate for the ultimate DNA-damaging agent is $\cdot OH$, which is known to be formed from H_2O_2 by Fe^{2+}. When H_2O_2 migrates into the nucleus, it may be reduced in situ to $\cdot OH$ by metal ions chelated to DNA or by the proteins of chromatin. DNA breaks that are caused by this type of interaction are termed site specific (Halliwell and Gutteridge, 1986; Chevion, 1988). Although it seems that $\cdot OH$ or $\cdot OH$-like species are ultimately responsible for the DNA damage, the damaging process is initiated by H_2O_2 because it is stable and unreactive enough to travel into the nucleus.

2. Formation of H_2O_2 and Oxidized DNA Bases

2.1. By Tumor Promoter-Stimulated PMNs

I will now discuss the formation of H_2O_2 by human PMNs stimulated with tumor promoters and the formation of oxidized thymine residues in DNA exposed to the activated PMNs. We and others have shown that $\cdot OH$ derived from Fe^{2+}-reduced H_2O_2 cause formation of 5-hydroxymethyl-2'-deoxyuridine (HMdU) and thymidine glycol (dTG) in co-incubated DNA (Troll et al., 1984;

Frenkel et al., 1986a; Frenkel and Chrzan, 1987b), and we and others have shown the presence of 8-hydroxyl-2'-deoxyguanosine (8-HdG) in the DNA of PMNs (Floyd et al., 1986; Bhimani et al., 1992).

It is well accepted that the tumor-initiating properties of carcinogens correlate with the formation of certain types of adducts with DNA bases (Jeffrey et al., 1977; Feldman et al., 1978; Ashurst et al., 1983; DiGiovanni et al., 1986; Trush and Kensler, 1991; Ji and Marnett, 1992). However, the mechanism of tumor promotion is not as yet clearly understood. In the last decade, the hypothesis of a multistage process of promotion, proposed by Boutwell in 1964, has received experimental support (Slaga et al., 1980, 1982; Fürstenberger et al., 1981, 1983; Kinzel et al., 1986; O'Connell et al., 1986). As of now, there seem to be two recognizable stages of promotion followed by a progression stage from benign to malignant tumors. It has long been assumed that modification of genetic material occurs only at the initiation stage. However, more recent evidence shows that if the so-called first-stage promoters are applied either after or even before an initiating agent, tumor growth can be induced by applying the second-stage promoters weeks later (Fürstenberger et al., 1983; Kinzel et al., 1986). These findings suggest that the first-stage promotional processes involve heritable DNA modification. A few years ago, we postulated that the tumor promoter-induced formation of H_2O_2 in vitro may be related to the in vivo first-stage promoting activity of the agents used for stimulation of PMNs, particularly because H_2O_2 itself is known to be a first-stage tumor promoter (Frenkel and Chrzan, 1987a,b). We further proposed that H_2O_2 generated by activated PMNs causes oxidative DNA damage, some of which can be responsible (at least in part) for the "memory" effects of the first-stage tumor promoters.

To test this hypothesis, tumor promoters differing in their first-stage activity were chosen (Frenkel and Chrzan, 1987b). These were: phorbol ester TPA (12-O-tetradecanoylphorbol-13-acetate), a complete tumor promoter with a potent first-stage activity, RPA (12-O-retinoylphorbol-13-acetate), a retinoyl derivative of TPA with a weak first-stage activity except in SENCAR mice, and mezerein (Mez), whose first-stage activity lies between those of TPA and RPA (Fürstenberger et al., 1981; Slaga et al., 1982; Fischer et al., 1985). Phorbol, a nonpromoting parent of TPA, was used as a control. All three tumor promoters caused formation of increasing amounts of H_2O_2 when increasing concentrations of tumor promoters were used (Frenkel and Chrzan, 1987a,b; Frenkel, 1989). However, using the same concentrations, TPA was the most active and RPA the least active in H_2O_2 formation at all concentrations tested (Table I). When PMNs were incubated with tumor promoters at the concentrations that caused maximal H_2O_2 formation, again, TPA was the most effective and RPA the least effective over the lifetime of the oxidative burst, whereas phorbol, a nonpromoter, was totally inactive.

Since the most important characteristic of first-stage tumor promoters seems to be an induction of heritable DNA damage, we have decided to determine

Table I. Percent Formation of H_2O_2,
HMdU, and dTG by Human PMNs
Activated with Mez or RPA,
in Comparison with TPA-Mediated
Activation[a]

Tumor promoter	H_2O_2	HMdU	dTG
	No plasma		
TPA	100	100	100
Mez	75	70	45
RPA	30	25	5
	10% autologous plasma		
TPA	100	100	100
Mez	70	50	40
RPA	30	30	20

[a]Reprinted with permission from Frenkel and Chrzan (1987a).

whether ROS generated by tumor promoter-activated PMNs are capable of causing modification of DNA bases. The modification of DNA was measured by formation of HMdU and dTG (Frenkel *et al.*, 1986a). The results of the experiments, in which DNA was co-incubated with tumor promoter-stimulated PMNs in the absence or presence of autologous plasma, paralleled those of H_2O_2 production (Table I) (Frenkel and Chrzan, 1987a,b). We have found that in the absence of plasma, the Fe/EDTA complex must be present in the reaction mixture in order to obtain comparable amounts of oxidized bases (Frenkel *et al.*, 1986a). In both the absence and presence of plasma, activation of PMNs by TPA was the most effective, since HMdU and dTG were formed in the highest amounts, and activation by RPA was the lowest (Frenkel, 1989). We have also found that formation of these oxidized bases is abolished by catalase. This finding points to the H_2O_2 as being a necessary intermediate of the tumor promoter-induced PMN-mediated DNA damage. It therefore appears that there may be a cause-and-effect relationship between the ability of first-stage tumor promoters to induce H_2O_2 formation and the consequent oxidative modification of DNA bases.

   In order to determine whether exogenously produced H_2O_2 is capable of damaging the DNA of neighboring cells, we looked for the formation of HMdU in the DNA of HeLa cells co-incubated with TPA-stimulated human PMNs in the presence of autologous plasma (Frenkel and Chrzan, 1987a). HMdU was indeed formed in HeLa cells DNA and its formation was dependent on the amount of TPA used to activate the cells (Table II). Some HMdU was formed in HeLa cells

Table II. TPA-Induced Formation
of HMdU in DNA of HeLa Cells in the
Presence or Absence of Human PMNs

TPA/10⁶ cells (pmole)	HMdU/10⁵ dT
In the presence of PMNs	
6	11
10	14
40	28
In the absence of PMNs	
12.5	2.2
50.0	4.4
250	6.0
500[a]	1.8

[a]This amount of TPA was toxic (12%) as determined by
trypan blue exclusion.

even in the absence of PMNs. This formation of HMdU in the HeLa cell DNA in
the absence of PMNs was also proportional to the concentration of TPA, until the
point at which it was too toxic to the cells. This finding is very important because
it indirectly shows that even in the absence of an exogenous source of H_2O_2, such
as PMNs, tumor promoters can induce intracellular formation of ROS. We have
recently found using spectrofluorometric methods that H_2O_2 is actually formed
by HeLa cells treated with TPA (Fig. 1) (Frenkel and Gleichauf, 1991). Such
"oxidative activation" of cells by a tumor promoter results in the modification of
DNA bases, formation of which can be enhanced by the action of stimulated
phagocytic cells.

2.2. By Hepatic Microsomes

It has not been established as yet what constitutes the promoting activity of
complete carcinogens such as PAHs. It has been suggested that PAHs also induce
formation of ROS as do tumor promoters (Ide *et al.*, 1984; Frenkel *et al.*, 1988a;
Frenkel, 1992; Wei and Frenkel, 1992a), particularly since antioxidants were
shown to reduce the carcinogenic effects of benzo(*a*)pyrene [B(*a*)P], as shown by
Wattenberg (1980), and of 7,12-dimethylbenz(*a*)anthracene (DMBA), as shown
by Dipple *et al.*, (1984) and McCormick *et al.* (1984). We have found that rat
hepatic microsomes are capable of H_2O_2 formation when incubated with B(*a*)P
(Frenkel *et al.*, 1988a), benzo(*e*)pyrene [B(*e*)P], DMBA, anthracene, and
3-methylcholanthrene (3MC) (Fig. 2) (Frenkel *et al.*, 1988b). H_2O_2 was generated in linearly increasing amounts with increased doses of PAHs. What was also
interesting was that pyrene, a noncarcinogenic parent of B(*a*)P, did not cause

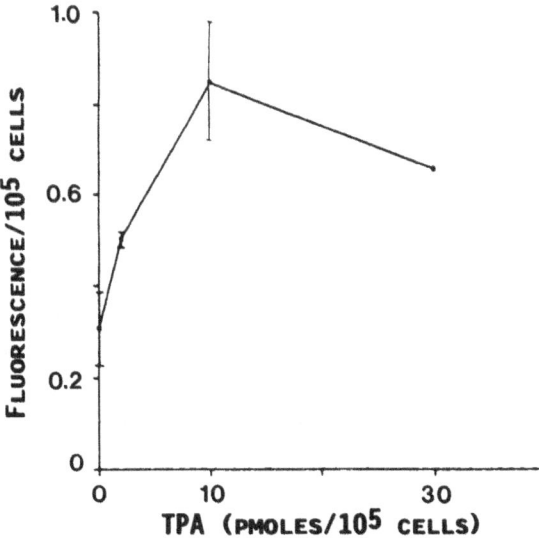

Figure 1. TPA-induced formation of H_2O_2 in HeLa cells. HeLa cells (5×10^5/ml PBS) were preincubated with 6% human plasma and 25 mM azide for 5 min, then with 0.5 μM 2',7'-dichlorofluorescin diacetate for 15 min, followed by treatment with TPA for 45 min. Cells were sonicated and fluorescence of the supernatants determined at λ_{exc} = 475 nm and λ_{emiss} = 525 nm (Frenkel and Gleichauf, 1991).

formation of H_2O_2 (Frenkel *et al.*, 1988a). Table III shows that when DNA was co-incubated with microsomes in the presence of B(*a*)P, HMdU was formed in that DNA. Moreover, its formation was decreased by catalase to a level below those formed in the control DNA in the absence of B(*a*)P. Again, this last finding points to the involvement of H_2O_2 in the formation of oxidized DNA bases in response to treatment with this PAH.

It was previously estimated that oxidative damage to the DNA of B(*a*)P-treated cells was about 20-fold higher than formation of adducts with DNA bases (Ide *et al.*, 1984), and that thymine glycol was part of that oxidative damage (Leadon, 1987). That formation of oxidized bases may be a more general result of treatment with complete carcinogens is shown by the presence of thymine glycol in the DNA of cells incubated not only with B(*a*)P but also with *N*-hydroxy-2-naphthylamine, 2-nitropropane, and in the UV- and ionizing radiation-treated cells (Table IV) (Cerutti, 1976; Frenkel *et al.*, 1981; Fiala *et al*, 1987; Leadon, 1987). 8-Hydroxyguanine is formed in cells incubated with 4-nitroquinoline-*N*-oxide and in γ-irradiated cells (Kasai *et al.*, 1986; Kohda *et al.*, 1986). We know that HMdU is formed through the action of γ radiation, 2-nitropropane, and, now, also by B(*a*)P (Teebor *et al.*, 1984; Frenkel *et al.*,

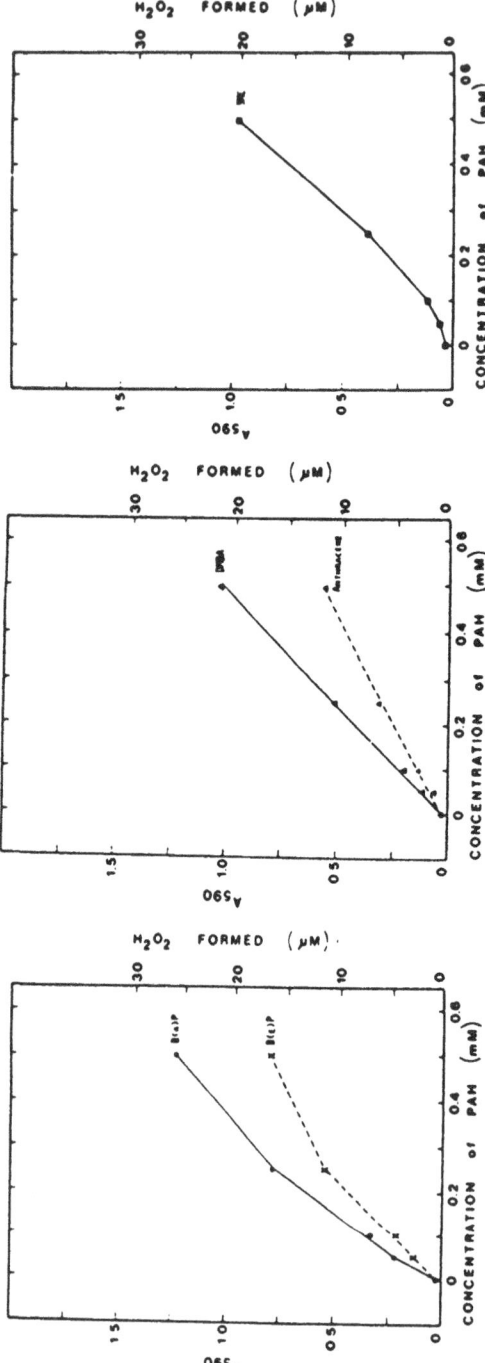

Figure 2. Formation of H_2O_2 by rat liver microsomes incubated with B(a)P (●) and B(e)P (X) (left panel), DMBA (▲) and anthracene (△) (middle panel), and 3MC (■) (right panel). Microsomes (50 μg) were treated with PAHs in the presence of 100 μg phenol red, 50 μg horseradish peroxidase, and NADPH regenerating system. After incubation at 37°C for 30 min, particulates were removed by centrifugation, supernatants made alkaline with NaOH, and absorbance determined at 590 nm against blanks containing boiled microsomes. (According to Frenkel *et al.*, 1988a.)

1985, 1986b, 1988a; Fiala et al., 1987). In the last few years a number of initiating and promoting carcinogens were shown to cause oxidation of DNA bases in vivo at the target sites. These include induction of 8-HdG in rat liver DNA by peroxisome proliferators (Kasai et al., 1989) and 2-nitropropane (Fiala et al., 1989), in rat kidney DNA by nickel acetate (Kasprzak et al., 1990), ferric nitrilotriacetate (Umemura et al., 1990), potassium bromate (Kasai et al., 1987), and other carcinogenic metals (Klein et al., 1991), and in mouse skin by TPA (Floyd et al., 1987). HMdU is formed in vivo in rat hepatic DNA by the actions of γ radiation, diethylnitrosamine, 2-acetylaminofluorene, and peroxisome proliferator ciprofibrate (Srinivasan and Glauert, 1990). Our laboratory identified all three oxidized base derivatives (HMdU, dTG, and 8-HdG) in epidermal DNA of SENCAR mice treated with either TPA (Frenkel et al., 1991a; Wei and Frenkel, 1991) or DMBA (Wei and Frenkel, 1992a). Thus, it appears that the same oxidized DNA bases are formed in DNA exposed to intra- as well as intercellularly generated ROS. Now that we know the identity of some of the DNA-damaging ROS, we have to find ways to either prevent their formation or counteract their action.

3. Inhibition of H_2O_2 Formation by Stimulated PMNs

There have been a few types of agents identified as being capable of decreasing oxidant formation by tumor promoter-activated PMNs or inhibiting progression of inflammatory diseases. These include protease inhibitors (PIs) and retinoids (Goldstein et al., 1979; Kitagawa et al., 1979; Witz et al., 1980; Fantone and Ward, 1982; Frenkel et al., 1987; Gensler et al., 1987; Troll et al., 1987). Recently, another class of compounds, sarcophytols (Sarp), were found to act as antitumor promoters (Fujiki et al., 1989). Sarps A and B were very effective in the inhibition of tumor formation, whereas all-trans retinoic acid, which has some structural similarity to open-ring Sarp, was totally ineffective. Since retinoic acid acts as an antioxidant due to its scavenging capabilities, the antitumor activity of Sarp is probably due to its other properties. We previously found that a certain type of PI inhibits generation of H_2O_2 by tumor promoter-activated human PMNs (Frenkel et al., 1987; Frenkel, 1989) and, now, we show that Sarp A is capable of similar inhibition patterns (Zhong et al., 1991; Wei and Frenkel, 1992b).

Stimulated phagocytic cells generate ROS that are known to contribute to inflammatory diseases, necrosis of surrounding tissues, mutagenicity, and carcinogenicity (Fantone and Ward, 1982; Freeman and Crapo, 1982; Weitzman and Stossel, 1982; Weitzman et al., 1985; Barak et al., 1983; Vuillaume, 1987; Weitzman and Gordon, 1990; Frenkel, 1992). It is apparent that the normal cellular antioxidant defenses can be overwhelmed and that other agents must be utilized if the damaging effects of ROS are to be contained. Formation of ROS is

Table III. Effect of B(a)P on HMdU Formation in DNA Co-incubated with or without Rat Liver Microsomes

Source of rat microsomes	Number of HMdU residues/10^4 dT			
	Control	B(a)P	B(a)P + catalase	H$_2$O$_2$ + Fe(II)/EDTA
Sprague–Dawley	0.5	3.1	—	—
Fisher 344	9.8	44.8	—	—
Fisher 344	22.5	36.5	5.4	—
—[a]	0.8	—	—	3.7

[a]No microsomes were used.

dependent on the activation of NADPH (reduced nicotinamide adenine dinucleotide phosphate) oxidase, which is present in the PMN membrane in a dormant state (Badwey and Karnovsky, 1980; Klebanoff, 1980; Fantone and Ward, 1982). Upon stimulation of PMNs, NADPH oxidase is rapidly activated and in this state it can catalyze formation of $\cdot O_2^-$ from molecular oxygen. NADPH serves as an electron donor and, in the process, it is oxidized to NADP$^+$. NADPH is regenerated from NADP$^+$ by a chain of reactions in which

Table IV. Carcinogen-Induced Formation of Oxidized DNA Bases

Carcinogen	5-Hydroxymethyl uracil	Thymine glycol	8-Hydroxyguanine	Refs.[a]
Benzo(a)pyrene	+	+	nd[b]	1, 2
7,12-Dimethylbenz(a)anthracene	+	+	+	3
N-hydroxy-2-naphthylamine	nd	+	nd	2
Diethylnitrosamine	+	nd	nd	4
2'-Acetylaminofluorene	+	nd	nd	4
4-Nitroquinoline-N-oxide	nd	nd	+	5
2-Nitropyrene	+	+	+	6
UV radiation	nd	+	nd	2
Ionizing radiation	+	+	+	4, 7
Tumor promoters/PMNs	+	+	+	8
Tumor promoters/mouse skin	+	+	+	3, 9
Nickel acetate	nd	nd	+	10
Peroxisome proliferators	+	nd	+	4, 11

[a]1, Frenkel *et al.* (1988a); 2, Leadon (1987); 3, Wei and Frenkel (1991, 1992a); 4, Srinivasan and Glauert (1990); 5, Kohda *et al.* (1986); 6, Fiala *et al.* (1987, 1989); 7, Cerutti (1976), Frenkel *et al.* (1981, 1985, 1986b), Teebor *et al.* (1984), Kasai *et al.* (1986); 8, Troll *et al.* (1984), Frenkel *et al.* (1986a, 1991b), Frenkel and Chrzan (1987a,b), Floyd *et al.* (1986); 9, Floyd *et al.* (1987); 10, Kasprzak *et al.* (1990); 11, Kasai *et al.* (1989).
[b]nd, not determined.

glucose serves as a substrate acted on by enzymes of the hexose monophosphate shunt. Interference with any of the enzymatic steps involved in the activation of NADPH oxidase may potentially lead to the inhibition of the oxidative burst.

3.1. Inhibition by Protease Inhibitors

It has been previously shown that some PIs can block formation of $\cdot O_2^-$ (Goldstein et al., 1979; Troll et al., 1987). However, a suggestion was made that the decrease in the $\cdot O_2^-$ levels was not due to the inhibition of $\cdot O_2^-$ formation but instead was due to the dismutation of $\cdot O_2^-$ by contaminating SOD (Abramowitz et al., 1983). In order to avoid this uncertainty and, at the same time, to determine whether PIs can inhibit the oxidative burst, we decided to use generation of H_2O_2 as its measure (Frenkel et al., 1987). Monitoring H_2O_2 formation has some advantages over that of $\cdot O_2^-$. The most important of them is that if a contaminating SOD is present in the preparation of PIs, there would be an increase in H_2O_2 levels over those formed in the absence of PIs, not a decrease, and addition of exogenous SOD should be without effect.

In the experiments to be described, H_2O_2 was determined using phenol red as a substrate for the horseradish peroxidase-mediated oxidation (Frenkel et al., 1987). The amount of oxidized phenol red (which is a measure of H_2O_2 formation) was determined spectrophotometrically at 590 nm, at which wavelength, oxidized phenol red has a severalfold higher absorbance than unoxidized phenol red. PMNs were stimulated with 25 nM TPA, a concentration that ensures formation of maximal levels of H_2O_2 (Frenkel and Chrzan, 1987b). To determine the influence of PIs on H_2O_2 production by TPA-activated PMNs, PIs of varying concentrations were added to human PMNs, phenol red, and horseradish peroxidase just prior to activation with TPA, and the complete mixtures were incubated at 37°C for 30 min (Frenkel et al., 1987).

The following PIs were used in these experiments: potato inhibitors 1 (PtI-1) and 2 (PtI-2), a chymotrypsin-inhibitory fragment of PtI-2 (PCI-2), chicken ovoinhibitor (COI), turkey ovomucoid ovoinhibitor (TOOI), Bowman–Birk inhibitor (BBI), lima bean inhibitor (LBI), and soybean (Kunitz) trypsin inhibitor (SBTI). These inhibitors were selected because they occur naturally in vegetables, such as potatoes, tomatoes, and beans, as well as in eggs. They include PIs that are specific either for chymotrypsin (PtI-1 and PCI-2) or for trypsin (SBTI). Moreover, several of these PIs are bifunctional, since they contain both chymotrypsin- as well as trypsin-inhibitory regions.

As is obvious from Fig. 3, PtI-1, a chymotrypsin inhibitor, was the most effective of the PIs used and SBTI, a trypsin inhibitor, was the least effective in the inhibition of H_2O_2 formation over all of the concentrations tested. The bifunctional PIs exhibited intermediate effects. At 10 μM, PtI-1 decreased H_2O_2 levels by 90%, PCI-2 by a little over 40%, and PtI-2 a little under 40%. Of the other PIs tested, the inhibitory activity of COI approached that of PtI-2 when

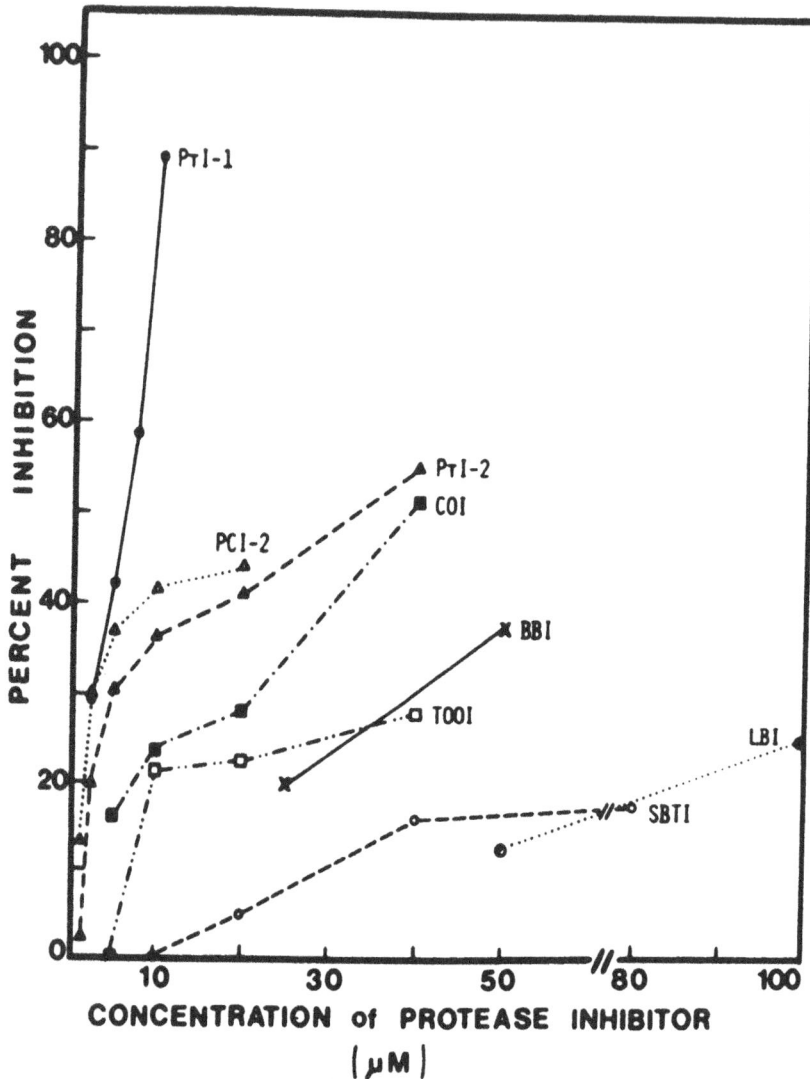

Figure 3. PI-mediated inhibition of H_2O_2 formation by TPA-activated human PMNs. PMNs (1 × 10^5/ml) were stimulated with 25 nM TPA in the presence or absence of PIs. After incubation at 37°C for 30 min, the mixture containing 100 μg phenol red and 50 μg horseradish peroxidase was treated with 50 μg catalase, centrifuged, made alkaline with NaOH, and absorbance of the supernatants determined at 590 nm. (Reprinted with permission from Frenkel *et al.*, 1987.)

used at 40 μM. PCI-2, a chymotrypsin-inhibitory fragment derived from PtI-2, is more inhibitory than its bifunctional parent PtI-2 when used at concentrations of up to 20 μM.

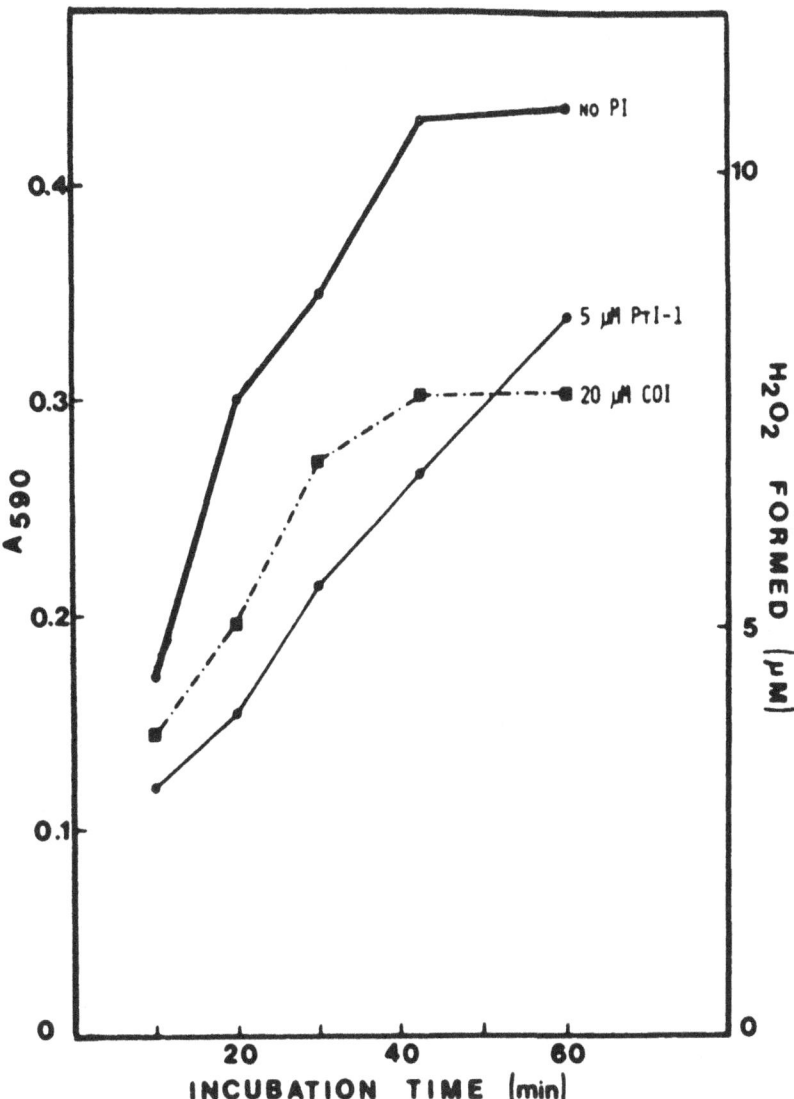

Figures 4 and 5. Formation of H_2O_2 in the absence (●) or presence of 5 μM PtI-1 (———) and 20 μM COI (—·—) (Fig. 4), or 5 μM PCI-2 (·····) and 10 μM PtI-2 (---) (Fig. 5) by TPA-activated human PMNs. Cells (1 × 10⁵/ml) were stimulated with 25 nM TPA and incubated at 37°C for 10–60 min, followed by determination of H_2O_2 formation as described in the caption of Fig. 3. (Reprinted with permission from Frenkel *et al.*, 1987.)

Figure 4 shows the time-dependent formation of H_2O_2 in the presence of constant concentrations of PIs. In the absence of inhibitors, the amount of H_2O_2 formed leveled off by 45 min incubation time. In the presence of 5 μM PtI-1

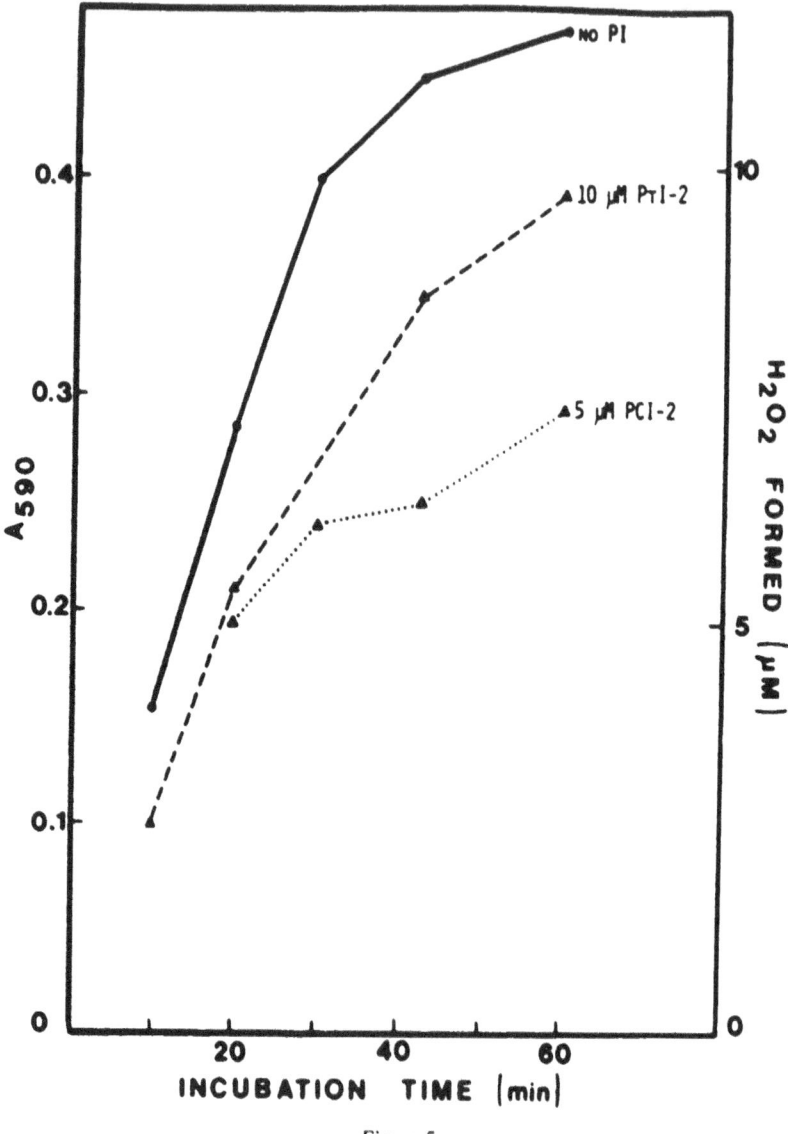

Figure 5

there was a linear increase in the formation of H_2O_2 through the 60 min incubation time point, but the amount of H_2O_2 produced at each of the incubation time
points was decreased by an average of 35% relative to the H_2O_2 formed in its
absence. At 20 μM, COI inhibited by an average of 30%, whereas TOOI inhibited by 10% (TOOI results are not shown). It is interesting that after a 30 min
incubation, COI totally inhibited further H_2O_2 formation, whereas PtI-1 had no
such effect.

Figure 5 shows the production of H_2O_2 in the presence of 5 μM PCI-2 and

Table V. Effectiveness of PIs in Inhibiting H_2O_2
Formation by TPA-Activated Human PMNs

Protease inhibitor	Protease specificity	Average inhibition by 10 μM PIs (%)
PCI-2	Chymotrypsin	77
PtI-1	Chymotrypsin	71
PtI-2	Chymotrypsin/trypsin	30
COI	Chymotrypsin/trypsin	15
SBTI	Trypsin	5

10 μM PtI-2 during 10–60 min incubation at 37°C. There are different rates of H_2O_2 formation by these two related PIs, as evidenced by the differences in the slopes. Overall, PCI-2 appears to be two to four times more effective than its parent PtI-2 in inhibiting H_2O_2 formation over the lifetime of the oxidative burst. PCI-2 also became more inhibitory at longer incubation times, which is similar to the effect shown by COI. If we normalized the effects of the PIs used at different concentrations and incubated them for 10–60 min, then we could use the average inhibition of H_2O_2 formation as a measure of the ability of PIs to decrease the TPA-induced oxidative burst of PMNs. By this measure, using a 10 μM concentration as a standard, PCI-2 might be the most effective of all PIs evaluated followed closely by PtI-1, both of which are chymotrypsin inhibitors (Table V), whereas SBTI, a trypsin inhibitor, would be the weakest of all inhibitors evaluated.

Inclusion of SOD in the incubation mixture caused a 20–30% increase in the formation of H_2O_2 by TPA-activated PMNs in the absence of PIs (not shown). Although in the presence of SOD there was overall more H_2O_2 formed than in its absence, PIs still caused a similar inhibition pattern. Conversely, these results show that even in the presence of PIs, SOD can cause an additional formation of H_2O_2 and that degree of such an increase is about the same as in the absence of PIs. Such results prove that the effects seen with PIs are due to them and not due to the contaminating SOD.

The fact that the two chymotrypsin-specific PIs are the most potent in inhibiting H_2O_2 formation and that the trypsin inhibitor is the least effective points to a chymotrypsin-like protease as being involved in the process(es) leading to the activation of NADPH oxidase. These findings also indicate that excessive inflammation might possibly be brought under control using exogenously applied PIs. This conclusion is strengthened by our recent finding that COI (one of the bifunctional PIs) as well as Sarp A (see below) suppress formation of HMdU and dTG in DNA co-incubated with TPA-activated PMNs (Frenkel *et al.*, 1991b).

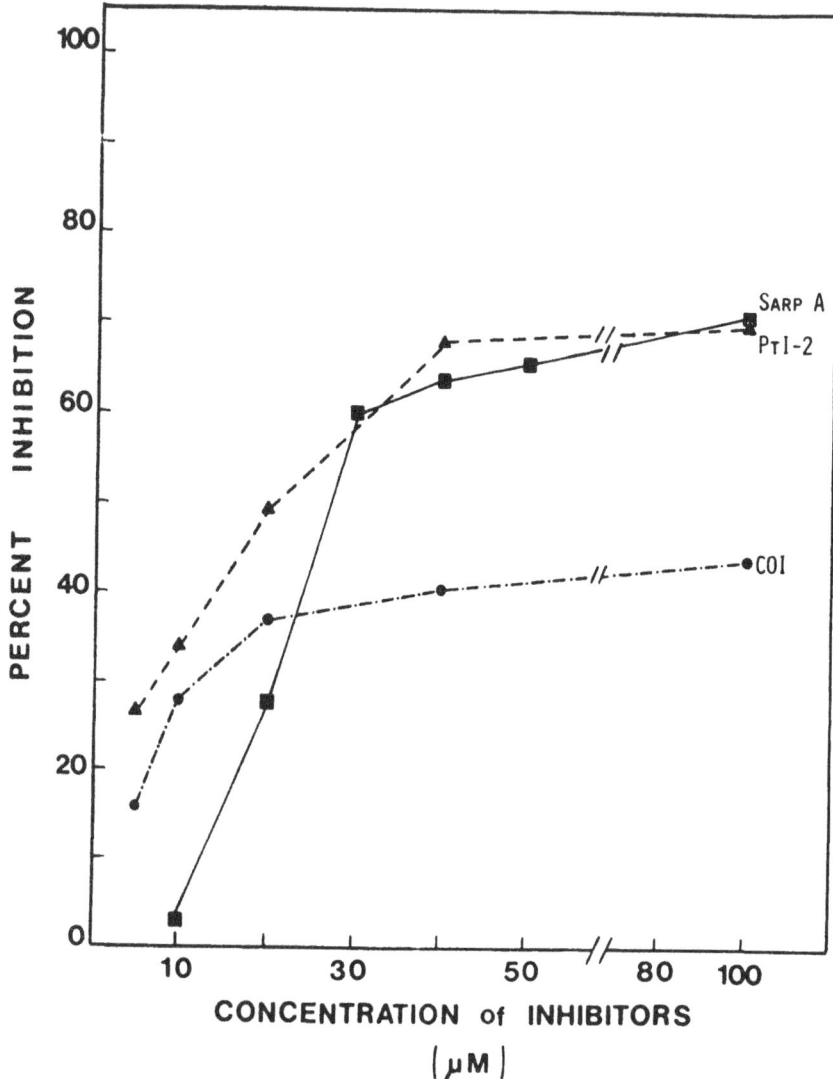

Figure 6. Effects of Sarp A and PIs on H_2O_2 formation by TPA-activated human PMNs. Cells (2.5 × 10^5/ml) were stimulated with 25 nM TPA in the absence or presence of Sarp A (■), PtI-2 (▲), and COI (●), and incubated at 37°C for 30 min. Assays were carried out as described in the caption of Fig. 3.

3.2. Inhibition by Sarcophytol A

Sarp A is a naturally occurring substance isolated from the marine soft coral *Sarcophyton glaucum*. It was found by Fujiki *et al.* (1989) to counteract the activity of the tumor promoter when applied to the DMBA-initiated and teleocidin-promoted mouse skin, as well as the activities of other tumor promoters such as TPA, aplysiatoxin, and okadaic acid. When present in the diet, it inhibited methylnitrosourea-induced large bowel cancer in rats (Narisawa *et al.*, 1989). Sarp A was found to be nontoxic even in the range of grams per kilogram body weight (Fujiki *et al.*, 1989), so it appears to be a good candidate for use as a chemopreventive agent. For all of these reasons, but particularly since it seems to act as an antitumor promoter, we have decided to test whether it can inhibit H_2O_2 formation by TPA-stimulated human PMNs. For comparison, two PIs were simultaneously tested as well. The preliminary results, shown in Fig. 6, indicate that Sarp A is capable of inhibiting H_2O_2 formation by PMNs (Zhong *et al.*, 1991; Frenkel *et al.*, 1991b). The effectiveness of Sarp A seems to be comparable to those of protease inhibitors COI and PtI-2, being less potent than PIs at lower concentrations and more effective at higher concentrations. The differences in the inhibitory activity of PtI-2, shown in Figs. 3 and 6, are probably due to the fact that samples of PtI-2 were obtained from different sources. At this point, all we know is that Sarp A does not act like PIs and, therefore, it must interfere with the generation of H_2O_2 by inhibiting a different step of PMN activation. However, inhibition of PMN activation suggests that Sarp A, in addition to its other anti-tumor-promoting effects, may effectively decrease inflammation as well, which would contribute to the anticarcinogenic properties of Sarp A. In fact, we recently found that Sarp A suppresses infiltration of PMNs *in vivo*, H_2O_2 production in mouse epidermis, as well as formation of HMdU, dTG, and 8-HdG in epidermal DNA of TPA-treated SENCAR mice (Wei and Frenkel, 1992b). That inhibition occurred at a very low Sarp A dose which was equimolar to that of TPA (6.5 nmole). Even more importantly, when used in the two-stage experimental carcinogenesis model, at 6.5 nmole Sarp A inhibited tumor formation and its multiplicity (Fujiki *et al.*, 1989). Cumulatively, it appears that Sarp A suppresses the action of a tumor promoter by suppressing PMN infiltration and activation, which results in decreased H_2O_2 production and a consequent decline in the levels of oxidized bases in the DNA of epidermal cells *in vivo*.

ACKNOWLEDGMENTS. The author is grateful to Dr. C. Ryan (Washington State University) for supplying PtI-1, -2, and PCI-2, to Dr. J. Yavelow (Rider College) for BBI, and to Dr. H. Fujiki (Japanese National Cancer Center Research Institute) for Sarp A. The PtI-2 used in the experiments shown in Fig. 6 was purchased from Kemin Industries (Des Moines, Ill.). The author thanks Mr. J. Karkoszka and Ms. Z. Zhong for their excellent technical assistance. This work was supported in part by PHS Grant CA 37858 from the National Cancer Institute, by NIEHS Cancer Center Grant ES 00260 and Superfund Grant 1 P42 ES 04895, and by American Cancer Society Cancer Center Grant SIG-9.

4. References

Abramowitz, A. S., Hong, J.-Y., and Randolph, V., 1983, Pseudo-inhibitors of neutrophils superoxide production: Evidence that soybean-derived polypeptides are superoxide dismutases, *Biochem. Biophys. Res. Commun.* **117**:22–29.

Ashurst, S. W., Cohen, G. M., Nesnow, S., DiGiovanni, J., and Slaga, T. J., 1983, Formation of benzo(a)pyrene/DNA adducts and their relationship to tumor-initiation in mouse epidermis, *Cancer Res.* **43**:1024–1029.

Aust, S. D., Morehouse, L. A., and Thomas, C. E., 1985, Role of metals in oxygen radical reactions, *J. Free Radical Biol. Med.* **1**:3–25.

Badwey, J. A., and Karnovsky, M. L., 1980, Active oxygen species and the functions of phagocytic leukocytes, *Annu. Rev. Biochem.* **49**:695–726.

Barak, M., Ulitzur, S., and Merzbach, D., 1983, Phagocytosis-induced mutagenesis in bacteria, *Mutat. Res.* **121**:7–16.

Bhimani, R., Zhong, Z., Stern, A., and Frenkel, K., 1992, Effects of red blood cells (RBCs) on formation of H_2O_2 and oxidized bases in DNA of human white blood cells (WBC) treated with the tumor promoter 12-*O*-tetradecanoylphorbol-13-acetate (TPA), *Proc. Am. Assoc. Cancer Res.* **33**:161.

Biemond, P., Swaak, A. J. G., Penders, J. M. A., Beindorff, C. M., and Koster, J. F., 1986, Superoxide production by polymorphonuclear leucocytes in rheumatoid arthritis and osteoarthritis: *In vivo* inhibition by the antirheumatic drug piroxicam due to interference with the activation of the NADPH-oxidase, *Ann. Rheum. Dis.* **45**:249–255.

Birnboim, H. C., 1983, Importance of DNA strand-break damage in tumor promotion, in: *Radioprotectors and Anticarcinogens* (O. F. Nygaard and M. G. Simic, eds.), Academic Press, New York, pp. 539–556.

Boutwell, R. K., 1964, Some biological aspects of skin carcinogenesis, *Prog. Exp. Tumor Res.* **4**:207–250.

Breimer, L. H., 1990, Molecular mechanisms of oxygen radical carcinogenesis and mutagenesis: The role of DNA base damage, *Mol. Carcinogenesis* **3**:188–197.

Burkhardt, H., Schwingel, M., Menninger, H., Macartney, H. W., and Tschesche, H., 1986, Oxygen radicals as effectors of cartilage destruction, *Arthritis Rheum.* **29**:379–387.

Byczkowski, J. Z., and Gessner, T., 1988, Minireview. Biological role of superoxide ion-radical, *Int. J. Biochem.* **20**:569–580.

Cadet, J., and Teoule, R., 1978, Comparative study of oxidation of nucleic acid components by hydroxyl radicals, singlet oxygen and superoxide anion radicals, *Photochem. Photobiol.* **28**:661–667.

Cerutti, P. A., 1976, Base damage induced by ionizing radiation, *Photochem. Photobiol. Nucleic Acids* **2**:375–401.

Chester, J. F., Gaissert, H. A., Ross, J. S., Malt, R. A., and Weitzman, S. A., 1986, Augmentation of 1,2-dimethylhydrazine-induced colon cancer by experimental colitis in mice: Role of dietary vitamin E, *J. Natl. Cancer Inst.* **76**:939–941.

Chevion, M., 1988, A site-specific mechanism for free radical induced biological damage: The essential role of redox-active transition metals, *Free Radical Biol. Med.* **5**:27–37.

de Mello-Filho, A. C., and Meneghini, R., 1985, Protection of mammalian cells by *o*-phenanthroline from lethal and DNA-damaging effects produced by active oxygen species, *Biochim. Biophys. Acta* **847**:82–89.

DiGiovanni, J., Sawyer, T. W., and Fisher, E. P., 1986, Correlation between formation of a specific hydrocarbon–deoxyribonucleoside adduct and tumor-initiating activity of 7,12-dimethylbenz(a)anthracene and its 9- and 10-monofluoroderivatives in mice, *Cancer Res.* **46**:4336–4341.

Dipple, A., Pigott, M. A., Bigger, A. H., and Blake, D. M., 1984, 7,12-Dimethylbenz(a)anthracene–DNA binding in mouse skin: Response of different mouse strains and effects of various modifiers of carcinogenesis, *Carcinogenesis* **5**:1087–1090.

D'Onofrio, C., Maly, F. E., Fischer, H., and Maas, D., 1984, Differential generation of chemiluminescence-detectable oxygen radicals by normal polymorphonuclear leukocytes challenged with sera from systemic lupus erythematosus and rheumatoid arthritis patients, *Klin. Wochenschr.* **62**:710–716.

Dunham, L. J., 1972, Cancer in man at a site of prior benign lesion of skin or mucous membrane: A review, *Cancer Res.* **32**:1359–1374.

Dutton, D. R., and Bowden, G. T., 1985, Indirect induction of a clastogenic effect in epidermal cells by a tumor promoter, *Carcinogenesis* **6**:1279–1284.

Fantone, J. C., and Ward, P. A., 1982, Role of oxygen-derived free radicals and metabolites in leukocyte-dependent inflammatory reactions, *Am. J. Pathol.* **107**:397–418.

Feldman, G., Ramsen, J., Shinohara, K., and Cerutti, P., 1978, Excisability and persistence of benzo(a)pyrene DNA adducts in epithelial human lung cells, *Nature* **274**:796–798.

Fiala, E. S., Conaway, C. C., Biles, W. T., and Johnson, B., 1987, Enhanced mutagenicity of 2-nitropropane nitronate with respect to 2-nitropropane—Possible involvement of free radical species, *Mutat. Res.* **179**:15–22.

Fiala, E. S., Conaway, C. C., and Mathis, J. E., 1989, Oxidative DNA and RNA damage in the livers of Sprague–Dawley rats treated with the hepatocarcinogen 2-nitropropane, *Cancer Res.* **49**:5518–5522.

Fischer, S. M., Hardin, L., Klein-Szanto, A., and Slaga, T., 1985, Retinoyl-phorbol-acetate is a complete skin tumor promoter in SENCAR mice, *Cancer Lett.* **27**:323–327.

Fletcher, D. S., Osinga, D., and Bonney, R. J., 1986, Role of polymorphonuclear leukocytes in connective tissue breakdown during the reverse passive Arthus reaction, *Biochem. Pharmacol.* **35**:2601–2606.

Floyd, R. A., Watson, J. J., Harris, J., West, M., and Wong, P. K., 1986, Formation of 8-hydroxydeoxyguanosine, hydroxyl free radical adduct of DNA in granulocytes exposed to the tumor promoter, tetradecanoylphorbolacetate, *Biochem. Biophys. Res. Commun.* **137**:841–846.

Floyd, R. A., West, M., Jasheway, D., and Fischer, S. M., 1987, Occurrence of 8-hydroxyguanine, the hydroxyl free radical adduct, in mouse skin epidermal DNA during tumor promotion by phorbol ester, *Proc. Am. Assoc. Cancer Res.* **28**:162.

Freeman, B. A., and Crapo, J. D., 1982, Biology of disease. Free radicals and tissue injury, *Lab. Invest.* **47**:412–426.

Frenkel, K., 1989, Oxidation of DNA bases by tumor promoter-activated processes, *Environ. Health Perspect.* **81**:45–54.

Frenkel, K., 1992, Carcinogen-mediated oxidant formation and oxidative DNA damage, *Pharmacol. Ther.* **53**(1):127–166.

Frenkel, K., and Chrzan, K., 1987a, Radiation-like modification of DNA and H_2O_2 formation by activated human polymorphonuclear leukocytes (PMNs), in: *Anticarcinogenesis and Radiation Protection* (P. A. Cerutti, O. F. Nygaard, and M. G. Simic, eds.), Plenum Press, New York, pp. 97–102.

Frenkel, K., and Chrzan, K., 1987b, Hydrogen peroxide formation and DNA base modification by tumor promoter-activated polymorphonuclear leukocytes, *Carcinogenesis* **8**:455–460.

Frenkel, K., and Gleichauf, C., 1991, Hydrogen peroxide formation by cells treated with a tumor promoter, *Free Radical Res. Commun.* **12–13**:783–794.

Frenkel, K., Goldstein, M. S., and Teebor, G. W., 1981, Identification of the *cis*-thymine glycol moiety in chemically oxidized and γ-irradiated deoxyribonucleic acid by high-pressure liquid chromatography, *Biochemistry* **20**:7566–7571.

Frenkel, K., Cummings, A., Solomon, J., Cadet, J., Steinberg, J. J., and Teebor, G. W., 1985, Quantitative determination of the 5(hydroxymethyl)uracil moiety in the DNA of γ-irradiated cells, *Biochemistry* **24**:4527–4533.

Frenkel, K., Chrzan, K., Troll, W., Teebor, G. W., and Steinberg, J. J., 1986a, Radiation-like modification of bases in DNA exposed to tumor promoter-activated polymorphonuclear leukocytes, *Cancer Res.* **46**:5533–5540.

Frenkel, K., Cummings, A., and Teebor, G. W., 1986b, 5-Hydroxymethyl uracil: A product of ionizing radiation and tritium transmutation formed in DNA, in: *Radiation Carcinogenesis and DNA Alterations* (F. J. Burns, A. C. Upton, and G. Sillini, eds.), Plenum Press, New York, pp. 439–445.

Frenkel, K., Chrzan, K., Ryan, C. A., Wiesner, R., and Troll, W., 1987, Chymotrypsin-specific protease inhibitors decrease H_2O_2 formation by activated human polymorphonuclear leukocytes, Carcinogenesis 8:1207–1212.

Frenkel, K., Donahue, J. M., and Banerjee, S., 1988a, Benzo(a)pyrene-induced oxidative DNA damage: A possible mechanism for promotion by complete carcinogens, in: Oxy-Radicals in Molecular Biology and Pathology (P. A. Cerutti, I. Fridovich, and J. M. McCord, eds.), Liss, New York, pp. 509–524.

Frenkel, K., Karkoszka, J., Donahue, J., and Banerjee, S., 1988b, Polycyclic aromatic hydrocarbon (PAH)-induced formation of H_2O_2 and of oxidized thymines in DNA by rat liver microsomes, Proc. Am. Assoc. Cancer Res. 29:151.

Frenkel, K., Zhong, Z., Wei, H., Karkoszka, J., Patel, U., Rashid, K., Georgescu, M., and Solomon, J. J., 1991a, Quantitative high-performance liquid chromatography analysis of DNA oxidized in vitro and in vivo. Anal. Biochem. 196:126–136.

Frenkel, K., Zhong, Z., Rashid, K., and Fujiki, H., 1991b, Sarcophytols and protease inhibitors suppress H_2O_2 formation and oxidative DNA damage, in: Anticarcinogenesis and Radiation Protection. 2: Strategies in Protection from Radiation and Cancer (O. F. Nygaard, ed.), Plenum Press, New York, pp. 357–366.

Fujiki, H., Suganuma, M., Suguri, H., Yoshizawa, S., Takagi, K., and Kobayashi, S., 1989, Sarcophytols A and B strongly inhibit tumor promotion by teleocidin in two-stage carcinogenesis in mouse skin, J. Cancer Res. Clin. Oncol. 115:25–28.

Fürstenberger, G., Berry, D. L., Sorg, B., and Marks, F., 1981, Skin tumor promotion by phorbol esters is a two-stage process, Proc. Natl. Acad. Sci. USA 78:7722–7726.

Fürstenberger, G., Sorg, B., and Marks, F., 1983, Tumor promotion by phorbolesters in skin: Evidence for a memory effect, Science 220:89–91.

Gensler, H. L., Watson, R. R., Moriguchi, S., and Bowden, G. T., 1987, Effects of dietary retinyl palmitate or 13-cis-retinoic acid on the promotion of tumors in mouse skin, Cancer Res. 47:967–970.

Goldstein, G. D., Witz, G., Amoruso, M., and Troll, W., 1979, Protease inhibitors antagonize the activation of polymorphonuclear leukocyte oxygen consumption, Biochem. Biophys. Res. Commun. 88:854–860.

Halliwell, B., and Gutteridge, J. M. C., 1986, Oxygen free radicals in relation to biology and medicine: Some problems and concepts, Arch. Biochem. Biophys. 246:501–514.

Ide, M. L., Kaneko, M., and Cerutti, P. A., 1984, Benzo(a)pyrene and ascorbate-$CuSO_4$ induce DNA damage in human cells by indirect action, in: Protective Agents in Cancer (D. C. H. McBrien and T. F. Slater, eds.), Academic Press, New York, pp. 125–140.

Jeffrey, A. M., Weinstein, I. B., Jennette, K. W., Grzeskowiak, K., Nakanishi, K., Autrup, H., and Harris, C., 1977, Structures of benzo(a)pyrene nucleic acid adducts formed in human and bovine bronchial explants, Nature 269:348–350.

Ji, C., and Marnett, L. J., 1992, Oxygen radical-dependent epoxidation of (7S,8S)-dihydroxy-7,8-dihydrobenzo[a]pyrene [(+)-BP-7,8-diol] in mouse skin in vivo: Stimulation by phorbol esters and inhibition by antiinflammatory steroids, J. Biol. Chem. 267:17842–17848.

Kasai, H., Crain, P. F., Kochino, Y., Nishimura, S., Ootsuyama, A., and Tanooka, H., 1986, Formation of 8-hydroxyguanine moiety in cellular DNA by agents producing oxygen radicals and evidence for its repair. Carcinogenesis 7:1849–1851.

Kasai, H., Nishimura, S., Kurakawa, Y., and Hayashi, Y., 1987, Oral administration of the renal carcinogen, potassium bromate, specifically produces 8-hydroxydeoxyguanosine in rat target organ DNA, Carcinogenesis 8:1959–1961.

Kasai, H., Okada, Y., Nishimura, S., Rao, M. S., and Reddy, J. K., 1989, Formation of 8-hydroxydeoxyguanosine in liver DNA of rats following long-term exposure to a peroxisome proliferator, Cancer Res. 49:2603–2605.

Kasprzak, K. S., Diwan, B. A., Konishi, N., Misra, M., and Rice, J. M., 1990, Initiation by nickel acetate and promotion by sodium barbital of renal cortical epithelial tumors in male F344 rats, *Carcinogenesis* 11:647–652.

Kinzel, V., Fürstenberger, G., Loehrke, H., and Marks, F., 1986, Three-stage tumorigenesis in mouse skin: DNA synthesis as a prerequisite for the conversion stage induced by TPA prior to initiation, *Carcinogenesis* 7:779–782.

Kitagawa, S., Takaku, F., and Sakamoto, S., 1979, Possible involvement of proteases in superoxide production by human polymorphonuclear leukocytes, *FEBS Lett.* 99:275–278.

Klebanoff, S. J., 1980, Oxygen metabolism and the toxic properties of phagocytes, *Ann. Intern. Med.* 93:480–489.

Klein, C. B., Frenkel, K., and Costa, M., 1991, The role of oxidative processes in metal carcinogenesis, *Chem. Res. Toxicol.* 4:592–604.

Kohda, K., Tada, M., Kasai, H., Nishimura, S., and Kawazoe, Y., 1986, Formation of 8-hydroxyguanine residues in cellular DNA exposed to the carcinogen 4-nitroquinoline 1-oxide, *Biochem. Biophys. Res. Commun.* 139:626–632.

Leadon, S. A., 1987, Production of thymine glycols in DNA by radiation and chemical carcinogens as detected by a monoclonal antibody, *Br. J. Cancer* 5:(Suppl. 8):113–117.

Leadon, S. A., Stampfer, M. R., and Bartley, J., 1988, Production of oxidative DNA damage during the metabolic activation of benzo(a)pyrene in human mammary epithelial cells correlates with cell killing, *Proc. Natl. Acad. Sci USA* 85:4365–4368.

McCord, J. M., 1974, Free radicals and inflammation: Protection of synovial fluid by superoxide dismutase, *Science* 185:529–531.

McCormick, D. L., Major, N., and Moon, R. C., 1984, Inhibition of 7,12-dimethylbenz(a)anthracene-induced rat mammary carcinogenesis by concomitant or postcarcinogen antioxidant exposure, *Cancer Res.* 44:2858–2863.

Meneghini, R., 1988, Genotoxicity of active oxygen species in mammalian cells, *Mutat. Res.* 195:215–230.

Narisawa, T., Takahashi, M., Niwa, Y., and Fujiki, H., 1989, Inhibition of methylnitrosourea-induced large bowel cancer development in rats by sarcophytol A, a product from a marine soft coral *Sarcophyton glaucum, Cancer Res.* 49:3287–3289.

O'Brien, P. J., 1988, Radical formation during the peroxidase catalyzed metabolism of carcinogens and xenobiotics: The reactivity of these radicals with GSH, DNA, and unsaturated lipid, *Free Radical Biol. Med.* 4:169–183.

Ochi, T., and Kaneko, M., 1989, Active oxygen contributes to the major part of chromosomal aberrations in V79 Chinese hamster cells exposed to N-hydroxy-2-naphthylamine, *Free Radical Res. Commun.* 5:351–358.

O'Connell, J. F., Klein-Szanto, A. J. P., DiGiovanni, D. M., Fries, J. W., and Slaga, T. J., 1986, Enhanced malignant progression of mouse skin tumors by the free-radical generator benzoyl peroxide, *Cancer Res.* 46:2863–2865.

Rice-Evans, C., Omorphos, S. C., and Baysal, E., 1986, Sickle cell membranes and oxidative damage, *Biochem. J.* 237:265–269.

Schacter, L. P., 1986, Generation of superoxide anion and hydrogen peroxide by erythrocytes from individuals with sickle trait or normal hemoglobin, *Eur. J. Clin. Invest.* 16:204–210.

Scholes, G., 1983, Radiation effects on DNA, *Br. J. Radiol.* 56:221–231.

Shacter, E., Beecham, E. J., Covey, J. M., Kohn, K. W., and Potter, M., 1988, Activated neutrophils induce prolonged DNA damage in neighboring cells, *Carcinogenesis* 9:2297–2304.

Shasby, D. M., Shasby, S. S., and Peach, J. J., 1983, Granulocytes and phorbol myristate acetate increase permeability to albumin of cultured endothelial monolayers and isolated perfused lungs, *Am. Rev. Respir. Dis.* 127:72–76.

Simon, R. H., Scoggin, C. H., and Patterson, D., 1981, Hydrogen peroxidase causes the fatal injury to human fibroblasts exposed to oxygen radicals, *J. Biol. Chem.* 256:7181–7186.

Slaga, T. J., Fisher, S. M., Nelson, K., and Gleason, G. L., 1980, Studies on the mechanism of skin tumor promotion: Evidence for several stages of promotion, *Proc. Natl. Acad. Sci. USA* **77**:3659–3663.

Slaga, T. J., Fisher, S. M., Weeks, C. E., Nelson, K., Mamrack, M., and Klein-Szanto, A. J. P., 1982, Specificity and mechanism(s) of promoter inhibitors in multistage promotion, in: *Carcinogenesis*, Volume 7 (E. Hecker, W. Kuntz, N. E. Fusenig, F. Marks, and H. W. Thielmann, eds.), Raven Press, New York, pp. 19–34.

Srinivasan, S., and Glauert, H. P., 1990, Formation of 5-hydroxymethyl-2′-deoxyuridine in hepatic DNA of rats treated with γ-irradiation, diethylnitrosamine, 2-acetylaminofluorene or the peroxisome proliferator ciprofibrate, *Carcinogenesis* **11**:2021–2024.

Teebor, G. W., Frenkel, K., and Goldstein, M., 1984, Ionizing radiation and tritium transmutation both cause formation of 5-hydroxymethyl-2′-deoxyuridine in cellular DNA, *Proc. Natl. Acad. Sci. USA* **81**:318–321.

Teebor, G. W., Boorstein, R. J., and Cadet, J., 1988, The repairability of oxidative free radical mediated damage to DNA: A review, *Int. J. Radiat. Biol.* **54**:131–150.

Troll, W., Frenkel, K., and Teebor, G. W., 1984, Free oxygen radicals: Necessary contributors to tumor promotion and cocarcinogenesis: in: *Cellular Interactions by Environmental Tumor Promoters* (H. Fujiki, E. Hecker, R. E. Moore, T. Sugimura, and I. B. Weinstein, eds.), Japan Scientific Societies Press, Tokyo, pp. 207–218.

Troll, W., Wiesner, R., and Frenkel, K., 1987, Anticarcinogenic action of protease inhibitors, *Adv. Cancer Res.* **49**:265–283.

Trush, M. A., and Kensler, T. W., 1991, An overview of the relationship between oxidative stress and chemical carcinogenesis, *Free Radical Biol. Med.* **10**:201–209.

Umemura, T., Sai, K., Takagi, A., Hasegawa, R., and Kurakawa, Y., 1990, Formation of 8-hydroxydeoxyguanosine (8-OH-dG) in rat kidney DNA after intraperitoneal administration of ferric nitrilotriacetate (Fe-NTA), *Carcinogenesis* **11**:345–347.

Vercellotti, G. M., van Asbeck, B. S., and Jacob, H. S., 1985, Oxygen radical-induced erythrocyte hemolysis by neutrophils; critical role of iron and lactoferrin, *J. Clin. Invest.* **76**:956–962.

Vuillaume, M., 1987, Reduced oxygen species, mutation, induction and cancer initiation, *Mutat. Res.* **186**:43–47.

Wallace, S., 1988, AP endonucleases and DNA glycosylases that recognize oxidative DNA damage, *Environ. Mol. Mut.* **12**:431–477.

Washburn, P. C., and Di Giulio, R. T., 1988, Nitroaromatic stimulation of superoxide production in three species of freshwater fish, *Mar. Environ. Res.* **24**:291–294.

Wattenberg, L. W., 1980, Inhibition of chemical carcinogenesis by antioxidants, in: *Carcinogenesis*, Volume 5 (T. J. Slaga, ed.), Raven Press, New York, pp. 85–98.

Wei, H., and Frenkel, K., 1991, *In vivo* formation of oxidized DNA bases in tumor promoter-treated mouse skin, *Cancer Res.* **51**:4443–4449.

Wei, H., and Frenkel, K., 1992a, 7,12-Dimethylbenz(a)anthracene (DMBA)-mediated *in vivo* induction of oxidative events and oxidative DNA damage in SENCAR mice, *Proc. Am. Assoc. Cancer Res.* **33**:180.

Wei, H., and Frenkel, K., 1992b, Suppression of tumor promoter-induced oxidative events and DNA damage *in vivo* by sarcophytol A: A possible mechanism of anti-promotion, *Cancer Res.* **52**:2298–2303.

Weitzman, S. A., and Gordon, L. I., 1990, Inflammation and cancer: Role of phagocyte-generated oxidants in carcinogenesis, *Blood* **76**:655–663.

Weitzman, S. A., and Stossel, T. P., 1982, Effects of oxygen radical scavengers and antioxidants on phagocyte-induced mutagenesis, *J. Immunol.* **128**:2770–2772.

Weitzman, S. A., Weitberg, A. B., Clark, E. P., and Stossel, T. P., 1985, Phagocytes as carcinogens: Malignant transformation produced by human neutrophils, *Science* **227**:1231–1233.

Witz, G., Goldstein, B. D., Amoruso, M., Stone, D. S., and Troll, W., 1980, Retinoid inhibition of superoxide anion radical production by human polymorphonuclear leukocytes stimulated with tumor promoters, *Biochem. Biophys. Res. Commun.* **97**:883–888.

Zhong, Z., Tius, M., Troll, W., Fujiki, H., and Frenkel, K., 1991, Inhibition of H_2O_2 formation by human polymorphonuclear leukocytes (PMNs) as a measure of anti-carcinogenic activity, *Proc. Am. Assoc. Cancer Res.* **32:**127.

Zvillich, M., Kol, R., Riklis, E., and Sarov, I., 1988, Induction of DNA strand scissions in HeLa cells by human polymorphonuclear leucocytes activated by *Chlamydia trachomatis* elementary bodies, *J. Gen. Microbiol.* **134:**2405–2412.

15

Protease Inhibitor Suppression of ras Oncogene-Induced Transformation

SEYMOUR J. GARTE, LYDIA COX, DIANE C. CURRIE, JOAN MOTZ, and WALTER TROLL

1. Introduction

As discussed in several chapters of this book, support for an active role of proteases and protease inhibitors in carcinogenesis and anticarcinogenesis has come from multiple observations that protease inhibitors suppress transformation *in vitro* and in several animal models (Belman and Garte, 1985; Troll and Wiesner, 1984; Corasanti *et al.*, 1982; Kennedy and Little, 1978; Yavelow *et al.*, 1983). Treatment of various cells and tissues with phorbol ester tumor promoters induces proteases including plasminogen activator (Quigley, 1979), and the promoting activity of phorbol ester is inhibited by protease inhibitors *in vivo* and *in vitro* (see Belman and Garte, 1985, for review). The mechanism of action of protease inhibitors as anticarcinogens is not well understood, and is probably complex. We thought it would be of interest to determine whether such agents could affect transformation of cells caused by a single purified activated oncogene, as opposed to radiation or chemical carcinogens. We therefore adapted the standard NIH3T3 transfection focus assay with an activated human H-*ras* oncogene to assess the effects of protease inhibitors (and other chemopreventive agents) on oncogene-induced cell transformation.

DNA-mediated gene transfer or transfection has proven to be a useful tech-

SEYMOUR J. GARTE, LYDIA COX, DIANE C. CURRIE, JOAN MOTZ, and WALTER TROLL • Department of Environmental Medicine, New York University Medical Center, New York, New York 10016.

Protease Inhibitors as Cancer Chemopreventive Agents, edited by Walter Troll and Ann R. Kennedy. Plenum Press, New York, 1993.

nique for identification and study of dominant transforming genes. In particular, the NIH3T3 mouse fibroblast cell line has been extremely valuable in the detection of activated *ras* and other oncogenes in human and animal tumor DNA (Weinberg, 1985; Balmain and Brown, 1988). The biochemical and molecular properties of the *ras* family of cellular oncogenes have been extensively studied in recent years (Barbacid, 1987). The point mutational mechanism of activation of proto-*ras* (Tabin *et al.*, 1982; Reddy *et al.*, 1982) has been well established and the biochemical consequences of activation, especially related to reduced GTPase activity, have also been examined (Sweet *et al.*, 1984; Gibbs *et al.*, 1984). In yeast, the *ras* homologous genes apparently code for signal transducing proteins involved in the adenylate cyclase induction pathway (Powers *et al.*, 1984). In mammalian cells the precise function of proto-*ras* is not as clear, although some evidence suggests a role for the *ras* gene product, p21, in signal transduction.

The mechanism by which activated oncogenes produce cell transformation is not known, even when the function of the gene product is known, as in the case of tyrosine kinase genes like *src* or growth factor genes like *sis*, *erb-b*, or *fms*. Although it has been known for many years that infection of certain cells with a retrovirus containing a single oncogene is sufficient to produce transformation, it appears that activation of a single cellular oncogene rarely, if ever, is a sufficient cause of transformation in normal diploid primary cell cultures. The *ras* oncogene, for example, by itself does not transform primary rat or mouse embryo fibroblasts that have not undergone establishment and immortalization (Land *et al.*, 1983; Ruley, 1983) unless it is linked to strong enhancers (Spandidos and Wilkie, 1984), or cotransfected with a second oncogene such as *myc* (Land *et al.*, 1983). We have observed concurrent activation *in vivo* of the K-*ras* and c-*myc* oncogenes in a panel of radiation-induced rat skin tumors (Sawey *et al.*, 1987). These results are entirely consistent with the multistage theory of carcinogenesis including the two-stage initiation–promotion paradigm (Boutwell, 1974). In fact, the correlation of *ras* gene activation with an initiation-type event has been demonstrated using the classical tumor promoter 12-*O*-tetradecanoyl 13-phorbol acetate (TPA) *in vivo* (Brown *et al.*, 1986) and *in vitro* (Hsiao *et al.*, 1984; Dotto *et al.*, 1985). The fact that mutationally activated *ras* genes are able to fully transform immortal lines such as NIH3T3 has been interpreted to indicate that such cell lines have already undergone one or more alterations corresponding to stages of neoplasia, and only require expression of a single active *ras* oncogene, to be fully transformed. In the case of the NIH3T3 line, which is exquisitely sensitive to *ras*-induced transformation, the cells appeared to be "primed" for transformation by *ras*, as the last missing step in a transformation pathway.

Results from our laboratory suggest that even for NIH3T3 cells, transformation by *ras* may be a multistage process in at least a large fraction of the cells. Our results further suggest that events occurring during cell division play a critical role in the transformation process, and that one or more of these events are inhibitable by protease inhibitors (Garte *et al.*, 1987).

2. Methods

2.1. Cell Culture and DNA Isolation

NIH3T3 cells were seeded from frozen stocks and subcultured every 3 days at 3×10^5 cells/26-cm^2 flask. The cells were grown in Dulbecco's modified Eagle medium supplemented with 10% fetal bovine serum. Cells were grown in Corning plastic culture flasks in a 5% CO_2 37°C humid incubator. A frozen vial of NIH3T3 cells was thawed and seeded for each transfection experiment. The pEJ (Parada *et al.*, 1982), pSVneo (Southern and Berg, 1982), and pAGT (Spandidos and Wilkie, 1984) plasmids containing the activated human H-*ras*, *aph*, and H-*ras* with *aph* genes, respectively, were grown, and DNA purified by standard methods (Maniatis *et al.*, 1982). For isolation of DNA from cells, frozen cell pellets were ground to a fine powder in a stainless steel mortar and pestle in liquid nitrogen.

2.2. DNA-Mediated Transfection

The calcium phosphate–DNA coprecipitate method of Wigler *et al.* (1979) was followed. Forty-eight hours after treatment, each flask was trypsinized and subcultured into three 25-cm^2 flasks. Medium was changed twice a week for 3 weeks, at which time foci were picked and/or flasks were fixed with methanol for 1 min and stained with 2% Giemsa for 30 min. Scoring was done by microscopic evaluation of foci to distinguish spontaneous overgrowths and type I foci from transformed type III foci. All transfections included controls, which were treated with normal mouse DNA. All experiments were scored double-blind with prior randomization of flasks at the time of subculture. Experiments were done with three to five flasks per treatment group, including controls.

When selection for G418 resistance was the endpoint in transfection experiments, cells were transfected with plasmid containing the neo or *aph* gene (Spandidos and Wilkie, 1984), as above; however, cells were subcultured at 1:3 at 30 hr after transfection, at which time they were fed with medium containing 0.7 mg/ml geneticin (Gibco). Each lot of geneticin was assayed for cell killing to determine the optimal concentration. After 2 weeks, colonies of resistant cells were isolated with cloning cylinders or stained for counting as described above.

2.3. Characterization of Transformed Phenotype

Cells were tested for anchorage independence by growth in soft agar. A base layer of 0.5% agar in MEM with 10% fetal bovine serum and 10% tryptose

(Gibco) was added (7 ml) to a 60-mm plastic culture dish. A suspension of 5×10^4 cells in 1.5 ml growth medium containing 0.33% agar was layered onto each base layer. Once a week, dishes were fed 1 ml liquid growth medium. Colonies were scored after 3 weeks of incubation at 37°C in a CO_2 incubator.

2.4. Southern Blot Hybridization

The DNA was digested to completion with one of several restriction endonucleases. After resuspension in Tris-borate buffer, pH 8.0, DNA was applied (10–30 mg) to a 0.8% agarose horizontal slab gel. Gel electrophoresis was performed according to McDonnell *et al.*, (1977). After electrophoresis, the DNA fragments were transferred to a nitrocellulose filter according to the method of Southern (1975), and Maniatis *et al.* (1982). Gels were denatured in 0.5 M NaOH, 1.5 M NaCl, rinsed in 1 M Tris, 3 M NaCl, and placed on a paper wick dipped in 20× standard saline citrate (SSC). A nitrocellulose filter was placed directly over the gel, and several layers of paper placed over the filter. After 16–24 hr, the filter was rinsed and baked at 80°C under vacuum for 2 hr and stored under vacuum until use. Probe DNA molecules were radiolabeled to a specific activity of $3–10 \times 10^9/\mu g$ DNA by nick translation in the presence of $[\alpha\text{-}^{32}P]dCTP$ (Rigby *et al.*, 1977). Filters were hybridized with radiolabeled probes in the presence of dextran sulfate using a modification of the procedure of Wahl *et al.* (1979), washed in 0.5× SSC–0.1% SDS at 65°C to remove nonspecifically bound probe molecules, dried, and subjected to autoradiography at −70°C using XRA-5 film (Kodak) and Cronex Lighting Plus intensifying screens (DuPont).

2.5. Northern Blot Hybridization

Northern Blot Analysis. RNA was isolated from cell pellets prepared from subconfluent cultures (~ 20×10^6 cells). RNA was extracted from pellets using the RNAzol method (Cinna/Biotecx, Friendswood, Tex.). RNA samples (10 μg) were glyoxalated according to the procedure of Williams and Mason (1985) and separated on 1.0% agarose gel. RNA was transferred onto Zetabind (Cuno, Meriden, Conn.) membranes overnight and baked for 1.5 hr at 80°C. Filters were washed at 65°C for 0.5 hr in 0.1× SSC (0.15 M NaCl and 0.015 M trisodium citrate) and 0.5% SDS. Prehybridization and hybridization of membranes were performed as described above for Southern blots. After hybridization with oncogene probes, filters were stripped in boiling double-distilled water and rehybridized to actin for standardization purposes. Common standards were included on blots to allow interblot comparisons.

Probes. DNA probes were prepared from pEJ (H-*ras*); pBS4, the *Pst*I fragment from the third exon of rat c-*myc* which was a gift from P. Tsichlis; and pHFBA-1, the 2.0-kb *Xho*I fragment of human B actin obtained from ATCC

(Rockville, Md.). Probes were nick-translated to a specific activity of 10^7–10^8 cpm/μg using [^{32}P]dCTP (New England Nuclear, Wilmington, Del.) according to the procedure of Maniatis *et al.* (1982).

Data Analysis. Southern blots were scanned by laser densitometry. Only those bands of 6.6 kb (the size of the H-*ras* insert in the pEJ plasmid) or greater were quantified. Gene copy number was determined relative to that of the normal human fibroblast cell line, MRC-5. Gene expression on Northern blots was quantified by laser densitometry and values were standardized by actin expression. Differences were analyzed for statistical significance using a one-tailed student's *t*-test.

3. Results

3.1. Dose Response of Protease Inhibitors on ras Transformation

The NIH3T3 focus assay can provide quantitative information for analysis of the biochemical events associated with *ras* oncogene-induced cellular transformation. The number of easily scored transformed foci is linearly related to the concentration of *ras* gene transfected into cell monolayers (Garte *et al.*, 1987). Inhibition of pEJ [a plasmid containing the mutationally activated human H-*ras* oncogene (Parada *et al.*, 1982)] transformation by the protease inhibitors antipain and ϵ-aminocaproic acid as well as retinoic acid occurred in a concentration-dependent manner as seen in Table I. The active agents shown in Table I, as well as protease inhibitors leupeptin and α-antitrypsin all exhibit a maximum inhibition of approximately 50% of control.

Table I. Dose Response for Inhibition
of Focus Formation

Agent	Dose	Foci (% of control)
Antipain	30 μm	84
	80 μm	44
	160 μm	53
	400 μm	44
Retinoic acid	3 μm	96
	10 μm	49
	30 μm	42
	100 μm	58
Epsilon amino	2.3 mM	109
Caproic acid	7.6 mM	76
	15 mM	63
	30 mM	44

3.2. Effects on aph Gene Transfection

In order to determine whether a general effect of the inhibitors on the incorporation or expression of exogenous genes in the gene transfer assay was responsible for the inhibition of *ras* transformation, we repeated these experiments using the neomycin-resistant plasmid pSVneo and scored G418 (geneticin)-resistant colonies. There was no significant depression in the number of G418-resistant colonies by either 50 or 100 mg/ml antipain. Similar results were obtained using α-antitrypsin. Further experiments were done using NIH3T3 cells transfected with pAGT, a plasmid containing both active *ras* and *aph*, a gene that confers resistance to G418. The number of pAGT-induced foci (in the absence of selection) was reduced by 50% with antipain relative to pEJ, but the number of G481 colonies was not only not reduced, but in fact was doubled. This surprising result could be explained by a possible toxic effect of *ras* expression on cells. Inhibition of *ras* expression would therefore allow for the survival of more G418–resistant colonies. Consistent with this possibility was our observation that the number of colonies in control plates produced by pSVneo was about 10 times higher than that seen with pAGT. In order to test this possibility, an experiment using antipain on cells cotransfected with pEJ and pSVneo in different proportions was performed. If antipain did in fact suppress *ras*-induced toxicity, then at high ratios of pEJ to pSVneo, antipain treatment should increase the number of colonies. Although we did observe a trend toward lower colony numbers with increasing pEJ/pSVneo ratios, in no case did antipain treatment have any effect. The explanation for the reproducible stimulatory effect of antipain on G418 resistance in pAGT-transfected NIH3T3 cells is therefore still unknown. However, whatever the mechanism for this effect is, it is certainly clear that the results on inhibition of H-*ras* transformation by antipain cannot be explained solely by effects on the cellular uptake or stable genomic integration of exogenous genes.

3.3. Time Course Studies

In order to examine the time of antipain activity, antipain was added to the medium during various periods of the 19-day transformation protocol. When antipain was present only during the first 2 days (before the 1 : 3 subculture step), no effect on transforming efficiency was seen. On the other hand, when antipain was present only after the subculture step on day 3, the complete inhibitory effect was seen. It appears that the early stage of this phase is susceptible to the effects of antipain since addition of the inhibitor starting on day 9 had no effect on transformation. This suggests that antipain is unable to reverse the transformed phenotype once it has been established. In order to further test the ability of antipain to revert H-*ras*-transformed cells to a normal phenotype, the T110 line of NIH3T3 cells (Garte, 1985) previously transformed by transfection with the

H-*ras* oncogene was treated at low seeding density with antipain (50 mg/ml) for 2 weeks. No morphological evidence of reversion to the normal phenotype was seen.

3.4. Influence of Cell Proliferation

The period of antipain efficacy in inhibition of NIH3T3 cell transformation corresponds to a period of cell proliferation after the 1:3 subculture step at day 3. The possibility that protease inhibitor action involves the growth stage following subculture was tested further. When cells were not subcultured 3 days after transfection, the yield of foci was dramatically reduced compared with that seen following the normal protocol of 1:3 subculture, and antipain exerted no inhibition of transformation. These findings support the idea that protease inhibitors act during cell proliferation and only block transformation of that fraction of cells which require division in order to express the transformed phenotype. Neither antipain nor α-antitrypsin had any effect on the viability or proliferation rate of NIH3T3 cells as measured by tritiated thymidine incorporation during and after log-phase growth. Furthermore, neither antipain nor retinoic acid had any effect on the growth rate of 608-ID cells, a clone of NIH3T3 transformed by transfection with pAGT.

3.5. Subculture and Serum Conditions

Since subculture involves use of trypsin, and antipain is added directly after replating of trypsinized cells, it is formally possible that some residual trypsin activity is responsible for enhanced transformation, and this is blocked by the inhibitors. This seems unlikely since cells are exposed to minimal levels of trypsin for only 3 min, and any residual trypsin activity should be halted by the protease inhibitors present in serum. When cells were subcultured using elastase instead of trypsin, no difference in transformation efficiencies was observed in either control or antipain-treated cultures. In order to further elucidate the potentially confounding effect of serum on our results, we performed a transfection experiment using cells grown in 10, 5, and 1% serum. The control number of foci was unchanged, and antipain exerted the same 50% inhibition in all three serum concentrations.

The observation that subculture and concomitant cell division increased transformation efficiency after transfection of NIH3T3 cells with a single active *ras* oncogene resembles effects described by Kennedy and others of x-ray- and chemically induced transformation in other cell systems (Kennedy and Little, 1984). We extended this observation by comparing the transfection efficiency of the *ras* gene in NIH3T3 cells subcultured at different densities. Splitting cells at day 3 to lower cell densities (resulting in a greater number of cell divisions) yielded increased numbers of foci per μg DNA.

3.6. Reversibility

Cell lines that had taken up the H-*ras* oncogene but whose transformation was suppressed by antipain (AP) treatment (see below) were grown in the presence and absence of AP (50 mg/ml) to determine whether the suppression of the transformed phenotype was reversible. Two different cell lines remained nontransformed (as determined by their inability to grow in soft agar) when grown in the presence of AP. However, when these same cells were switched to medium without AP, a rapid change in their phenotype, including increased growth rate, morphological alterations, and anchorage independence, occurred within 2–3 weeks. We conclude that the effect of AP on suppression of *ras*-induced transformation is readily reversible, and requires the continuous presence of AP.

3.7. ras Gene Expression

In order to study gene expression and incorporation in *ras*-transfected cells as a function of inhibitor treatment, we have isolated a number of cell lines derived from pEJ and pSVneo cotransfected G418-resistant colonies. Each of five untreated colonies was anchorage independent, as expected. Six of the ten AP-treated colonies failed to grow in soft agar, while the other four exhibited the transformed phenotype of soft agar growth. Southern blot analysis revealed that two of the six nontransformed lines had failed to incorporate the *ras* oncogene. However, the other four cell lines which were exposed to AP and were negative for transformation had on average a similar number of copies of the transfected EJ gene as the four positive lines which were exposed to AP and the five positive lines which served as untreated controls. Northern blot analyses of mRNA levels of the transfected H-*ras* gene in untreated and AP-exposed cell lines showed that H-*ras* expression was similar in all transformed cell lines whether untreated or AP-exposed. In contrast, levels of H-*ras* mRNA were decreased approximately fourfold in the AP-treated cell lines whose transformed phenotype was suppressed ($p < 0.05$) (Cox *et al.*, 1991a).

Northern blot analyses of mRNA levels of the c-*myc* gene in untreated and AP-exposed cell lines revealed that all transformed cell lines expressed comparable levels of c-*myc* independent of AP treatment. The level of c-*myc* expression in nontransformed AP-treated cell lines was approximately 2.5 times lower than in their transformed counterparts ($p < 0.10$). These results suggest that transformation by H-*ras* involves an increase in expression of the endogenous c-*myc* gene. Furthermore, when such transformation is inhibited by AP there is a concomitant suppression of c-*myc* expression to control levels (Cox *et al.*, 1991a).

3.8. Retinoic Acid Effects

We expanded our studies to determine whether other known chemopreventive or anticarcinogenic agents might have similar effects to the protease inhibitors. Indomethacin, an inhibitor of prostaglandin synthesis, with antipromoting activity in mouse skin had no effect on *ras* transformation of NIH3T3 cells at concentrations of 10–100 mM. Retinoic acid, which is a well-known inhibitor of tumor promotion and other models of carcinogenesis, inhibited focus formation at concentrations of 1 to 10 µg/ml. As was seen for antipain, the maximum inhibition was around 40–50% of control (Cox *et al.*, 1991b).

We have observed that reduction of the number of foci in retinoic acid-treated cells is not the only effect of this agent. The foci that appear after transfection with either pEJ or pAGT exhibit morphological characteristics strikingly different from control foci. Foci from retinoic acid-treated cultures are less tightly packed, more diffuse, the cells stain less intensely, and the edges of the focus are poorly defined. This phenomenon has been consistently observed in all foci from retinoic acid-treated plates, but has never been seen with AP. Other evidence also suggests that the inhibitory action by retinoic acid and AP are due to different mechanisms. In a time course experiment, the maximal inhibition of foci (38% of control) was obtained by treatment from day 0 to day 3 of transfection, whereas treatment during the proliferation phase after subculture (days 3–6) reduced the focus yield only to 65% of control. Treatment from days 6 to 19 produced only marginal inhibition. Only the late-stage treatment with retinoic acid yielded the anomalous focus morphology result. It appears that the inhibition of H-*ras* transforming efficiency by retinoic acid may be disassociated from its effects on focus morphology. Experiments using pSVneo indicate that retinoic acid inhibition of focus formation is in fact due to a nonspecific block of transfection and not inhibition of transformation. This result is consistent with the time course data, and further differentiates the mechanism of action of retinoic acid from that of protease inhibitors (Cox *et al.*, 1991b).

4. Discussion

Our data suggest that multistep mechanisms including cell proliferation are involved in a significant fraction of NIH3T3 cells transformed by the *ras* oncogene. Furthermore, protease inhibitors appear to block this proliferation-associated process. Three lines of evidence argue against interference by protease inhibitors with the uptake or expression of the exogenous gene during transfection. First, the transfection efficiency of another, nontransforming gene was not affected by AP in independent experiments using pSVneo, as well as in experiments where both *aph* and *ras* genes were present in the same transfected plasmid DNA. Second, AP present only 4 hr before, during, and 48 hr after transfection did not inhibit transformation. In contrast, when AP was present during the period of cell proliferation following subculture, focus formation was reproducibly suppressed. Finally, the direct analysis of *ras* gene copy number by Southern blot hybridization confirmed that AP treatment had no effect on the incorporation of the exogenously transfected activated H-*ras* gene.

The unexpected finding of a maximal inhibition at 50% of the normal transformation efficiency of H-*ras* by AP suggests the possibility that there are two populations of potential transformed cells. It may be hypothesized that some fraction of the cells which have taken up and expressed the activated *ras* gene require no further mechanistic steps to proceed to transformation and focus formation, or that if other steps are required, they are not affected by protease inhibitors. Another fraction of *ras*-transfected cells apparently does require the involvement of other events (which our data indicate occur during cell proliferation) for complete transformation and one or more of these events are protease inhibitor sensitive. The 50% maximum inhibition value would suggest that half of the transfected cells are in the "complete transformation" pathway. The experiments on subculture show that elimination of the cell proliferation phase following subculture indeed results in a 50% reduction of foci per flask scored. However, when the data are corrected for transformation efficiency per µg DNA transfected, the decrease is closer to only 20% of the control (1 : 3 subculture) value. This apparent inconsistency may be explained by the fact that from one to two rounds of cell division occur between transfection of the subconfluent cultures on day 1 and the subculture step 48 hr later. This will result in a two to fourfold expansion of the transfected cells. When these cells are trypsinized, mixed, and reseeded, the ultimate number of foci in the scored flasks will depend on the degree of cell division between transfection and subculture. If an average of 1.5 cell divisions are assumed to occur during this time, then in order to compare transfection efficiencies in subcultured versus nonsubcultured cells (in which such division will not yield new foci, since the cells are never reseeded) the latter value must be corrected by a factor of 3 (that is, 2×1.5). If this is done, the actual number of originally transformed cells in the nonsubculture experiment is one-half that of the subcultured cells. The value of 1.5 cell divisions is a reasonable approximation based on growth curves.

The mechanism of action of protease inhibitors on *ras*-induced transformation is not known. AP has been shown to inhibit expression of the c-*myc* oncogene in C3H10T1/2 fibroblasts (Chang *et al.*, 1985) and selective DNA amplification through inactivation of DNA polymerase-α in SV40-transformed Chinese hamster ovary cells (Heilbronn *et al.*, 1985). It was reported that 3T3 cells transformed by *ras* oncogenes contain a metalloprotease that has cytolytic activity (DiStefano *et al.*, 1988). The report by Diamond *et al.* (1989) that ADPRT inhibitors also suppress the transformation by several oncogenes of NIH3T3 cells lends support to the idea that this assay could provide a useful way to detect anticarcinogenic agents. The relationship between the mechanisms of action of protease and ADPRT inhibitors is of considerable interest, and should be further explored.

AP-induced suppression of oncogenic transformation of NIH3T3 cells is associated with alterations in expression of both the exogenously transfected H-*ras* oncogene and the endogenous c-*myc* oncogene. The effect of AP on gene expression was seen in those colonies whose transformation phenotype was inhibited by AP, but no decrease in expression was seen in treated cells that escaped the antineoplastic effects of AP. This lends strong evidence to a mechanistic connection between AP-induced suppression of both gene expression and transformation.

The decrease in expression of both H-*ras* and c-*myc* is of particular interest, since these oncogenes are complementary in their action on the transformation of primary cells (Land *et al.*, 1983). An approximate 2.5-fold enhancement of c-*myc* expression was found in the transformed cell lines in comparison to NIH3T3 cells or the transfected cell lines which did not take up the transforming gene. Although the mechanism by which *ras* transformation results in enhanced expression of c-*myc* in NIH3T3 cells is not known, the enhanced c-*myc* expression may be necessary for the maintenance of the transformed phenotype. This idea is supported by the data which show that the suppression of the transformed phenotype which occurs upon exposure to AP is associated with a decrease in c-*myc* levels to levels found in NIH3T3 parent cells or transfected control cells.

The idea that *ras*-induced transformation of NIH3T3 cells may be a multistep process resembles what is known about multiple stages in carcinogenesis *in vivo*. If the proliferation of NIH3T3 cells during transfection has a promoterlike effect on transformed focus production, then inhibition of transformation by protease inhibitors may involve mechanisms similar to those exerted by these agents *in vivo* and in cell transformation systems. Further elucidation of the specific biochemical mechanisms by which protease inhibitors suppress transformation by an activated *ras* oncogene should provide important information regarding the carcinogenic process.

5. References

Balmain, A., and Brown, K., 1988, Oncogene activation in chemical carcinogenesis, *Adv. Cancer Res.* **51**:147–182.

Barbacid, M., 1987, ras genes, *Annu. Rev. Biochem.* **56**:779–827.

Belman, S., and Garte, S. J., 1985, Proteases and cyclic nucleotides, in: *Arachidonic Acid Metabolism and Tumor Promotion* (S. M. Fischer and T. J. Slaga, eds.), Martinus Nijhoff, Boston, pp. 199–253.

Boutwell, R. K., 1974, The function and mechanism of promoters of carcinogenesis, *CRC Crit. Rev. Toxicol.* **2**:419–443.

Brown, K., Quintanilla, M., Ramsden, M., Kerr, I. B., and Balmain, A., 1986, v-ras genes from Harvey and BALB murine sarcoma viruses can act as initiators of two-stage mouse skin carcinogenesis, *Cell* **46**:447–456.

Chang, J. D., Billings, P. C., and Kennedy, A. R., 1985, C-myc expression is reduced in antipain-treated proliferating C3H 10T1/2 cells, *Biochem. Biophys. Res. Commun.* **133**:830–835.

Corasanti, J. G., Hobika, G. H., and Markus, G., 1982, Interference with dimethylhydrazine induction of colon tumors in mice by epsilon-amniocaproic acid, *Science* **216**:1020–1021.

Cox, L. R., Motz, J., Troll, W., and Garte, S. J., 1991a, Antipain-induced suppression of oncogene expression in H-ras transformed cells, *Cancer Res.* **51**:4810–4814.

Cox, L., Motz, J., Troll, W., and Garte, S. J., 1991b, Effects of retinoic acid on NIH3T3 cell transformation by the H-*ras* oncogene, *J. Cancer Res. Clin. Oncol.* **117**:926–932.

Diamond, A. M., Der, C. J., and Schwartz, J. L., 1989, Alterations in transformation efficiency by the ADPRT-inhibitor 3-aminobenzamide are oncogene specific, *Carcinogenesis* **10**:383–385.

DiStefano, J. F., Cotto, C. A., and Hagag, N., 1988, Oncogene ras p21- and v-src pp60-transformed cells exhibit altered expression of proteases, *Cancer Invest.* **6**:487–498.

Dotto, G. P., Parada, L. F., and Weinberg, R. A., 1985, Specific growth response of ras-transformed embryo fibroblasts to tumour promoters, *Nature* **318**:472–475.

Garte, S. J., 1985, Differential effects of phorbol ester on the β-adrenergic response of normal and ras-transformed NIH3T3 cells, *Biochem. Biophys. Res. Commun.* **133**:702–708.

Garte, S. J., Currie, D. C., and Troll, W., 1987, Inhibition of H-ras oncogene transformation of NIH3T3 cells by protease inhibitors, *Cancer Res.* **47**:3159–3162.

Gibbs, J. B., Sigal, I. S., and Scolnick, E. M., 1984, Intrinsic GTPase activity distinguishes normal and oncogenic ras p21 molecules, *Proc. Natl. Acad. Sci. USA* **81**:5704–5708.

Heilbronn, R., Schlehofer, J. R., and Zur Hausen, H., 1985, Selective DNA-amplification induced by carcinogens (initiators): Evidence for a role of proteases and DNA polymerase alpha, *Int. J. Cancer* **36**:85–91.

Hsiao, W. L., Gattoni-Celli, S., and Weinstein, I. B., 1984, Oncogene-induced transformation of C3H 10T1/2 cells is enhanced by tumor promoters, *Science* **226**:552–555.

Kennedy, A. R., and Little, J. B., 1978, Protease inhibitors suppress radiation-induced malignant transformation in vitro, *Nature* **276**:825–826.

Kennedy, A. R., and Little, J. B., 1984, Evidence that a second event in X-ray-induced oncogenic transformation in vitro occurs during cellular proliferation, *Radiat. Res.* **99**:228–248.

Land, H., Parada, L. F., and Weinberg, R. A., 1983, Cellular oncogenes and multistep carcinogenesis, *Science* **222**:771–778.

McDonnell, M. W., Simon, M. N., and Studier, R. W., 1977, Analysis of restriction fragments of T7 DNA and determination of molecular weights by electrophoresis in neutral and alkaline gels, *J. Mol. Biol.* **110**:119–146.

Maniatis, T., Fritsch, E. F., and Samibrook, J., 1982, *Molecular Cloning,* Cold Spring Harbor Laboratory, Cold Spring Harbor, N.Y.

Parada, L. F., Tabin, C. J., Shih, C., and Weinberg, R. A., 1982, Human EJ bladder carcinoma oncogene is homologue of Harvey sarcoma virus *ras* gene, *Nature* **297**:474–478.

Powers, S., Kataoka, T., Fasano, O., Goldfarb, M., Strathern, J., and Wigler, M., 1984, Genes in S. cerevisiae encoding proteins with domains homologous to the mammalian ras proteins, *Cell* **36**:607–612.

Quigley, J. P., 1979, Phorbol ester-induced morphological changes in transformed chick fibroblasts: Evidence for direct catalytic involvement of plasminogen activator, *Cell* **17**:131–141.

Reddy, E. P., Reynolds, R. K., and Barbacid, M., 1982, A point mutation is responsible for the acquisition of transforming properties by the T24 human bladder carcinoma oncogene, *Nature* **300**:149–152.

Rigby, P. W. J., Dieckmann, M., Rhodes, C., and Berg, P., 1977, Labeling deoxyribonucleic acid to high specific activity in vitro by nick translation with DNA polymerase I, *J. Mol. Biol.* **113**:237–251.

Ruley, H. E., 1983, Adenovirus early region 1A enables viral and cellular transforming genes to transform primary cells in culture, *Nature* **304**:602–606.

Sawey, M. J., Hood, A. T., Burns, F. J., and Garte, S. J., 1987, Activation of c-*myc* and c-K-*ras* oncogenes in primary rat tumors induced by ionizing radiation, *Mol. Cell Biol.* **7**:932–935.

Southern, E. M., 1975, Detection of specific sequences among DNA fragments separated by gel electrophoresis, *J. Mol. Biol.* **98**:503–517.

Southern, P. J., and Berg, P., 1982, Transformation of mammalian cells to antibiotic resistance with a bacterial gene under control of the SV40 early region promoter, *J. Mol. Appl. Genet.* **1**:327–341.

Spandidos, D. A., and Wilkie, N. M., 1984, Malignant transformation of early passage rodent cells by a single mutated human oncogene, *Nature* **310**:469–475.

Sweet, R. W., Yokoyama, S., Kamata, T., Feramisco, J. R., and Gross, M., 1984, The product of ras is a GTPase and the T24 oncogenic mutant is deficient in this activity, *Nature* **311**:273–275.

Tabin, C. J., Bradley, S. M., Bargmann, C. I., Weinberg, R. A., Papageorge, A. G., Scolnick, E. M., Dhar, R., and Chang, E. H., 1982, Mechanism of activation of a human oncogene, *Nature* **300**:143–149.

Troll, W., and Wiesner, R., 1984, Protease inhibitors as anticarcinogens, *J. Natl. Cancer Inst.* **73**:1245–1250.

Wahl, G. M., Stern, M., and Stark, G. R., 1979, Efficient transfer of large DNA fragments from agarose gels to diazobenzyloxymethyl-paper and rapid hybridization by using dextran sulfate, *Proc. Natl. Acad. Sci. USA* **76**:3683–3687.

Weinberg, R. A., 1985, The action of oncogenes in the cytoplasm and nucleus, *Science* **230**:770–776.

Wigler, M., Pellicer, A., Silverstein, S., Axel, R., Urlaub, G., and Chasin, L., 1979, DNA-mediated transfer of the adenine phosphoribosyltransferase focus into mammalian cells, *Proc. Natl. Acad. Sci. USA* **76**:1373–1376.

Williams, J. G., and Mason, P. J., 1985, Hybridization in the analysis of RNA, in: *Nucleic Acid Hybridization: A Practical Approach* (B. D. James and S. J. Higgins, eds.), IRL Press, Oxford, pp. 139–148.

Yavelow, J., Finlay, T. H., and Troll, W., 1983, Bowman–Birk soybean protease inhibitor as an anticarcinogen, *Cancer Res.* **43**:2454s–2459s.

16

Suppression of c-myc by Anticarcinogenic Protease Inhibitors

JANICE D. CHANG and ANN R. KENNEDY

1. Introduction

Malignant transformation *in vitro* and *in vivo* can be prevented by treating carcinogen-exposed cells or animals with a variety of microbial and plant protease inhibitors. As one approach to studying the nature by which protease inhibitors may be preventing malignant transformation, we have performed studies on the effects of protease inhibitors on c-*myc* expression in proliferating normal and transformed mouse fibroblast cells. Our experiments were designed with the aim of understanding the way in which protease inhibitors might be working in the cell to prevent malignant transformation and determining whether the protease inhibitor effect of reducing transformation yields could be related to the reduction in c-*myc* RNA levels by protease inhibitors. Additional experiments were also performed, examining the role of c-*myc* in the cell cycle and determining the effect of antipain on the stability of the c-*myc* message.

2. The Oncogene c-myc and Malignant Transformation

The normal c-*myc* gene is found on chromosome 8 of man and consists of three exons and two introns. Determination of the nucleotide sequence of this gene shows that c-*myc* is highly conserved, suggesting an important role for this

JANICE D. CHANG • Department of Biology, Massachusetts Institute of Technology, Cambridge, Massachusetts 02139.   *ANN R. KENNEDY* • Department of Radiation Oncology, School of Medicine, University of Pennsylvania, Philadelphia, Pennsylvania 19104.

Protease Inhibitors as Cancer Chemopreventive Agents, edited by Walter Troll and Ann R. Kennedy. Plenum Press, New York, 1993.

gene in normal cellular metabolism. The 5' end of this gene containing exon 1 is noncoding and not translated; this region has no translatable initiation codons in the 550-base-long segment and contains multiple termination codons in all three reading frames (Watt *et al.*, 1983). Two active promoters are also encoded within exon 1. The second two exons are translated and code for a protein homologous to the *myc* domain of the viral p100 *gag-myc* protein (Gazin *et al.*, 1984); the c-*myc* product is a nuclear protein that binds to double-stranded DNA (Donner *et al.*, 1982; Persson and Leder, 1984; Watt *et al.*, 1985). This section will review some of the background of the c-*myc* oncogene and its role in malignant transformation.

2.1. Activation of c-myc

Alterations of c-*myc* have been found in a variety of human neoplasias and tumor cell lines. Activated or amplified forms of c-*myc* have been found in a wide range of tumors; those of B-cell origin have been most widely studied. In these types of tumors, proviral insertion or chromosomal translocation is clearly linked to the activation of c-*myc* and tumor formation. Integration of the avian leukosis virus in close juxtaposition to the cellular c-*myc* gene results in chicken B-cell lymphomas (Hayward *et al.*, 1981). Chromosomal translocations have been found in human Burkitt lymphomas (Taub *et al.*, 1982; Erikson *et al.*, 1983) and in mouse plasmacytomas (Shen-Ong *et al.*, 1982; Marcu *et al.*, 1983). Examples of neoplasias in cells of T-cell origin activated by retroviral insertion have also been found (Steffen, 1984; Corcoran *et al.*, 1984). c-*myc* amplification and enhanced c-*myc* expression have been found in other human tumors such as HL-60 cells (human myeloid leukemias) (Collins and Groudine, 1982; Dalla-Favera *et al.*, 1982a,b), small cell lung cancer cells (Little *et al.*, 1983), neuroendocrine tumor cell lines of colon origin, APUDomo Colo 320 cells (Alitalo *et al.*, 1983), and osteosarcoma cells induced in mice by infection with polyoma virus (Schwab *et al.*, 1985).

The exact nature by which c-*myc* is activated is not clearly understood. In plasmacytomas and Burkitt lymphomas, the translocated allele is transcriptionally active while the normal c-*myc* allele is inactive. It appears that the protein coding sequences of the activated oncogene are similar to those of the normal cellular *myc* gene (Stanton *et al.*, 1983; Battey *et al.*, 1983), suggesting that the same protein is produced in both the activated and normal genes. *myc* is most likely not activated by mutations in its coding exons, since mutations are not found in the translocated *myc* nor are there breaks in either exon 2 or 3 in Burkitt lymphomas (Battey *et al.*, 1983).

A model of overexpression of the c-*myc* gene has been hypothesized as playing a role in the oncogenesis of a tumor (Erikson *et al.*, 1983; Marcu *et al.*, 1983; Mushinski *et al.*, 1983). The observations that the c-*myc* gene in Burkitt lymphoma and murine plasmacytoma cells is translocated into the region of the immunoglobulin heavy chain locus (Taub *et al.*, 1982), and that the ALV provirus integrates in the vicinity of the c-*myc* gene (Hayward *et al.*, 1981) have led to speculation that the increased c-*myc* expression observed in these cases results from new control elements which regulate the expression of the c-*myc* gene.

However, the insertion of new control elements in juxtaposition to the normal c-*myc* gene, which results in increased c-*myc* expression, may not be the complete picture. High levels of c-*myc* expression have been observed in non-Burkitt lymphoma B-cell lines and other tissues (Rabbits *et al.*, 1983a,b; Hamlyn and Rabbits, 1983), and c-*myc* expression levels in mouse plasmacytoma tumor cells have been found to be similar to those of normal proliferating cells (Keath *et al.*, 1984a,b). In addition, a transcription enhancer near the immunoglobulin heavy chain locus has not been found on the 14q+ chromosome in the case of t(8:14), and therefore cannot control c-*myc* gene transcription in this translocated event (Rabbits *et al.*, 1983a,b).

Other models to explain increases in c-*myc* expression have also been proposed. For example, proviruses contributing their 3' LTR end for a more efficient transcription of downstream host sequences in a gene could explain increased expression of c-*myc*. However, this model is not without problems; it has also been shown that ALV proviruses can be in the vicinity downstream on the 3' side of c-*myc*, or opposite that of c-*myc* on the 5' side (i.e., located in positions such that there is no linkage between viral and c-*myc* RNA) and still lead to increased c-*myc* expression (Varmus, 1982). Activation of c-*myc* may occur through mechanisms other than the use of the viral LTR as a strong promoter. Other models which have been suggested to identify the critical change in c-*myc* expression have been the deregulation of c-*myc* in the cell cycle (Leder *et al.*, 1983; Campisi *et al.*, 1984), and the hypothesis that translocation of c-*myc* results in increased translational efficiency of the gene (Saito *et al.*, 1983).

2.2. Function of the Normal c-myc Gene

It is widely believed that the c-*myc* gene is involved in immortalization and plays a role in the regulation of cell division and proliferation. Although *c-myc* expression is intimately associated with cell proliferation and growth, the exact function of the c-*myc* gene product remains controversial.

DNA transfection studies, as described by Land *et al.* (1983a,b), have shown that transformation of rat secondary fibroblasts can occur with the co-transfection of c-*myc* attached to a viral promoter along with mutant *ras* genes. Altered *ras* alone can transform NIH 3T3 cells, a line of established, immortalized cells. The similarities between *myc* in this experimental system and the E1A transforming gene of adenovirus and large T antigen of polyoma virus, both of which immortalize cells without transforming them (Ruley, 1983; Land *et al.*, 1983a,b), have suggested that the c-*myc* gene may be involved in immortalization.

The role that the c-*myc* gene plays in immortalization, however, is not clear. Immortalization is a prerequisite for transformation by a mutated *ras* gene, as shown by the transforming ability of EJ c-Ha-*ras*-1 in fibroblasts immortalized by carcinogens (Newbold and Overell, 1983). Establishment or immortality appears to be a necessary but not a sufficient prerequisite for transformation of cells by *ras*. REF52, a line of established, immortalized rat cells, is not stably transformed by overexpressed rat oncogenes (Franza *et al.*, 1986) and transformation in other established cell lines, such as mouse C3H10T1/2 cells, cannot be brought about by *ras* alone; however, in these cells, transformation can be potentiated by transfection of a *gag-myc* oncogene with *ras* (Taparowsky *et al.*, 1987). Immortalization of nonestablished rat or hamster cells can be brought about when *ras* genes are attached to a transcriptional enhancer and transfected into these nonestablished cells (Spandidos and Wilkie, 1984). Thus, all immortalization functions may not be equal and the categorization of c-*myc* as an immortalization gene is a purely operational one since there is no direct evidence that c-*myc* immortalizes cells. Although immortalization is thought to be a prerequisite for malignant transformation, the genes involved in immortalization have not been clearly defined.

Evidence that the expression of c-*myc* occurs at a specific stage in the cell cycle and that c-*myc* is tightly coupled to the growth state, has led to the hypothesis that c-*myc* has a critical role in the regulation of cell division. Kelly *et al.* (1983) have shown that c-*myc* is an inducible gene modulated by specific growth factors, and is expressed in a cell-cycle-dependent manner. Campisi *et al.* (1984) have also shown that chemically transformed cells have levels of c-*myc* RNA which are only slightly elevated when compared with normal proliferating cells; however, whereas c-*myc* RNA levels are cell cycle dependent in normal cells and will decrease when proliferation declines, c-*myc* is constitutively expressed in the transformed cells. When c-*myc* expression is reduced in many cell lines, there is a corresponding decrease in proliferation (Campisi *et al.*, 1984; Billings *et al.*, 1987). c-*myc* is normally expressed in logarithmically growing cells *in vitro* and decreases as cells reach confluence (Kelly *et al.*, 1983; Campisi *et al.*, 1984; Billings *et al.*, 1986). There is also a strong correlation between c-*myc* expression and cellular proliferative activity *in vivo*, as has been shown in human placentas (Pfeifer-Ohlsson *et al.*, 1984).

Reduction in c-*myc* transcripts has been associated with G_0/G_1 growth arrest in interferon-treated Daudi Burkitt lymphoma cells (Einat *et al.*, 1985), in HL-60 cells treated with 1,25-dihydroxy vitamin D_3 (Reitsma *et al.*, 1983), and in HL-60 cells terminally differentiated with DMSO and retinoids (Westin *et al.*, 1982). Expression of the c-*myc* gene under the influence of a promoter reduces the requirement of cells for growth factors, and allows cells to respond to EGF in the absence of PDGF, suggesting the acquisition of competence in cell cycle progression (Armelin *et al.*, 1984).

Evidence suggesting that c-*myc* is involved in the control of cell proliferation comes from the observation that microinjection of the c-*myc* protein into 3T3 cells induces DNA synthesis if cells are exposed to platelet-poor plasma after the microinjection (Kaczmarek *et al.*, 1985); it has been hypothesized that c-*myc* may be acting as a competence factor allowing cells to progress through the S phase of the cell cycle. It has been shown that addition of c-*myc* antibodies reversibly inhibits DNA synthesis and polymerase activity in purified nuclei (Studzinski *et al.*, 1986); these observations suggest that c-*myc* may play a role in the elongation of nascent DNA chains in isolated nuclei. However, when c-*myc* antibodies are injected directly into the nuclei of living cells, ongoing DNA synthesis is not inhibited under conditions when an antibody against DNA polymerase α will inhibit DNA replication (Kaczmarek *et al.*, 1986). Thus, the observation that DNA synthesis can be inhibited in purified nuclei by antibodies to c-*myc* may not be relevant to the role of c-*myc* in intact cells. It has been shown recently that addition to the culture media of antisense oligodeoxynucleotides complementary to regions coding for c-*myc* RNA induces differentiation and decreases proliferation in human promyelocytic leukemia HL-60 cells; c-*myc* protein expression is also reduced when antisense oligomers are added (Heikkila *et al.*, 1987). Heikkila *et al.* (1987) also show that entry into the S phase of the cell cycle is inhibited but not the progression from the G_0 to the G_1 stage. These results from experiments utilizing the malignant HL-60 cell line are consistent with the evidence that c-*myc* is involved in DNA synthesis.

It is highly suggestive that c-*myc* has a role in the regulation of cell proliferation; however, work in other experimental systems has shown that c-*myc* expression and cell proliferation are not always related. c-*myc* oncogene protein synthesis has been shown to be independent of the cell cycle in human and avian fibroblasts (Hann and Eisenman, 1984). In addition, although c-*myc* expression can be rapidly modulated during the G_0 to G_1 transition, c-*myc* RNA levels do not change throughout the cell cycle in growing cells (Thompson *et al.*, 1985; Rabbits *et al.*, 1985). Continuous expression of c-*myc* does not prevent differentiation in chronic lymphocytic leukemia cells (unlike HL-60 cells), and increased expression of c-*myc* does not result in proliferation (Larsson *et al.*, 1987). Mitotically and meiotically dividing germ cells proliferate with very few *myc* transcripts (Stewart *et al.*, 1984). In the *Xenopus* species, an unfertilized egg (a cell which does not divide) expresses *myc* RNA at least 10^5-fold over the level which is observed in proliferating cells (Taylor *et al.*, 1986; Godeau *et al.*, 1986). Estrogen-induced proliferation of cells in the chick oviduct results in decreased steady-state levels of c-*myc* RNA, suggesting that c-*myc* is not necessary for cell proliferation under these conditions (Cohrs *et al.*, 1988). As discussed in Section 4, our own results suggest that elevated c-*myc* expression is not required for the initiation of DNA synthesis (Chang and Kennedy, 1988). Thus, these results suggest that c-*myc* expression can be dissociated from DNA synthesis and cell division.

2.3. Mechanism of c-myc Regulation

Knowledge of the mechanism(s) by which c-myc is regulated normally should help in the determination of its role in the malignant transformation of a cell. Studies done in a variety of experimental systems suggest that control of c-myc expression is under the regulation of both transcriptional and post-transcriptional mechanisms.

The observation that c-myc can be superinduced by the protein synthesis inhibitor cycloheximide (Kelly et al., 1983) has suggested that c-myc is regulated by a labile protein. It has been hypothesized that the c-myc gene is normally repressed and that this labile protein controls the transcription of the c-myc gene which is normally repressed (Leder et al., 1983). This has led to the proposal that the first exon has a regulatory function in the control of myc gene expression; this region could be a binding site for a transcriptional repressor (Leder et al., 1983).

A model for the regulation of c-myc expression by a transcriptional repressor implies that quiescent cells (which do not express high levels of c-myc) have a low basal rate of transcription. This is not the case in Chinese hamster lung fibroblasts; c-myc is transcribed at a high rate in these cells when maintained in a G_0-arrested state (Blanchard et al., 1985). In addition, growth factors which dramatically induce high levels of c-myc RNA levels have little or no effect on nuclear transcription rates (Kelly et al., 1983; Greenberg and Ziff, 1984). The c-myc message has been found to be unstable, with a half-life of around 10 to 20 min (Dani et al., 1984; Knight et al., 1985; Piechaczyk et al., 1985). These observations suggest that expression of c-myc may also be regulated via post-transcriptional mechanisms. In support of this model are the observations that c-myc expression is reduced in interferon-treated Daudi cells, but that the rate of transcription in nuclei of cells treated with or without interferon does not differ (Knight et al., 1985). In addition, truncated c-myc RNA in plasmacytoma cells can accumulate at higher levels than normal-sized transcripts even when their genes are transcribed at a slightly slower rate (Piechaczyk et al., 1985).

3. c-myc Expression Is Reduced in Protease Inhibitor-Treated Proliferating Mouse Fibroblasts

Certain protease inhibitors have the ability to suppress transformation yields when added to proliferating cells after carcinogen treatment (reviewed by Kennedy, 1984). Although protease inhibitors can still be effective anticarcinogenic agents when added at long time intervals after the carcinogen exposure, they must be present while cells are proliferating to work as anticarcinogenic agents (Kennedy, 1985). This observation that cell proliferation is critical for the effectiveness of the protease inhibitors as anticarcinogenic agents led to the focusing of our efforts on the oncogene c-myc. At the time these experiments were begun, it was widely interpreted that c-myc was involved in the regulation of cell division and proliferation, as described in the previous section. It was our hypothesis that the anticarcinogenic action of protease inhibitors could result from an effect on an oncogene, such as c-myc, which was thought to play an important role in cell proliferation.

Our previous work showing that steady-state c-myc RNA levels are reduced in cells grown in a variety of different protease inhibitors as observed by both Northern and dot blotting has been described elsewhere (Chang et al., 1985; Chang and Kennedy, 1988). Briefly summarized, our results showed that several of the protease inhibitors which have the ability to reduce transformation yields in carcinogen-exposed cells reduced c-myc RNA levels to a greater extent than several of the protease inhibitors which do not have anticarcinogenic activity. Under conditions in which there is a reduction in c-myc RNA expression, RNA synthesis, growth rate, or saturation density are not affected.

The protease inhibitors antipain, leupeptin, and Bowman–Birk inhibitor [which all have anticarcinogenic activity, as they are capable of suppressing transformation in vitro (reviewed by Kennedy, 1984)] all reduced c-myc RNA expression by approximately 50% or greater, as determined by densitometric analysis, with antipain being the most effective of the protease inhibitors at reducing c-myc expression. Elastatinal and α_1-antitrypsin, which do not have the ability to reduce transformation yields, reduced c-myc expression by 11%. The effect of antipain on c-myc RNA transcripts was observed to be dose-dependent. When antipain was added at a concentration of 10 μg/μl in the medium, c-myc RNA levels were reduced only slightly, by approximately 18%, in comparison with an approximately 70% reduction when concentrations of 25 μg/ml or higher were used. Antipain and the Bowman–Birk inhibitor, which are effective at reducing transformation yields in carcinogen-exposed cells, reduced c-myc RNA levels in the radiation (F-17) and methylcholanthrene (Cl 16)-transformed cell lines to a much lower extent than observed in normal proliferating fibroblasts. It is noteworthy that, while capable of suppressing transformation (the conversion of a cell to the malignant state), the protease inhibitors discussed here do not have the ability to convert transformed cells back into normal cells.

It has been hypothesized that protease inhibitors are capable of reversing an early step in the transformation process (Kennedy, 1985). It is possible that the activation of c-myc could be such an early event in the carcinogenic process. Malignant transformation is thought to involve at least two steps, the first being a high-frequency event which is heritable, and a later event which is rare and mutationlike (Kennedy et al., 1980, 1984). Transfection of oncogenes into normal diploid cells also suggests a minimum of two steps which contribute to the transformed state since at least two oncogene alterations (overexpressed myc and a mutated ras gene) must be present for transformation to occur in diploid fibroblasts; established NIH 3T3 cells, which are immortal, can be transformed into a tumorigenic state by altered ras alone (Land et al., 1983a,b). The changes in c-*myc* expression brought about by protease inhibitors are assumed to be a general effect observed in the majority of cells since a rare event in only a few cells would not be detectable by the methods utilized in our studies.

Transformation of normal Syrian hamster cells with altered *ras* requires the transfection of the mutated *ras* gene into cells which have been newly immortalized with carcinogens (Newbold and Overell, 1983). Thus, the carcinogen-induced immortalized state, occurring as an early event, may predispose cells to further progression toward malignancy. One could further speculate that the alteration of *myc*, which contributes to the immortalized state as an early event, precedes the activation of *ras* as a subsequent step in carcinogenesis. From our studies, we hypothesize that the anticarcinogenic protease inhibitors suppress c-*myc* expression, which is involved in an early step in the transformation process, such that a subsequent step, which leads directly to the malignant state, does not occur.

4. Cells Progress through the Cell Cycle in the Absence of an Increase in c-myc RNA Levels

Our observations that steady-state levels of c-*myc* RNA could be reduced in mouse fibroblasts without a corresponding decrease in proliferation suggested to us that previous observations of others, showing decreases in c-*myc* transcripts when cell proliferation was inhibited, could be a consequence rather than a cause of the inhibition of cell proliferation. In order to test the hypothesis that changes in c-*myc* expression were not necessary for progression of cells through the cell cycle, c-*myc* RNA levels were determined at various time points after confluent serum-starved cells were stimulated with serum in the presence or absence of the protease inhibitor antipain. In these studies, the ability of cells to progress through the cell cycle, from G_0/G_1 to the S phase, was measured by [^{3}H]thymidine incorporation. As c-*myc* RNA levels were reduced by antipain, but cells continued to progress through the cell cycle, we concluded from our studies that the rise in levels of c-*myc* RNA was not sufficient for cell cycle progression. As part of these studies, we observed that both C3H10T1/2 and 3T3 cells grown in the presence of antipain to a density-inhibited, confluent state did not show an increase in c-*myc* RNA to levels which are normally seen after confluent cells are stimulated to divide (Chang and Kennedy, 1988). c-*myc* RNA levels at time points of 15 min and 1, 2, 5, and 24 hr after serum stimulation in antipain-treated cells remained at about the same levels as in the unstimulated confluent cells. Cells continued to progress from the G_0/G_1 phase to the S phase in the absence of an increase in c-*myc* RNA. The kinetics of [^{3}H]thymidine incorporation after serum stimulation were comparable to those observed in cells in which c-*myc* RNA levels rise after serum stimulation. Superinduction of c-*myc* RNA with serum and cycloheximide also did not occur when cells were grown in the

Table I. Summary of the Densitometric Scanning Analysis of the Suppression
of c-*myc* RNA Levels by Antipain in Cells Which Have Been Grown
to Confluence in the Presence or Absence of Antipain and Stimulated
with Serum under Different Conditions[a]

Description of experiment	Percent reduction in c-*myc* RNA levels
10T1/2 cells grown in antipain	72%
10T1/2 cells grown to confluence in antipain; stimulated with serum for 15 min	74%
10T1/2 cells grown to confluence in antipain; stimulated with serum for 1 hr	83%
10T1/2 cells grown to confluence in antipain; stimulated with serum for 2 hr	81%
10T1/2 cells grown to confluence in antipain; stimulated with serum for 5 hr	76%
10T1/2 cells grown to confluence in antipain; stimulated with antipain included in the serum for 1 hr	94%
10T1/2 cells grown to confluence without antipain; stimulated with antipain included in the serum for 1 hr	26%
10T1/2 cells grown to confluence without antipain; antipain added to cells while confluent; stimulated with serum for 1 hr	32%
3T3 cells grown to confluence in antipain; stimulated with serum for 1 hr	90%
3T3 cells grown to confluence in antipain; stimulated with cycloheximide included in the serum for 1 hr	87%

[a]The results obtained represent a comparison between the Northern blots, prepared as described in Chang and Kennedy (1988). The percent reduction in c-*myc* RNA levels is compared with control cells not treated with antipain.

presence of antipain. The percent reduction (when various treatments are compared with untreated cells), as determined by densitometric analysis, is summarized in Table I.

Our results showing that resting cells enter S phase in the absence of an increase in c-*myc* RNA levels suggest that elevated c-*myc* expression is not required for the initiation of DNA synthesis and can be dissociated from cell division; thus, the increase in c-*myc* RNA levels observed after cells are stimulated to divide with serum may not be causally related to the initiation of DNA synthesis. A direct role for c-*myc* in cell division has not been demonstrated. The rise in c-*myc* RNA levels occurring before DNA synthesis, as a response to growth factors (Kelly *et al.*, 1983; Campisi *et al.*, 1984), is a temporal relationship which only suggests that a causal relationship may exist. The response of c-*myc* to growth factors, although relative rapid (c-*myc* RNA levels increase 1–2 hr after serum stimulation), is not an immediate response to serum factors. There are other cellular events which could be taking place in the 1–2 hr after serum stimulation which then result in the rise in c-*myc* RNA levels which are observed. In addition, DNA synthesis does not occur until about 16 hr after cells are stimulated to divide with serum; this is a long lag time during which many other events could be contributing to the synthesis of DNA. The increase in c-*myc* RNA levels which precede DNA synthesis could be a secondary event resulting from other events which directly trigger the initiation of DNA synthesis.

The observation that cell cycle progression occurs in the absence of a rise in c-*myc* RNA levels, however, does not "prove" that c-*myc* expression has no role in the regulation of cell division. It is possible that antipain could be stabilizing the *myc* protein while at the same time reducing c-*myc* RNA levels. The *myc* protein could perhaps have a feedback effect on *myc* RNA levels, such that when the concentration of *myc* protein reached a certain threshold level, *myc* RNA levels were affected by being reduced. It has not yet been shown that cell cycle progression occurs in the absence of or in reduced levels of the *myc* protein; the expression of the c-*myc* protein under conditions when c-*myc* RNA levels were reduced could not be determined accurately in our studies since antipain appeared to inhibit proteolytic degradation of proteins which took place in the cell fractionation procedure (Chang and Kennedy, unpublished results). Future studies are planned to determine whether the c-*myc* protein levels are reduced in parallel with c-*myc* RNA levels.

5. Antipain Increases the Half-Life of the c-myc Message

The observation that protease inhibitors have the ability to reduce c-*myc* expression in proliferating fibroblasts led to experiments to gain further insight into the mechanism by which these inhibitors could regulate c-*myc* RNA levels. Experiments were performed to determine whether protease inhibitors could interfere with the degradation of a putative repressor protein, and thus increase its levels and prevent the transcription of c-*myc* RNA. A model of a labile protein regulating the level of c-*myc* RNA has been suggested by the observation that c-*myc* can be induced by cycloheximide and superinduced by cycloheximide plus mitogen (Kelly *et al.*, 1983). If protease inhibitors were to interfere with the degradation of a regulatory protein, one might expect that the addition of a protease inhibitor to serum-starved cells stimulated with cycloheximide and mitogen would prevent the transient increase in c-*myc* expression observed after serum stimulation. The stability of the c-*myc* message in cells grown in the presence or absence of antipain was also determined by performing an actinomycin chase experiment with or without cycloheximide. An effect of protease inhibitors on the stability of the c-*myc* message would suggest other mechanisms (i.e., posttranscriptional control of c-*myc*) by which protease inhibitors could regulate c-*myc* expression.

We have studied the stability of the c-*myc* message in cells grown in the presence or absence of antipain by performing an actinomycin D chase experiment (Chang et al., 1990). In these experiments we showed that antipain decreases the steady-state c-myc RNA levels and increases the half-life of the message by about fourfold. The protein synthesis inhibitor cycloheximide superinduces c-myc expression in response to growth factors and further stabilizes the c-myc message in the presence of antipain; these results suggest that a labile protein is involved in the regulation of c-myc RNA levels.

The observation that antipain increases the half-life of the c-myc message while at the same time decreasing the steady-state myc RNA levels, suggests that antipain could be decreasing the synthesis of the c-myc message. However, we found that the rate of c-myc transcription was not significantly different in cells grown in the presence or absence of antipain, as determined by nuclear runoff experiments (Chang et al., 1990). Reduction in the c-myc message does not result from a decreased rate in transcription.

6. Possible Mechanisms by Which Protease Inhibitors Regulate c-myc Expression

Potential control points and possible protease steps which may be important in controlling and regulating the expression of c-myc will be discussed in this section. The proposed regulatory schemes as described below take into account the observations that steady-state c-myc RNA levels are decreased and the stability of the message increases when cells are grown in the presence of antipain. Antipain may be regulating c-myc expression through a combination of transcriptional and posttranscriptional mechanisms. Our observation that c-myc RNA levels can be reduced by protease inhibitors such as antipain suggests that proteases may be involved in the regulation of c-myc RNA levels.

One of the simplest models to propose regarding the role of proteases in regulating c-myc expression is the negative regulation of myc by a repressor protein which prevents transcription of the c-myc message; this repressor protein could be sensitive to degradation or cleavage by a cellular protease. It can be hypothesized that protease inhibitors prevent the cleavage or degradation of the repressor protein which, when absent, would allow myc transcription to take place. An example of such a system is the inhibition of SOS repair in E. coli by antipain; in this system, antipain has been shown to prevent lambda repressor inactivation (Meyn et al., 1977). However, it has been shown that the rate of c-myc transcription (Blanchard et al., 1985), but not c-myc expression (Kelly et al., 1983; Campisi et al., 1984; Billings et al., 1986), is similar in proliferating and quiescent cells, and that c-myc transcription rates have been found to be comparable in both antipain- and non-antipain-treated cells (Chang et al., 1990). These observations suggest that a regulatory scheme based purely on transcriptional control through a repressor is probably not likely.

The observation that the c-*myc* message is unstable ($t_{1/2} \sim 10$ min) suggests that steady-state levels of c-*myc* could be regulated through posttranscriptional mechanisms. When cells have been grown in the presence of antipain, the *myc* message is stabilized ($t_{1/2}$ increases to 40 min); cycloheximide further increases the stability of the *myc* message. It can be hypothesized that antipain inhibits the enzymes that degrade c-*myc* RNA. In addition, the increase in c-*myc* stability when cells are treated with cycloheximide could be accounted for by the decreased production of enzymes which degrade c-*myc* RNA.

This model proposes that a "turnover protein" signals the specific degradation of the *myc* message, perhaps by binding to *myc* RNA. This "turnover protein" could be under the control of a positive regulatory protein. It can be hypothesized that antipain prevents the cleavage of the regulatory protein which, when present, allows the "turnover protein" to be produced, thus signaling *myc* RNA degradation. This type of mechanism has been proposed because the rate of *myc* transcription alone cannot account for differences in steady-state c-*myc* RNA levels observed in proliferating and quiescent cells, and the c-*myc* message is unstable ($t_{1/2} \sim 10$ min); these data indirectly support a posttranscriptional regulatory mechanism of *myc* regulation. This proposed model also takes into account a labile protein which regulates *myc* RNA levels.

Steady-state levels of c-*myc* RNA could also be regulated in a homeostatic fashion by a protein which has a feedback effect on the message, resulting in reduced *myc* RNA levels. Such a protein could be the *myc* protein or other regulatory protein. Antipain could be inhibiting the enzymes involved in the turnover of a regulatory protein such that protein degradation is inhibited, resulting in a more stable protein which could then have the effect of reducing c-*myc* RNA levels.

Other potential mechanisms of *myc* regulation cannot be excluded at this time. There is evidence that a mitogenic protein is present in the membrane of human and mouse fibroblasts which can be cleaved by both exogenous and endogenous proteases (Scott, 1987). Proteases could have a role in releasing the mitogenic protein which would then result in an increase in c-*myc* expression; protease inhibitors could conceivably prevent such an event from occurring. In addition, there are other mechanisms which could also contribute to the steady-state level of *myc* RNA; e.g., alterations in splicing efficiency and nuclear dwell time of pre-mRNAs or in the transport of mature derivatives to the cytoplasm.

7. Concluding Remarks

In summary, we have shown that: (1) several of the protease inhibitors which have the ability to reduce transformation yields in carcinogen-exposed cells also reduce c-*myc* RNA expression, (2) c-*myc* RNA levels are not reduced by the anticarcinogenic protease inhibitors to as great an extent in transformed cells as they are in normal proliferating cells, (3) the protease inhibitors do not have an effect on cell growth, total RNA synthesis, or saturation density, and (4) cell cycle progression in confluent resting cells stimulated to divide with serum can occur under conditions when c-*myc* RNA levels are reduced (when cells are grown to confluence in the presence of a protease inhibitor). Our studies suggest the possibility that protease inhibitors could be suppressing carcinogenesis through an effect on c-*myc* expression.

8. References

Alitalo, K., Schwab, M., Lin, C. C., Varmus, H. E., and Bishop, J. M., 1983, Homogeneously staining chromosomal regions contain amplified copies of an abundantly expressed cellular oncogene c-myc in malignant neuroendocrine cells from a human colon carcinoma, *Proc. Natl. Acad. Sci. USA* **80**:1707–1711.

Armelin, H. A., Armelin, M. C. S., Kelly, K., Steward, T., Leder, P., Cochran, B. H., and Stiles, C. D., 1984, Functional role for c-myc in mitogenic response to platelet-derived growth factor, *Nature* **310**:655–700.

Battey, J., Moulding, C., Taub, R., Murphy, W., Stewart, T., Potter, H., Lenoir, G., and Leder, P., 1983, The human c-myc oncogene: Structural consequences of translocation into the IgH locus in Burkitt lymphoma, *Cell* **34**:779–787.

Billings, P. C., Shuin, T., Lillehaug, J., Miura, T., Roy-Burman, P., and Landolph, J. R., 1987, Enhanced expression and state of the c-myc oncogene in chemically and X-ray transformed C3H10T1/2 cl 8 mouse embryo fibroblasts, *Cancer Res.* **47**:3643–3649.

Blanchard, J. M., Piechaczyk, M., Dani, C., Chambard, J. C., Franchi, A., Pouoyssegur, J., and Jeanteur, P., 1985, C-myc gene is transcribed at high rate in G$_0$-arrested fibroblasts and is post-transcriptionally regulated in response to growth factors, *Nature* **317**:443–445.

Campisi, J., Gray, H. E., Pardee, A. B., Dean, M., and Sonenshein, G. E., 1984, Cell cycle control of c-myc but not c-ras expression is lost following chemical transformation, *Cell* **36**:241–247.

Chang, J. D., and Kennedy, A. R., 1988, Cell cycle progression of C3H10T1/2 and 3T3 cells in the absence of an increase in c-myc RNA levels, *Carcinogenesis* **9**:17–20.

Chang, J. D., Billings, P. C., and Kennedy, A. R., 1985, C-myc expression is reduced in antipain-treated proliferating C3H10T1/2 cells, *Biochem. Biophys. Res. Commun.* **133**:830–835.

Chang, J. D., Li, J. H., Billings, P. C., and Kennedy, A. R., 1990, Effects of protease inhibitors on c-myc expression in normal and transformed C3H10T1/2 cell lines, *Mol. Carcinogenesis* **3**:226–232.

Cochran, B. H., Zullo, J., Verma, I. M., and Stiles, C. D., 1984, Expression of the c-fos gene and of fos-related gene is stimulated by platelet-derived growth factor, *Science* **226**:1080–1082.

Cohrs, R. J., Goswami, B. B., and Sharma, O. K., 1988, Down regulation of c-myc, c-fos and erb-B during estrogen induced proliferation of the chick oviduct, *Biochem. Biophys. Res. Commun.* **150**:82–88.

Collins, S., and Groudine, M., 1982, Amplification of endogenous myc-related DNA sequences in a human myeloid leukaemia cell line, *Nature* **298**:679–681.

Corcoran, L. M., Adams, J. M., Dunn, A. R., and Cory, S., 1984, Murine T lymphomas in which the cellular myc oncogene has been activated by retroviral insertion, *Cell* **37**:113–122.

Dalla Favera, R., Bregni, M., Erikson, J., Patterson, D., Gallo, R. C., and Croce, C. M., 1982a, Human c-myc onc gene is located on the region of chromosome 8 that is translocated in Burkitt lymphoma cells, *Proc. Natl. Acad. Sci. USA* **79**:7824–7827.

Dalla Favera, R., Wong-Staal, F., and Gallo, R. C., 1982b, Onc gene amplification in promyelocytic leukaemia cell line HL-60 and primary leukaemic cells of the same patient, *Nature* **299**:61–63.

Dani, C., Blanchard, J. M., Piechaczyk, M., Sabouty, S. E., and Jeanteur, P., 1984, Extreme instability of myc mRNA in normal and transformed human cells, *Proc. Natl. Acad. Sci. USA* **81**:7046–7050.

Dean, M., Levine, R. A., Ran, W., Kindy, M. S., Sonenshein, G. E., and Campisi, J., 1986, Regulation of c-myc transcription and mRNA abundance by serum growth factors and cell contact, *J. Biol. Chem.* **261**:9161–9166.

Donner, P., Greiser-Wilke, I., and Moelling, K., 1982, Nuclear localization and DNA binding of the transforming gene product of avian myelocytomatosis virus, *Nature* **305**:112–116.

Einat, M., Resnitzky, D., and Kimchi, A., 1985, Close link between reduction of c-myc expression by interferon and G_0/G_1 arrest, *Nature* **313**:597–600.

Erikson, J., Ar-Rushdi, A., Drwinga, H. L., Nowell, P. C., and Croce, C. M., 1983, Transcriptional activation of the translocated c-myc oncogene in Burkitt lymphoma, *Proc. Natl. Acad. Sci. USA* **80**:820–824.

Franza, B. R., Maruyama, K., Garrels, J. I., and Ruley, H. E., 1986, *In vitro* establishment is not a sufficient prerequisite for transformation by activated ras oncogenes, *Cell* **44**:409–418.

Gazin, C., Dupont de Dichenin, S., Hampe, A., Masson, J. M., Martin, P., Stehelin, D., and Galibert, F., 1984, Nucleotide sequence of the human c-myc locus: Provocative open reading frame within the first exon, *EMBO J.* **3**:383–388.

Godeau, F., Persson, H., Gray, H. E., and Pardee, A. B., 1986, C-myc expression is dissociated from DNA synthesis and cell division in Xenopus oocyte and early embryonic development, *EMBO J.* **5**:3517–3577.

Greenberg, M. E., and Ziff, E. B., 1984, Stimulation of 3T3 cells induces transcription of the c-fos proto-oncogene, *Nature* **311**:433–438.

Hamlyn, P. H., and Rabbits, T. H., 1983, Translocation joins c-myc and immunoglobulin gamma-1 genes in a Burkitt lymphoma revealing a third exon in the c-myc oncogene, *Nature* **304**:135–139.

Hann, S. R., and Eisenman, R. N., 1984, Proteins encoded by the human c-myc oncogene: Differential expression in neoplastic cells, *Mol. Cell. Biol.* **4**:2486–2497.

Hayward, W. S., Neel, B. G., and Astrin, S., 1981, Activation of a cellular onc gene by promoter insertion in ALV-induced lymphoid leukosis, *Nature* **290**:475–479.

Heikkila, R., Schwab, G., Wickstrom, E., Loke, S. L., Pluznik, D. H., Watt, R., and Neckers, L. M., 1987, A c-myc antisense oligodeoxynucleotide inhibits entry into S phase but not progression from G_0 to G_1, *Nature* **328**:445–449.

Kaczmarek, L., Hyland, J. K., Watt, R. A., Rosenberg, M., and Baserga, R., 1985, Microinjected c-myc as a competence factor, *Science* **228**:1313–1315.

Kaczmarek, L., Miller, M., Hammond, R. A., and Mercers, W. E., 1986, A microinjected monoclonal antibody against human DNA polymerase-α inhibits DNA replication in human, hamster, and mouse cell lines, *J. Biol. Chem.* **261**:10802–10807.

Keath, E. J., Caimi, P. G., and Cole, M. D., 1984a, Fibroblast lines expressing activated c-myc oncogenes are tumorigenic in nude mice and syngeneic animals, *Cell* **39**:339–348.

Keath, E. J., Kelekar, A., and Cole, M. D., 1984b, Transcriptional activation of the translocated c-myc oncogene in mouse plasmacytomas: Similar RNA levels in tumor and proliferating normal cells, *Cell* **37**:521–528.

Kelly, K., Cochran, B. H., Stiles, C. D., and Leder, P., 1983, Cell-specific regulation of the c-myc gene by lymphocyte mitogens and platelet-derived growth factor, *Cell* **35**:603–610.

Kennedy, A. R., 1984, Promotion and other interactions between agents in the induction of transformation *in vitro* in fibroblasts, in: *Mechanisms of Tumor Promotion*, Volume III (T. J. Slaga, ed.), CRC Press, Boca Raton, Fla., pp. 13–55.

Kennedy, A. R., 1985, The conditions for the modification of radiation transformation *in vitro* by a tumor promoter and protease inhibitors, *Carcinogenesis* **6**:1441-1445.

Kennedy, A. R., Fox, M., Murphy, G., and Little, J. B., 1980, Relationship between x-ray exposure and malignant transformation in C3H 10T/2 cells, *Proc. Natl. Acad. Sci. USA* **77**:7262–7266.

Knight, E., Anton, E. D., Fahey, D., Friedland, B. K., and Jonak, G. J., 1985, Interferon regulates c-myc gene expression in Daudi cells at the post-transcriptional level, *Proc. Natl. Acad. Sci. USA* **82**:1151–1154.

Land, H., Parada, L. F., and Weinberg, W. A., 1983a, Cellular oncogenes and multistep carcinogenesis, *Science* **222**:771–778.

Land, H., Parada, L. F., and Weinberg, W. A., 1983b, Tumorigenic conversion of primary embryo fibroblasts requires at least two cooperating oncogenes, *Nature* **304**:596–606.

Larsson, L., Gray, H. E., Totterman, T., Petterson, U., and Nilsson, K., 1987, Drastically increased expression of myc and fos proto-oncogenes during *in vitro* differentiation of chronic lymphocytic leukemia cells, *Proc. Natl. Acad. Sci. USA* **84**:223–227.

Leder, P., Battey, J., Lenoir, G., Moulding, C., Murphy, W., Potter, H. T., and Taub, R., 1983, Translocations among antibody genes in human cancer, *Science* **222**:765–771.

Little, C. D., Nau, M. N., Carney, D. N., Gazdar, A. F., and Minna, J. F., 1983, Amplification and expression of the c-myc oncogene in human lung cancer cell lines, *Nature* **306**:194–196.

Marcu, K. B., Harris, L. J., Stanton, L. W., Erikson, J., Watt, R., and Croce, C. M., 1983, Transcriptionally active c-myc oncogene is contained within NIARD, a DNA sequence associated with chromosome translocations in B-cell neoplasia, *Proc. Natl. Acad. Sci. USA* **80**:519–523.

Meyn, M. S., Rossman, T., and Troll, W., 1977, A protease inhibitor blocks SOS functions in *Escherichia coli:* Antipain prevents λ repressor inactivation, ultraviolet mutagenesis, and filamentous growth, *Proc. Natl. Acad. Sci. USA* **74**:1152–1156.

Mushinski, J. F., Bauer, S. R., Potter, M., and Reddy, E. P., 1983, Increased expression of myc-related oncogene mRNA characterizes most BALB/c plasmacytomas induced by pristane or Abelson murine leukemia virus, *Proc. Natl. Acad. Sci. USA* **80**:1073–1077.

Newbold, R. F., and Overell, R. W., 1983, Fibroblast immortality is a prerequisite for transformation by EJ c-Ha-ras oncogene, *Nature* **304**:648–651.

Persson, H., and Leder, P., 1984, Nuclear localization and DNA binding properties of protein expressed by human c-myc oncogene, *Science* **225**:718–721.

Pfeifer-Ohlsson, S., Goustin, A. S., Rydnert, J., Wahlstrom, T., Bjersing, L., Stehelin, D., and Ohlsson, R., 1984, Spatial and temporal pattern of cellular myc oncogene expression in developing human placenta: Implications for embryonic cell proliferation, *Cell* **38**:585–596.

Piechaczyk, M., Yang, J. Q. Blanchard, J. M., Jeanteur, P., and Marcu, K. B., 1985, Post-transcriptional mechanisms are responsible for accumulation of truncated c-myc RNAs in murine plasma cell tumors, *Cell* **42**:589–597.

Rabbits, P. H., Watson, J. V., Lamond, A., Forster, A., Stinson, M. A., Evan, G., Fischer, W., Atherton, E., Sheppard, P., and Rabbits, T. H., 1985, Metabolism of c-myc gene products: c-myc mRNA and protein expression in the cell cycle, *EMBO J.* **4**:2009–2015.

Rabbits, T. H., Forster, A., Baer, R., and Hamlyn, P. H., 1983a, Transcriptional enhancer identified near the human C_μ immunoglobulin heavy chain gene is unavailable to the translocated c-myc gene in a Burkitt lymphoma, *Nature* **306**:806–809.

Rabbits, T. H., Hamlyn, P. H., and Baer, R., 1983b, Altered nucleotide sequences of a translocated c-myc gene in Burkitt lymphoma, *Nature* **306**:706–765.

Reitsma, P. H., Rothberg, P. G., Astrin, S. M., Trial, J., Bar-Shavit, Z., Hall, A., Teitelbaum, S. L., and Kahn, A. J., 1983, Regulation of myc gene expression in HL-60 leukaemia cells by a vitamin D metabolite, *Nature* **306**:492–494.

Ruley, H. E., 1983, Adenovirus early region IA enables viral and cellular transforming genes to transform primary cells in culture, *Nature* **304**:602–606.

Saito, H., Hayday, A. C., Wiman, K., Hayward, W. S., and Tonegawa, S., 1983, Activation of the c-myc gene by translocation: A model for translational control, *Proc. Natl. Acad. Sci. USA* **80**:7476–7480.

Schwab, M. F., Ramsay, G., Alitalo, K., Varmus, H. E. Bishop, J. M., Martinsson, T., Levan, G., and Levans, A., 1985, Amplification and enhanced expression of the c-myc oncogene in mouse SEWA tumour cells, *Nature* **315**:345–347.

Scott, G. K., 1987, Proteinases and eukaryotic cell growth, *Comp. Biochem. Physiol.* **87B:**1–10.

Shen-Ong, G. L. C., Keath, E. J., Piccoli, S. P., and Cole, M. D., 1982, Novel myc oncogene RNA from abortive immunoglobulin gene recombination in mouse plasmacytomas, *Cell* **31:**443–452.

Spandidos, D. A., and Wilkie, N. M., 1984, Malignant transformation of early passage rodent cells by a single mutated human oncogene, *Nature* **310:**469–475.

Stanton, L. W., Watt, R., and Marcu, K. B., 1983, Translocation, breakage and truncated transcripts of c-myc oncogene in murine plasmacytomas, *Nature* **303:**401–406.

Steffen, D., 1984, Proviruses are adjacent to c-myc in some murine leukemia virus-induced lymphomas, *Proc. Natl. Acad. Sci. USA* **81:**2097–2101.

Stewart, T. A., Bellve, A. R., and Leder, P., 1984, Transcription and promoter usage of the myc gene in normal somatic and spermatogenic cells, *Science* **226:**707–710.

Studzinski, G. P., Brelvi, Z. S., Feldman, S. C., and Watt, R. A., 1986, Participation of c-myc protein in DNA synthesis of human cells, *Science* **234:**467–470.

Taparowsky, E. J., Heaney, M. L., and Parson, J. T., 1987, Oncogene-mediated multistep transformation of C3H10T1/2 cells, *Cancer Res.* **47:**4125–4129.

Taub, R., Kirsch, I., Morton, C., Lenoir, G., Swan, D., Tronick, S., Aaronson, S., and Leder, P., 1982, Translocation of the c-myc gene into the immunoglobulin heavy chain locus in human Burkitt lymphoma and murine plasmacytoma cells, *Proc. Natl. Acad. Sci. USA* **79:**7837–7841.

Taylor, M. V., Gusse, M., Evans, G. I., Dathan, N., and Mechali, M., 1986, Xenopus myc protooncogene during development: Expression as a stable maternal mRNA uncoupled from cell division, *EMBO J.* **5:**3563–3570.

Thompson, C. B., Challoner, P. B., Neiman, P. E., and Groudine, M., 1985, Levels of c-myc oncogene mRNA are invariant throughout the cell cycle, *Nature* **314:**363–366.

Varmus, H. E., 1982, Form and function of retroviral proviruses, *Science* **216:**812–820.

Watt, R., Nishizuka, K., Sorrentino, J., Ar-Rushdi, A., Croce, C. M., and Rovera, G., 1983, The structure and nucleotide sequence of the 5' end of the human c-myc oncogene, *Proc. Natl. Acad. Sci. USA* **80:**6307–6311.

Watt, R. A., Shatzman, A. R., and Rosenberg, M., 1985, Expression and characterization of the human c-myc DNA binding protein, *Mol. Cell. Biol.* **5:**448–456.

Westin, E. H., Wong-Staal, F., Gelmann, E. P., Dalla-Favera, R., Papas, T. S., Lautenberger, J. A., Eva, A., Reddy, E. P., Tronick, S. R., Aaronson, S. A., and Gallo, R. C., 1982, Expression of cellular homologues of retroviral oncogenes in human hematopoietic cells, *Proc. Natl. Acad. Sci. USA* **79:**2490–2494.

17

A Role for Esterases in Steroid Hormone Turnover

MORTIMER LEVITZ, SILA BANERJEE, JOSEPH KATZ,
UMA RAJU, and THOMAS H. FINLAY

1. Introduction and Scope of the Chapter

Studies attempting to elucidate the physiological role of esterases have been complicated by their lack of specificity exhibited and the overall failure to identify specific substrates that may be targets for an esterase under study. The availability of naphthyl esters and azo dyes containing ester linkages, coupled with histochemical staining techniques that permitted the visualization of hydrolytic activities following electrophoretic separations, led to classifications according to substrate preference. However, the early broad classification of esterases in vertebrate plasma into three types by Augustinsson (1961)—carboxyl esterases (EC 3.1.1.1), aryl esterases (EC 3.1.1.2), and cholinesterases (EC 3.1.1.8)—must be viewed within the context of overlapping activities.

The concentrations of two important regulators of cell functions—cholesterol and choline—are controlled, to some extent, by the appropriate esterase activities, but reasons for the remarkably large number of esterases found in tissues and body fluids remain a mystery. An important role ascribed to carboxyl esterases is that of detoxification. In a review of the subject (Heymann, 1980), it is pointed out that deleterious drugs and insecticides are rendered innocuous by the action of esterases. On the other hand, biologically inert esters can be converted to their physiologically active forms by cleavage of the ester linkage,

MORTIMER LEVITZ, SILA BANERJEE, JOSEPH KATZ, UMA RAJU, and THOMAS H. FINLAY •
Department of Obstetrics and Gynecology, New York University Medical Center, New York, New
York 10016.

Protease Inhibitors as Cancer Chemopreventive Agents, edited by Walter Troll and Ann R. Kennedy.
Plenum Press, New York, 1993.

which is the case for steroid esters. This chapter will focus on steroid esters and the carboxyl esterases, for which they serve as potential substrates, and not on the general question of nonspecific esterases that has received extensive treatment in the literature (e.g., Heymann, 1980; Peters, 1982; Berning *et al.*, 1985; von Deimling *et al.*, 1985). Particular emphasis will be placed on the concentrations and properties of a novel esterase we have identified in human breast cyst fluid.

2. Endogenous Steroid Esters

2.1. Steroid Esters in Body Fluids

The earliest identification of steroid esters in body fluids culminated from the analysis of normal human blood. Although the quantification was crude, it was estimated that about 50% of circulating Porter–Silber chromogens were cortisol acetate and corticosterone acetate (Margraf *et al.*, 1963). Estradiol has also been detected in human serum in the esterified form, but in contrast to the above-mentioned study, long-chain fatty acids were involved in the linkages. In women, an approximately 50% increase in radioimmunoassayable estradiol resulted from the mild alkaline hydrolysis of serum extracts (Janocko and Hochberg, 1983). Nonpolar conjugates, presumably esters, of pregnenolone, dehydroepiandrosterone, and androstenediol have also been isolated from human plasma (Jones and James, 1985).

Human breast cyst fluid, aspirated from women with fibrocystic disease, is also rich in steroid esters. Long-chain fatty acid esters of androsterone have been identified by mass spectrometry. Ten specimens yielded concentrations of 0.56–3.79 ng/ml. The fatty acid moieties included: palmitoleate, arachidonate, linoleate, oleate, palmitate, and stearate. The compositions tended to vary among specimens, but the unsaturated acids predominated (Raju *et al.*, 1985).

2.2. Steroid Esters in Tissues

Extracts of steroidogenic tissues have yielded a variety of fatty acid ester derivatives of steroids. Thus, bovine corpora lutea contain significant concentrations of such esters of pregnenolone and 3β-hydroxy-5α-pregnan-20-one (Albert *et al.*, 1980). The major fatty acids identified were similar to those cited above for the breast cyst fluid studies. Although the analytical characterizations were somewhat less definitive, bovine adrenal glands were shown to contain fatty acid esters of pregnenolone derivatives and dehydroepiandrosterone (Hochberg *et al.*, 1979).

2.3. Steroid Fatty Acid Ester Production in Vitro

The identification of steroid esters in endocrine tissues raises the question of site of synthesis. Production *in situ* or accumulation from the blood of esters synthesized elsewhere are alternatives. The results of several *in vitro* studies demonstrate that tissues exhibiting high concentrations of steroid esters are rich in acyl-forming enzymes. Following incubation of labeled estradiol with slices of bovine endometrium, 11 fatty acid esters of the steroid were identified by mass spectrometry (Mellon-Nussbaum *et al.*, 1982). Roy and Belanger (1989) conducted *in vitro* studies and found that the high levels of pregnenolone esters in human follicular fluid can be attributed to synthesis *in situ*. The long-chain fatty acids esterified to pregnenolone were 80% unsaturated, the rest was virtually all palmitic acid. Concerning studies on human breast cancer, homogenates of breast tumor converted tritiated androsterone to esters in varying amounts, 3–48% (Raju *et al.*, 1981). Estradiol also serves as a substrate for conversion to nonpolar, presumably long-chain fatty acid esters, by human breast tumor slices, but the recorded yields have been less than 1% (Schatz and Hochberg, 1982). In the same study, the authors examined a variety of rat tissues for their ability to convert estradiol to its nonpolar esters. The yields for fat, liver, and heart were less than 1%, whereas the yields for kidney, induced breast tumors, and uterus were greater than 5%. The values for brain cortex and hypothalamus were in the 2–3% range. Abul-Hajj (1982) has confirmed the formation of fatty acyl esters of estradiol by human and rat mammary tumor tissue. The observation has been made that significant esterification and deesterification of estradiol occurs in cultures of MCF-7 and other breast tumor cell lines (Adams *et al.*, 1986). Interestingly, the MCF-7 cell line propagated in our laboratory following receipt from the Michigan Cancer Foundation, the original source of the cell line, exhibited virtually no esterification of incubated estradiol, although esterase activity toward estradiol esters was demonstrated. These divergent results dramatize the genetic lability of breast tumor cell lines maintained in culture.

3. Steroid Ester Metabolism: Physiological Implications

3.1. In Man

The literature records only one study in man in which the metabolism of estradiol fatty acid esters was compared with that of estradiol. The investigation focused on the rate of oxidation at carbon 17 of estradiol. Specifically, the rate of transfer of tritium to tritiated water from the 17α position of estradiol was compared with the rate of transfer when the 17α tritiated compound was esterified with stearic or arachidonic acids. The results in the five subjects studied indicated: (1) the rate of release of tritium from the free estradiol exceeded that of either ester; (2) the total extent of tritium release was greater for the esters; and (3) the extent of tritium release from the arachidonate exceeded that of the stearate. These results would predict prolonged and perhaps greater integrated estrogenic activity on the part of the steroid esters. Moreover, they point to the importance of carboxyl esterases in their metabolism (Hershcopf et al., 1985).

3.2. In MCF-7 Cells

Several years ago, our laboratory demonstrated the presence of intracellular carboxyl esterases in MCF-7 human breast cancer cells able to hydrolyze E_2-17β esters (Katz et al., 1987). The focus was on an estrogen-sensitive enzyme with a preference for esters of short-chain fatty acids. Apparent activity of this esterase increased two- to fourfold when MCF-7 cells were maintained in the presence of 10^{-8} M E_2. In a second study (Katz et al., 1991) aimed at establishing a possible role for the estrogen-sensitive esterase, we confirmed that it was located intracellularly and showed that it was not released into the media by MCF-7 cells growing in culture. Fractionation by sucrose density centrifugation suggested that the enzyme was not membrane-bound. Gel exclusion chromatography indicated an apparent mass of 45–50 kDa. Although the natural substrate of the MCF-7 cell esterase (or esterases) is unknown, we showed that it was able to cleave a variety of steroid esters with K_m's of approximately 10^{-7} M.

The experiments with MCF-7 cells indicated that both long- and short-chain fatty esters of E_2 were as effective as unesterified E_2 in stimulating protein and DNA synthesis (measured by [3H]thymidine incorporation). Although long-chain fatty acid esters of E_2 are poor substrates for the MCF-7 cells esterases, hydrolysis appears to proceed at a rate sufficient to provide enough free E_2 for activation of the estrogen receptor. It is possible that in normal (and malignant) breast epithelial cells a similar esterase could serve to generate E_2 from an exogenous lipoidal estrogen. If this were to be the case, then esterase levels might be of some value in predicting the outcome of certain hormonally sensitive cancers.

4. Esterification and Deesterification Enzymes

Barely more than a decade has elapsed since interest in steroid esters intensified. Most of the studies have been of a descriptive nature, concentrating on organ sites of biosynthetic activities and speculations on the possible physiological importance of these compounds. Accordingly, there is limited definitive information on the purity, and even less on the specificity, of the relevant enzymes. It is within this context and reservation that this section is presented.

Fatty Acid Transferases

Much of the stimulus for the investigation of esterifying enzymes stemmed from the recognition that the synthesis, transport, and disposition of cholesterol is intimately linked to the metabolism of its esters. An important enzyme that catalyzes cholesterol esterification is lecithin:cholesterol O-acyltransferase (EC 2.3.1.43). The enzyme is produced in the liver and secreted into plasma and lymph circulations. It utilizes the acyl group from carbon-2 of phosphatidylcholine as the fatty acid source. Electrophoretic homogeneity has been achieved for the enzyme (Chong *et al.*, 1981). Although the enzyme plays a crucial role in cholesterol metabolism, its impact on steroid esterification is virtually unknown. A plausible explanation is that steroid esters appear to be synthesized principally in tissues, whereas lecithin:cholesterol acyltransferase is present in plasma.

A second mechanism for producing steroid esters utilizes fatty acyl CoA as the fatty acid donor in a reaction catalyzed by acyl CoA:cholesterol O-acyltransferase (EC 2.3.1.26). Human mammary cancer cells grown in culture possess an enzyme activity that transfers the fatty acid of long-chain fatty acyl CoA to the 17β position of estradiol. The authors (Martyn *et al.*, 1987) have named the enzyme fatty acyl CoA:estradiol acyltransferase, an action premature considering that not even partial purification has been achieved and investigations into the properties were in the early stages. Nevertheless, interesting data on the properties of the enzyme have been forthcoming. The activity was mainly in the microsomal compartment following subcellular fractionation. Ester synthesis was enhanced by the addition of the CoA derivatives of oleic, linoleic, and palmitic acids; but competitively inhibited by testosterone, dehydroepiandrosterone, and 5-androstene-3β,17β-diol. The enzyme may play an important role in the turnover of estradiol esters in breast tumor tissue.

The potential importance of producing sterol esters is dramatized by the availability of a third mechanism for their production. Surprisingly, this pathway exploits the reversibility of the ester hydrolase. Thus, there is good reason to surmise that pregnenolone is esterified in bovine adrenal mitochondria by an enzyme analogous to cholesterol ester hydrolase (EC 3.1.1.13) (Mellon-Nussbaum *et al.*, 1979). Rather than the fatty acyl CoA derivative, the enzyme utilizes the free fatty acid as donor and the pH optimum for esterification of the two sustrates is similar, 5.0 (Norum, 1974).

5. Transesterification

Human breast cancer cell lines grown in culture manifest the enzymatic capability of converting estradiol to a variety of its long-chain fatty acid esters.

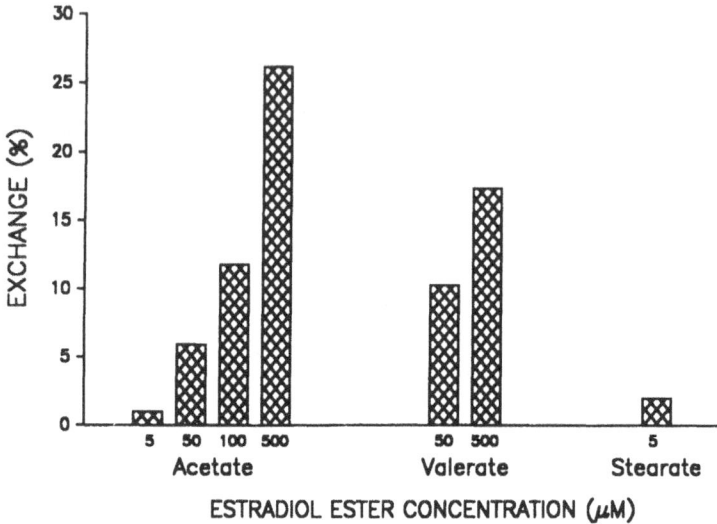

Figure 1. Transesterification of estradiol by MCF-7 cells. Tritiated estradiol (0.1 nM, 2×10^5 cpm) and radioinert estradiol ester were incubated 20 min in confluent MCF-7 cell cultures at optimum growth conditions. Media and sonicated cells were extracted with chloroform–methanol (2:1) and the dried extracts were chromatographed on Sephadex LH-20 to separate free and esterified estradiol. The fraction of total radioactivity in the estradiol ester zone indicated the extent of exchange.

These cultures, including the MCF-7 cell line, also exhibited esterase activity, so that when estradiol was removed from the culture medium, hydrolysis of the estradiol esters was the dominant process (Adams *et al.*, 1986). Cell cultures are notorious for undergoing mutation, as reflected by the absence of esterifying capability in the MCF-7 cells we obtained from the Michigan Cancer Foundation. In any event, we were afforded the opportunity to test whether our cell line possessed a transferase capable of transferring the fatty acid moiety of estradiol ester to another estradiol molecule. The experimental design was to incubate tritiated estradiol in cultures to which increasing amounts of various unlabeled estradiol esters were added. The data in Fig. 1 demonstrate the presence in MCF-7 cells of an enzyme activity capable of mediating transesterification.

The enzyme that exhibits transferase activity has not been isolated or identified. A likely candidate is an estrogen-responsive esterase present in the 100,000*g* supernate following subcellular fractionation of MCF-7 cells. A plausible mechanism for an esterase acting in the capacity of a transferase is depicted in Fig. 2. A technical problem arises on attempting to gain experimental support for the correctness of this mechanism. The poor solubility of steroid esters in aqueous media imposes a restriction on substrate concentrations that can be tested.

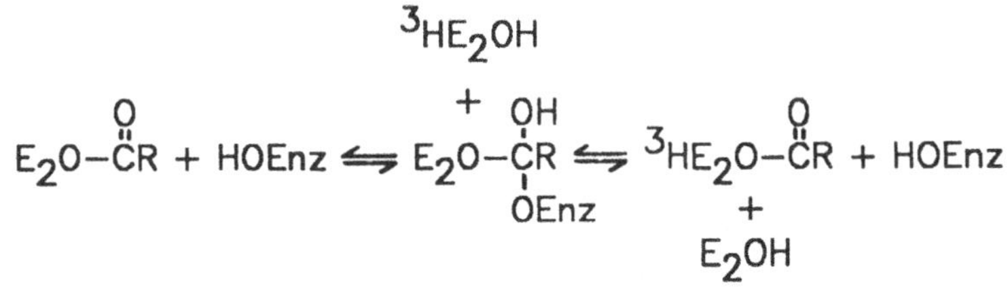

$$^{3}HE_{2}OH$$

$$E_2O-\overset{O}{\overset{\|}{C}}R + HOEnz \rightleftharpoons E_2O-\underset{OEnz}{\overset{+\ OH}{\overset{|}{C}}}R \rightleftharpoons {}^{3}HE_2O-\overset{O}{\overset{\|}{C}}R + HOEnz$$

$$+$$
$$E_2OH$$

Figure 2. Proposed scheme for an esterase in MCF-7 cells mediating transesterification. The esterase is a serine enzyme that can link covalently with substrate as shown. The reaction is reversible so that transesterification may result.

6. Breast Cyst Fluid Esterase

It was pointed out earlier in this chapter that steroid esters seem to be most concentrated in tissues that are targets for hormone action. Although esterase activity is requisite for converting these biologically inactive esters to the parent hormone, no systematic studies on the distribution of the relevant hydrolyzing enzymes have been forthcoming. We reasoned that fibrocystic disease of the breast would present an appropriate model for such a study. The breast, including the breast cyst compartment, accumulates steroid esters. Studies of this kind may be important because fibrocystic disease of the breast places the patient at risk, albeit small, for developing breast cancer (Haagensen, 1971), particularly where there is a familial history of breast carcinoma (Dupont and Page, 1985). Abnormal concentrations of enzymes or other active substances may serve to identify a subset of patients with this normally benign lesion who are at greater risk for developing breast cancer.

In a preliminary study we examined 19 breast cyst fluids (BCF) for esterase activity (Banerjee, *et al.*, 1990). It was found expedient to use estradiol-17-acetate labeled with tritium in the acetate moiety as substrate. The data in Fig. 3 indicate a wide range of activities in BCF, varying some 80-fold. There was no correlation between the esterase activities in BCF and plasma, but the log of the potassium ion concentration in BCF appeared to correlate inversely with that of the esterase level. Potassium ion levels were included in the study because this cation associates positively with concentrations of estrogens in BCF(Raju *et al.*, 1985), and in retrospective studies it was observed that patients with fibrocystic disease who subsequently developed breast cancer had relatively high potassium ion concentrations in their BCF (Fleisher *et al.*, 1984). This investigation has been extended to a study of some 400 specimens. The data analysis is highly complex, but it appears that the preliminary sampling (Banerjee *et al.*, 1990) was too small and not representative. Further work in this area is indicated.

Some BCF specimens exhibited sufficiently high esterase activity to permit

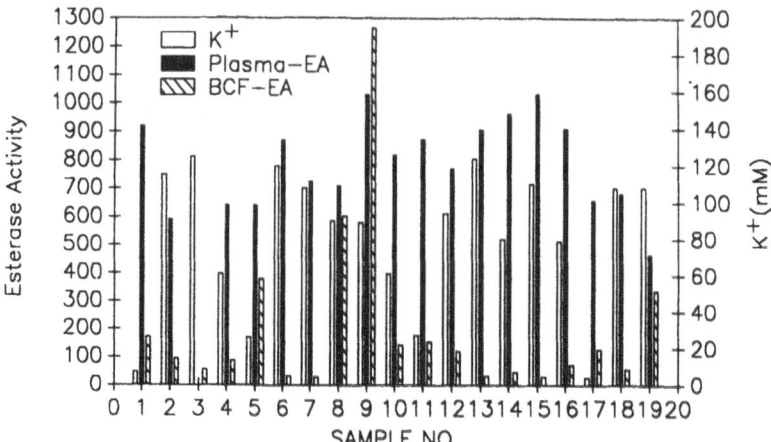

Figure 3. Esterase activity and potassium concentrations in human breast cyst fluid (BCF) and esterase activity in serum. Esterase activity was determined with estradiol-[³H]acetate and is reported as percent hydrolysis/30 min per 100 μl (serum) or per mg protein (BCF). (Reproduced from Banerjee *et al.*, 1990, with permission from the *Annals of the New York Academy of Sciences.*)

Table I. Substrates and Inhibitors of BCF Esterase[a]

		Activity	
Substrate	Inhibitor	pmole ester hydrolyzed/min per μg protein	% maximum
p-Nitrophenyl acetate		167	100
p-Nitrophenyl butyrate		889	
p-Nitrophenyl hexanoate		755	
p-Nitrophenyl caprate		267	
p-Nitrophenyl myristate		<30	
E₂-acetate		4.00	
E₂-valerate		0.021	
E₂-stearate		0.015	
	DIFP (10^{-4} M)		0
	DENPP (10^{-4} M)		0
	Ebelactone B (1 μg/ml)		11
	NaF (2×10^{-5} M)		14
	Antipain (10^{-4} M)		93
	Leupeptin (10^{-4} M)		100
	N-ethylmaleimide (10^{-4} M)		100
	Iodoacetic acid (10^{-4} M)		100

[a]Purified BCF esterase was assayed with 10^{-4} M nitrophenyl ester in 1 ml PBS or with 0.5 μM E₂-[³H]acetate. The assays with E₂-valerate and E₂-stearate employed [³H]-E₂-esters. The E₂-ester and free E₂ were separated by chromatography on Sephadex LH-20 as previously described (Katz *et al.*, 1987). Inhibition was determined with *p*-nitrophenyl at the concentrations indicated above. Activity in the absence of added inhibitor was considered to be 100%.

investigation of the physical and biochemical properties of the enzyme and to make comparisons with plasma esterases. The esterase from BCF, upon submission to ammonium sulfate precipitation, ion-exchange chromatography, and chromatography on octyl-Sepharose, displayed protein-staining bands on SDS-PAGE of 22 and 23 kDa (Banerjee et al., 1991). It is noteworthy that the electrophoretic mobility of the BCF esterase differs from either that in plasma or those in granulocytes, monocytes, and platelets, suggesting that the BCF esterase derives from the cyst rather than the blood compartment. Other properties that differentiated the BCF esterase from the blood esterases were the ability of only the former to hydrolyze α-naphthyl chloroacetate and α-naphthyl acetate (Dufer et al., 1984) and that only the BCF esterase was inhibited by ebelactone B, an esterase inhibitor produced by actinomycetes (Umezawa et al., 1980).

Studies of the substrate specificity and the inhibition profile shown in Table I indicate that the 22 to 23-kDa polypeptide(s) is indeed an esterase. This point is emphasized because a polypeptide of similar size (24 kDa), also isolated from BCF, has been reported to be a chymotrypsin-like protease (Kesner et al., 1988). Further intensifying interest in the latter polypeptide is its apparent ability to bind progesterone (Pearlman et al., 1973). A systematic study should be undertaken in order to characterize these polypeptides of close molecular weights.

7. Perspectives and Conclusions

Steroid esters have been located in the serum and in various intracellular compartments, but modes of transport and mechanisms for expression of biological activity have not been elucidated for these lipoidal substances. However, the results of several studies in the human and in rodents permit tentative conclusions to be drawn in these respects.

An important component in the consideration of steroid activity is the binding of the hormone to its receptor. In the standard assay using crude preparations, long-chain fatty acid esters of estradiol do not compete with estradiol for rabbit uterine cytosolic estrogen receptors, but estradiol-17-valerate and the acetate do compete (Janocko et al., 1984). Under the assay conditions, only the shorter-chain esters were hydrolyzed, suggesting that the esters had no intinsic binding capability. Indeed, when a purified uterine receptor preparation was employed, the esters did not compete with estradiol for estrogen binding sites. The acetate exhibited minor binding capability, but this was traced to residual esterase activity not dissociated from the uterine receptor. These observations are consistent with the relative esterase activities displayed by the purified BCF esterase. As shown in Table I, several orders of magnitude separate the rate of hydrolysis of the acetate from those of the valerate and stearate.

Although information on the intracellular transport of steroid esters is lacking, studies have been conducted, the results of which permit conjecture on possible modes of transport from the blood to target cells. Estradiol esters were shown not to bind to sex hormone binding globulin of human plasma or to α-fetoprotein in rat plasma (Larner *et al.*, 1987). Ultracentrifugation separations have been performed on plasma proteins in the human and in the rat after applying the appropriate equilibration with tritiated estradiol stearate. In the human, the ester was most concentrated in the low-density lipoprotein (LDL) fraction, whereas in the rat, the high-density lipoprotein HDL) fraction incorporated most of the estradiol stearate. This report may be particularly noteworthy since the internalization of cholesterol esters by the cell is mediated in the human and the rat by LDL and HDL receptors, respectively. Paradoxically, in the rat the blood clearance rate of estradiol stearate exceeds that of the corresponding C_{12} or C_{14} ester, although the overall metabolic clearance rate is lower for the stearate (Larner and Hochberg, 1985). A logical interpretation of these data is that the stearate, bound to HDL, is preferentially internalized, but its biological half-life is greater by virtue of being a poorer substrate for esterases. Esterases have also been localized on cell surfaces (Aoyagi *et al.*, 1978), but their role, if any, in the turnover of steroid esters is highly conjectural.

The fate of steroid esters, so internalized, is also unknown. Based on the information presented in this chapter, with the reservation that it has been accumulated from a variety of diverse experimental models and systems, a diagrammatic depiction of the fate of steroid esters is presented in Fig. 4. The mechanism

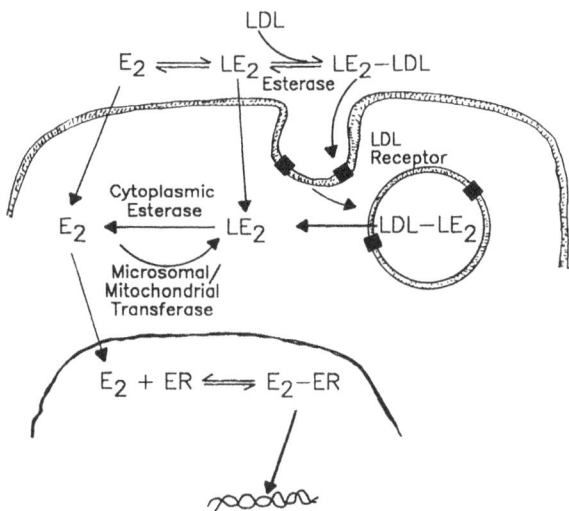

Figure 4. Proposed pathway for turnover of estradiol esters in target cells. LDL-LE_2 is depicted being internalized by a receptor-mediated mechanism and processed further in endosomes, either directly or after incorporation into lysosomes. A minor part of the LE_2 may traverse the plasma membrane by passive diffusion. E_2, estradiol; LDL, low-density lipoprotein; LE_2, estradiol long-chain fatty acid ester; ER, estradiol receptor, shown in the nucleus.

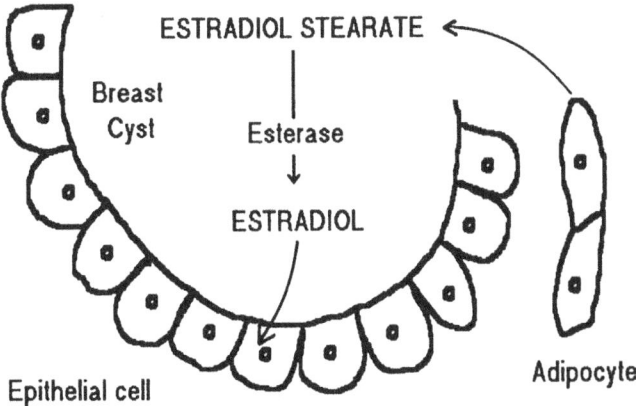

Figure 5. Proposed pathway for turnover of estradiol ester in breast cyst. The source of ester may be the adipocyte, but this is conjecture. The esterase appears to originate in the cyst compartment since its properties differ from those of blood esterases.

of the release of the internalized presumed LDL-bound ester is not known, but it serves to supplement intracellularly produced ester. The regeneration of the physiologically active steroid is mediated by esterase activity concentrated in the cytosolic fraction of the disrupted cell—as we have shown in the MCF-7 tumor cell line—or in other subcellular fractions, about which definitive information has not been forthcoming.

In contrast to the projected role that esterification–deesterification may play in a steroid hormone target cell, shown in Fig. 4, Fig. 5 focuses on the breast cyst compartment. Aspirated BCF contains four major proteins (Haagensen *et al.*, 1979), in a milieu intimately surrounded by epithelial cells of the cyst wall. The particulate matter is composed of sloughed epithelial cells, dead cells, and possibly macrophages. Figure 5 presents the origin of neither the steroid esters nor the esterase capable of effecting their hydrolysis because such information is not available. However, it bears repeating that the cyst fluid esterase exhibits physical properties and inhibition profiles distinct from those of leukocyte esterases. The logical implication is that the breast cyst esterase is not of blood origin.

It is apparent from the foregoing considerations that steroid esters and esterases exercise a measure of control on the endocrine milieu of a target tissue, that at the present state of knowledge cannot be quantified or even estimated. Theoretically, the inhibition of esterases directed at steroid esters would diminish hormonal activity at the target tissue level, but this supposition would be difficult to verify. An inhibitor amenable to testing in biological systems, ebelactone B, has been described (Umezawa *et al.*, 1980). It has very low toxicity and even enhances immune responses. As shown in Table I, it is a good inhibitor of steroid ester esterases. However, ebelactone also inhibits *N*-formylmethionine aminopeptidase activity. Such lack of specificity of inhibitors would complicate conclusions that could be drawn from endocrine changes mediated by their introduction into biological systems. Research in this area is at such a primitive stage that physiologic implications are best adduced from studies associating abnormal esterase activity with pathology. A case in point is our finding of enormous levels of an esterase, not of blood origin, in human BCF in less than 10% of specimens. It is too early to assess the association of this finding with the course of benign breast disease, but such studies are in progress.

8. References

Abul-Hajj, Y. J., 1982, Formation of estradiol-17β fatty acyl esters in mammary tumors, *Steroids* **40**:149–156.

Adams, J. B., Hall, R. T., and Nott, S., 1986, Esterification–deesterification of estradiol by human mammary cancer cells in culture, *J. Steroid Biochem.* **24**:1159–1162.

Albert, D. H., Ponticarvo, L., and Lieberman, S., 1980, Identification of fatty acid esters of pregnenolone and allopregnenolone from bovine corpora lutea, *J. Biol. Chem.* **255**:10618–10623.

Aoyagi, T., Nagai, M. Iwabuchi, M., Liaw, W. S., Andoh, T., and Umezawa, H., 1978, Aminopeptidase activities on the surface of mammalian cells and their alterations associated with transformation, *Cancer Res.* **38**:3505–3508.

Augustinsson, K.-B., 1961, Multiple forms of esterase in vertebrate blood plasma, *Ann. N.Y. Acad. Sci.* **94**:844–860.

Banerjee, S., Katz, J., Levitz, M., and Finlay, T. H., 1990, Identification of a novel esterase in human breast cyst fluid, *Ann. N.Y. Acad. Sci.* **586**:204–212.

Banerjee, S., Katz, J., Levitz, M., and Finlay, T. H., 1991, Purification and properties of an esterase from human breast cyst fluid, *Cancer Res.* **51**:1092–1098.

Berning, W., de Looze, S. M., and von Deimling, O., 1985, Identification and development of a genetically closely-linked carboxylesterase family of the mouse liver, *Comp. Biochem. Physiol.* **80B**:859–865.

Chong, K. S., Davidson, L., Huttash, R. G., and Lacko, A. G., 1981, Characterization of lecithin:cholesterol acyltransferase from human plasma: Purification of the enzyme, *Arch. Biochem. Biophys.* **211**:119–124.

Dufer, J., Trentesaux, C., and Desplaces, A., 1984, Differential effect of the serine protease inhibitor phenyl methyl sulfonyl fluoride on cytochemically detectable esterase in human leukocytes and platelets, *Scand. J. Haematol.* **32**:25–32.

Dupont, W. D., and Page, D. L., 1985, Risk factors for breast cancer in women with proliferative breast disease, *N. Engl. J. Med.* **312**:146–151.

Fleisher, M., Bradlow, H. L., Schwartz, M. K., and Breed, C. N., 1984, The anion gap in human breast cyst fluid (HBCF): A possible high risk indicator for breast cancer, *Clin. Chem.* **30**:940 (abstract #3).

Haagensen, C. D., 1971, *Diseases of the Breast,* Saunders, Philadelphia, p. 155.

Haagensen, D. E., Mazoujian, G., Dilley, W. G., Pedersen, C. E., Kister, S. J., and Wells, S. A., 1979, Breast gross cyst fluid analysis. 1. Isolation and radioimmunoassay for a major component, *J. Natl. Cancer Inst.* **62**:239–247.

Hershcopf, R. J., Bradlow, H. L., Fishman, J., Swaneck, G. E., Larner, J. M., and Hochberg, R. B., 1985, Metabolism of estradiol fatty acid esters in man, *J. Clin. Endocrinol. Metab.* **61**:1071–1075.

Heymann, E., 1980, Carboxylesterases and amidases, in: *Enzymatic Basis of Detoxification,* Volume 11 (W. B. Jacoby, eds.), Academic Press, New York, pp. 291–323.

Hochberg, R., Bandy, L., Ponticorvo, L., Welch, M., and Lieberman, S., 1979, Naturally occurring lipoidal derivatives of 3β-hydroxy-5-pregnen-20-one; 3β,17α-dihydroxy-5-prenen-20-one and 3β-hydroxy-5-androsten-17-one, *J. Steroid Biochem.* **11**:1333–1340.

Janocko, L., and Hochberg, R. B., 1983, Estradiol fatty acid esters occur naturally in human blood, *Science* **222**:1334–1336.

Janocko, L., Larner, J. M., and Hochberg, R. B., 1984, The interaction of C-17 esters of estradiol with the estrogen receptor, *Endocrinology* **114**:1180–1186.

Jones, D. L., and James, V. H. T., 1985, The identification, quantification and possible origin of non-polar conjugates in human plasma, *J. Steroid Biochem.* **22**:243–247.

Katz, J., Finlay, T. H., Banerjee, S., and Levitz, M., 1987, An estrogen-dependent esterase activity in MCF-7 cells, *J. Steroid Biochem.* **26**:687–692.

Katz, J., Levitz, M., Kadner, S. S., and Finlay, T. H., 1991, Estradiol esters can replace 17β-estradiol in the stimulation of DNA and esterase synthesis by MCF-7 cells: A possible role for the estrogen-sensitive MCF-7 cell esterase, *J. Steroid Biochem. Mol. Biol.* **38**:17–26.

Kesner, L., Wangshang, Y. H., Bradlow, H. L., Breed, C. N., and Fleisher, M., 1988, Proteases in cyst fluid from human gross cyst breast disease, *Cancer Res.* **48**:6379–6383.

Larner, J. M., and Hochberg, R. B., 1985, The clearance and metabolism of estradiol and estradiol-17-esters in the rate, *Endocrinology* **117**:1209–1214.

Larner, J. M., Rosner, W., and Hochberg, R. B., 1987, Binding of estradiol-17-fatty acid esters to plasma proteins, *Endocrinology* **121**:738–744.

Margraf, H. W., Margraf, C. O., and Weichselbaum, T. E., 1963, Isolation and identification of adrenocortical steroids in human peripheral blood, *Steroids* **2**:155–165.

Martyn, P., Smith, D. L., and Adams, J. B., 1987, Selective turnover of the essential fatty acid ester components of estradiol-17β lipoidal derivatives formed by human mammary cancer cells in culture, *J. Steroid Biochem.* **28**:393–398.

Mellon-Nussbaum, S. H., Ponticorvo, L., and Lieberman, S., 1979, Characterization of the lipoidal derivatives of pregnenolone prepared by incubation of the steroid with adrenal mitochondria, *J. Biol. Chem.* **254**:12500–12505.

Mellon-Nussbaum, S. H., Ponticorvo, L., Schatz, F., and Hochberg, R. B., 1982, Estradiol fatty acid esters, *J. Biol. Chem.* **257**:5678–5684.

Norum, K. R., 1974, The enzymology of cholesterol esterification, *Scand. J. Clin. Lab. Invest.* **33**(Suppl. 137):7–13.

Pearlman, W. H., Gueriguian, J. L., and Sawyer, M. E., 1973, A specific progesterone-binding component of human breast cyst fluid, *J. Biol. Chem.* **248**:5736–5741.

Peters, J., 1982, Nonspecific esterases of *Mus musculus*, *Biochem. Genet.* **20**:585–606.

Raju, U., Kadner, S., Levitz, M., Kaganowicz, A., and Blaustein, A., 1981, Glucosiduronidation and esterification of androsterone by human breast tumors *in vitro*, *Steroids* **37**:399–407.

Raju, U., Levitz, M., Banerjee, S., Bencsath, A., and Field, F. H., 1985, Androsterone long chain fatty acid esters in human breast cyst fluid, *J. Clin. Endocrinol. Metab.* **60**:940–946.

Roy, R., and Belanger, A., 1989, Formation of lipoidal steroids in follicular fluid, *J. Steroid Biochem.* **33**:257–262.

Schatz, F., and Hochberg, R. B., 1981, Lipoidal derivative of estradiol: The biosynthesis of a nonpolar estrogen metabolite, *Endocrinology* **109**:697–703.

Umezawa, H., Aoyagi, T., Uotani, K., Hamada, M., Takeuchi, T., and Takahashi, S., 1980, Ebelactone, an inhibitor of esterase, produced by actinomycetes, *J. Antibiot.* **33**:1594–1596.

von Deimling, O., Ronai, A., and de Looze, S., 1985, Nonspecific esterases of mammalian testis. Comparative studies on the mouse (*Mus musculus*) and rat (*Rattus norvegicus*), *Histochemistry* **82**:547–555.

18

Protease Inhibitors and Pancreatic Carcinogenesis

B. D. ROEBUCK and DANIEL S. LONGNECKER

1. Pancreatic Cancer

1.1. Human Disease

In the United States, pancreatic cancer is the fifth most common cause of death due to cancer, claiming over 25,000 lives annually (Silverberg and Lubera, 1989). Males are at a slightly higher risk than females (1.5:1) and for both sexes, the age-adjusted death rates have shown a steady increase from 1930 to 1970. Usually, diagnosis of pancreatic cancer is late in the course of disease development, thus precluding effective treatment. The mean survival following diagnosis is 4 to 6 months and the 5-year survival rate is one of the worst of any cancer being less than 5% of cases (Mack, 1982).

The etiology of pancreatic cancer is poorly understood. To date, an association of pancreatic cancer with the smoking of cigarettes is the strongest etiological relationship (Mack, 1982). Less convincing epidemiological evidence indicates a positive association of pancreatic cancer with the ingestion of high levels of fat (Carroll and Khor, 1975; Wynder, 1975; Durbec et al., 1983; Gold et al., 1985; Norell et al., 1986). Recent studies of a California Seventh-Day Adventist population indicate that a high consumption of vegetarian protein products as legumes (peas, beans, and lentils) as well as dried fruit is associated with a reduced incidence of pancreatic cancer (Mills et al., 1988). Legumes are rich

B. D. ROEBUCK • Department of Pharmacology and Toxicology, Dartmouth Medical School, Hanover, New Hampshire 03755.   *DANIEL S. LONGNECKER* • Department of Pathology, Dartmouth Medical School, Hanover, New Hampshire 03755.

Protease Inhibitors as Cancer Chemopreventive Agents, edited by Walter Troll and Ann R. Kennedy. Plenum Press, New York, 1993.

sources of protease inhibitors but these are also sources of a large array of other chemicals. Studies of the human diet, especially of the dietary patterns as surmised by retrospection, are fraught with difficulties and uncertainties. Clearly, the high intake of vegetable foods precludes the intake of other foods such as those high in fat. Nonetheless, these epidemiological studies are interesting and provocative though they do not indicate which specific chemicals and/or food components are protective. Considering the extremely complex nature of the usual human diet, it is highly likely that in any particular diet a balance of "good" and "bad" components is the key to the cancer outcome. Because of the dearth of clues as to causation of human pancreatic cancer, studies with experimental animal models assume great importance. For example, results from rodent models now indicate that dietary fats are causally related to pancreatic carcinogenesis, thus adding strength to that relatively weak body of epidemiological data (Roebuck, 1987).

1.2. Animal Models of Pancreatic Cancer

Animal models of human diseases obviously have limitations and such is the case for rodent models of pancreatic cancer. Important features of animal models are (1) a tumor type that mimics the human spectrum, (2) the ability to induce cancers with a single does of a carcinogen, and (3) the opportunity to enhance or inhibit tumor development and incidence by treatments either during or after exposure to the carcinogen. For studies of dietary constituents, it is critical that the animals tolerate the test diets. These important features are generally met by the two best characterized models of pancreatic cancer, namely, the Wistar or Lewis rat treated with azaserine to yield adenocarcinomas of primarily acinar cell phenotype (Longnecker, 1987) and the Syrian golden hamster treated with one of several nitrosamines to yield adenocarcinomas of ductlike phenotype (Pour and Wilson, 1980). While most human pancreatic cancers are classified as ductal adenocarcinomas, the total spectrum of histologic types is best matched by a combination of tumor types found in these two animal models. Important features of these two models are discussed briefly.

The predominant features in the rat model of pancreatic cancer are the appearance of atypical acinar cell foci and nodules and the subsequent development of adenocarcinomas possessing acinar cell characteristics (Longnecker, 1987). All evidence indicates that the cancers are of acinar cell origin. Foci of atypical acinar cells are observed as early as 1 month following a single dose of azaserine and these lesions have been shown to increase in number and/or size with time. Carcinomas *in situ* have been observed as early as 4 months and the incidence of rats with adenocarcinomas increases progressively from 12 to 18 months (Roebuck *et al.*, 1987a; Lhoste and Longnecker, 1987). Several studies have shown the utility of quantitatively measuring the number and size of the early putative preneoplastic lesions (foci and nodules) as an index of the ultimate incidence of neoplasms. This quantitative short-term model has been described in detail (Roebuck *et al.*, 1984; Roebuck, 1986a,b, 1987).

N-nitrosobis(2-oxopropyl)amine (BOP) and related nitrosamines induce a wide spectrum of tumors of hamsters, with pancreatic carcinomas being the dominant malignant neoplasm (Pour and Lawson, 1984). The most significant histological characteristic of pancreatic carcinogenesis in the hamster is the ductular morphology of the lesions. Carcinomas require approximately 16 to 21 months to develop, but with high doses they develop as early as 6 to 10 months following first exposure. Though not identified grossly, focal proliferative lesions have been identified histologically within the lobular ductular elements of the pancreas and have been termed pseudoductular hyperplasia or tubular ductal complexes. Intraductal epithelial hyperplasia also occurs. These lesions are commonly regarded as precursors to the carcinomas. BOP induces atypical acinar cell foci or nodules, but these lesions are apparently not precursors of pancreatic ductular carcinomas in the hamster and are less prominent than in the rat model (Birt *et al.*, 1981). Considerable controversy exists regarding the cell of origin of the pancreatic ductal adenocarcinoma in the hamster and in humans. Bell and Ray (1987) argue for a ductal cell origin in support of earlier reports (Moore *et al.*, 1983a,b). But, there is evidence of an acinar cell origin for these tumors of the hamster (Flaks *et al.*, 1982). Resolution of this issue is important for the reasons which will be discussed below.

1.3. Cholecystokinin Hypothesis

Cholecystokinin (CCK) has long been regarded as a major regulatory hormone for the pancreas of the rat (Green and Lyman, 1972) with considerably less known about its action in the hamster pancreas (see below). CCK in conjunction with a number of other hormones and neural stimuli controls pancreatic function in response to the ingestion of food in several species. Acinar cells secrete enzymes by exocytosis of the zymogen granules into the acinar lumen in response to cholinergic vagal nerve stimuli generated during feeding, or in response to specific circulating peptide hormones such as CCK for which the cells have receptors. CCK itself is secreted by cells of the proximal small intestine and secretion is under the control of a feedback loop that responds to an increase in the level of trypsin activity in the intestinal lumen (Green and Lyman, 1972). Recent evidence suggests that a peptide, currently called "monitor peptide," is secreted with the pancreatic juice and serves as a signal for CCK secretion by the intestinal mucosa (Miyasaka *et al.*, 1989). The data suggest that when there is no competing substrate or trypsin inhibitor in the intestinal lumen, the monitor peptide is destroyed by protease activity and CCK secretion decreases. Excess CCK secretion can be induced by the presence of trypsin inhibitor in the diet which presumably protects the monitor peptide from degradation.

2. Response of the Pancreas to Trypsin Inhibitors

The feeding of diets high in trypsin inhibitor content has been associated with hyperplasia of the pancreas in some species. It has been hypothesized and there are data to support the idea that CCK induces hypertrophy and hyperplasia of the acinar tissue of the pancreas as an adaptive response to demands for increased functional capacity of the pancreas. CCK also appears to stimulate the growth of the ductal elements of the pancreas (Morgan, 1987).

2.1. Soybean Products

The effect of trypsin inhibitors on the pancreas was first noted with raw or non-heat-treated soybean products and is, at present, best characterized with these products. Evidence that trypsin inhibitors are indeed the chemical component of major importance in these products is largely circumstantial. It is well known that the feeding of raw soybean products, particularly to chickens (Chernick et al., 1948) and rats (Booth et al., 1960; Melmed et al., 1976; Crass and Morgan, 1981), leads to a rapid and dramatic growth of the pancreas. This is due to both hypertrophy and hyperplasia of the acinar tissue. Research concerning whole soybean flour and its effects on the rat pancreas has been reviewed (McGuinness et al., 1984; Morgan, 1987). In non-carcinogen-treated rats, the long-term feeding to rats of soybean flour (McGuinness et al., 1980) resulted in hyperplastic lesions of the exocrine pancreas including adenomas and adenocarcinomas. The feeding of a diet containing a high content of raw, full-fat soybean flour or the proteinaceous isolate rich in trypsin inhibitor enhanced pancreatic carcinogenesis in rats when fed either concurrent with (Levison et al., 1979; McGuinness et al., 1981; Morgan et al., 1977) or following (Roebuck et al., 1987b) exposure to a known pancreatic carcinogen. These hypertrophic, hyperplastic, and carcinogenic effects on the acinar cells are largely abolished by heat treatment of the soybean flour (McGuinness et al., 1980, Folsch et al., 1974; Roebuck et al., 1987b). These growth stimulatory effects and the pancreatic carcinogenesis usually have been attributed to the proteinaceous trypsin inhibitor content of the soybean products. Evidence that the entire effect is due to the trypsin inhibitor protein activity is indirect and incomplete. Particularly with the soybean flour there is a high content of unsaturated fat which by itself is known to enhance pancreatic carcinogenesis (Roebuck et al., 1987b). A trypsin inhibitor-enriched, protein fraction of soybeans induced a dose-related increase of acinar cell adenomas in rats and the authors attributed the entire enhancement to the trypsin inhibitor content (Gumbmann et al., 1985).

2.2. Camostate (FOY-305)

The effect of CCK on pancreatic carcinogenesis in the rat model has been evaluated further using the synthetic trypsin inhibitor camostate (FOY-305) in

4-month nodule induction studies. Administration of this compound by gavage or in the diet stimulated nodule growth in azaserine-treated rats, presumably by the induction of excessive secretion of endogenous CCK (Lhoste *et al.*, 1988). This experiment was repeated and the results extended by demonstrating that enhanced nodule growth due to camostate could be partially blocked by lorglumide (CR-1409), a potent CCK receptor antagonist. These results strongly support the involvement of CCK (Douglas *et al.*, 1989a).

3. Carcinogenesis and Cholecystokinin

3.1. Rat Pancreas

Several reports provide support for the promoting role of exogenous CCK during pancreatic carcinogenesis in the rat. Repeated subcutaneous injection of exogenous CCK promoted the growth of preneoplastic foci in a 4-month study in the azaserine rat model (Douglas *et al.*, 1989b). The effect of exogenous CCK was blocked by the CCK receptor blocker lorglumide. In a similar study, injection of caerulein, a structural analogue of CCK that also induces pancreatic hyperplasia in rats, has stimulated the growth of azaserine-induced lesions in rats (Lhoste *et al.*, 1988). In the latter experiment, two rats developed carcinomas *in situ* whereas no such lesions were encountered in rats in studies of similar duration using camostate to stimulate the release of endogenous CCK. This observation raises the possibility that camostate has a dichotomous effect on pancreatic carcinogenesis in the rat. Camostate might promote the growth of early preneoplastic lesions by enhancing CCK secretion, and at the same time oppose expression of a malignant phenotype by virtue of its antiprotease activity within the pancreas subsequent to absorption from the intestine (Goke *et al.*, 1984). This intriguing possibility has not been evaluated by giving camostate in a long-term experiment in the rat model, but such a study would be of interest because camostate has been reported to inhibit carcinogenesis in other organs. Inhibition of skin carcinogenesis by feeding camostate was reported in mice (Ohkoshi and Fujii, 1983). In rats, liver carcinogenesis was inhibited by camostate (Yamauchi *et al.*, 1987) and mammary carcinogenesis was inhibited by a closely related compound (Yamamura *et al.*, 1978).

A larger fraction of the pancreas is occupied by foci and nodules in azaserine-treated rats after excess CCK stimulation than in the control groups that are subject only to physiologic cycles of CCK stimulation in association with eating (Douglas *et al.*, 1989b). Therefore, preneoplastic foci are stimulated to grow more than normal pancreas by CCK, indicating that the foci are more responsive to CCK than is the normal rat pancreas in regard to stimulation of growth.

3.2. Other Species Including Humans

Whether CCK can play a promoting role in other species including the human is an emerging issue in pancreatic carcinogenesis. There are marked differences in the response of various species to the presence of protease inhibitors in the diet. Relatively few species have been shown to develop pancreatic hyperplasia in response to dietary trypsin inhibitors such as those in soybeans (Folsch et al., 1974). In response to the feeding of raw soybean flour or soybean protein isolate, pancreatic enlargement is observed in the rat but not in the pig or monkey (Struthers et al., 1983). This suggests either that the duodenal mucosa fails to respond by secreting CCK or that CCK does not stimulate pancreatic growth in some species. Data are not clear with regard to the response of the hamster to soybean products. Some report pancreatic hypertrophy and hyperplasia (Douglas et al., 1989a) and others report no response (Pour et al., 1988). Administration of camostate has failed to induce elevation of plasma CCK in humans (Watanabe et al., 1986; Adler et al., 1986) and it is not known if CCK stimulates growth of the human pancreas. Data regarding the above issues are needed to evaluate the hypothesis that CCK modulates human pancreatic cancer development.

In hamsters treated with N-nitrosobis (2-hydroxypropyl) amine, the incidence of pancreatic carcinomas was similar in groups with or without camostate added to the diet (Egami et al., 1983; Yokoyama et al., 1985). Further studies are required to clarify the effect of CCK and its analogue, caerulein, in the hamster model because there are now discrepant reports in the literature claiming inhibition, promotion, and no effect on carcinogenesis (Johnson et al., 1983; Andren-Sandberg et al., 1984; Howatson and Carter, 1985; Pour et al., 1988; Satake et al., 1986). Thus, the effect of CCK as a promoter of carcinogenesis in acinar cells of the rat model is better established than in ductal cells of the hamster model.

4. Conclusion

Further work in animal models of pancreatic carcinogenesis is warranted because of the potential to examine several important questions regarding the ability of absorbable protease inhibitors to inhibit carcinogenesis in the pancreas and the ability of intraluminal protease inhibitors to promote carcinogenesis in species other than the rat. The trophic activity of CCK for the pancreas, the ability of dietary protease inhibitors to elicit CCK secretion in some species, and the resulting enhancement or promotion of pancreatic carcinogenesis, particularly in the rat, raise concerns regarding the use of protease inhibitors as general anticarcinogens in human populations.

5. References

Adler, G., Mullenhoff, A., Bozkurt, T., Koop, I., Goke, B., Beglinger, C., and Arnold, R., 1986, Pancreatic function and plasma CCK in humans after ingestion of a proteinase inhibitor (FOY-305), *Dig. Dis. Sci.* **31**:1123.

Andren-Sandberg, A., Dawiskiba, S., and Ihse, I., 1984, Studies of the effect of caerulein administration on experimental pancreatic carcinogenesis, *Scand. J. Gastroenterol.* **19**:122–128.

Bell, R. H., and Ray, M. B., 1987, Cytokeratin antigen in BOP-induced pancreatic tumors—Implications for histogenesis, *Carcinogenesis* **8**:1563–1566.

Birt, D. F., Salmasi, S., and Pour, P. M., 1981, Enhancement of experimental pancreatic cancer in Syrian golden hamsters by dietary fat, *J. Natl. Cancer Inst.* **67**:1327–1332.

Booth, A. N., Robbins, D. J., Ribelin, W. E., and Deeds, F., 1960, Effects of raw soybean meal and amino acids on pancreatic hypertrophy in rats, *Proc. Soc. Exp. Biol. Med.* **104**:681–683.

Carroll, K. K., and Khor, H. T., 1975, Dietary fat in relation to tumorigenesis, *Prog. Biochem. Pharmacol.* **10**:308–353.

Chernick, S. S., Lepkovsky, S., and Chaikoff, I. L., 1948, A dietary factor regulating the enzyme content of the pancreas: Changes induced in size and proteolytic activity of the chick pancreas by the ingestion of raw soy-bean meal, *Am. J. Physiol.* **155**:33–41.

Crass, R. A., and Morgan, R. G. H., 1981, Rapid changes in pancreatic DNA, RNA and protein in the rat during pancreatic enlargement and involution, *Int. J. Vitam. Nutr. Res.* **51**:85–91.

Douglas, B. R., Woutersen, R. A., Jansen, J. B. M. J., deJong, A. J. L., Rovati, L. C., and Lamers, C. B. H. W., 1989a, Modulation by CR-1409 (lorglumide), a cholecystokinin receptor antagonist, of trypsin inhibitor-enhanced growth of azaserine-induced putative preneoplastic lesions in rat pancreas, *Cancer Res.* **49**:2438–2441.

Douglas, B. R., Woutersen, R. A., Jansen, J. B. M. J., deJong, A. J. L., Rovati, L. C., and Lamers, C. B. H. W., 1989b, Influence of cholecystokinin antagonist on the effects of cholecystokinin and bombesin on azaserine-induced lesions in rat pancreas, *Gastroenterology* **96**:462–469.

Durbec, J. P., Chevillotte, G., Bidart, J. M., Berthezene, P., and Sarles, H., 1983, Diet, alcohol, tobacco and risk of cancer of the pancreas: A case–control study, *Br. J. Cancer* **47**:463–470.

Egami, T., Takai, A., Taniguchi, Y., Watanabe, A., Yano, M., Sasajima, K., Tanaka, N., Miki, M., Shirota, A., Asano, G., and Takubo, U., 1983, Effect of a protease inhibitor FOY-305 on experimental carcinoma of the pancreas induced by diisopropanol nitrosamine (DIPN), *Jpn. J. Gastroenterol.* **80**:2023–2033.

Flaks, B., Moore, M. A., and Flaks, A., 1982, Ultrastructural analysis of pancreatic carcinogenesis. VI. Early changes in hamster acinar cells induced by N-nitrosobis-(2-hydroxypropyl) amine, *Carcinogenesis* **3**:1063–1070.

Folsch, U. R., Winckler, K., and Wormsley, K. G., 1974, Effect of a soybean diet on enzyme content and ultrastructure of the rat exocrine pancreas, *Digestion* **11**:161–171.

Goke, B., Stockmann, F., Muller, R., Lankisch, P. G., and Creutzfeld, W., 1984, Effect of a specific serine protease inhibitor on the rat pancreas: Systemic administration of camostate and exocrine pancreatic secretion, *Digestion* **30**:171–178.

Gold, E. B., Gordis, L., Diener, M. D., Seltser, R., Boitnott, J. K., Bynum, T. E., and Hutcheon, D. F., 1985, Diet and other risk factors for cancer of the pancreas, *Cancer* **55**:460–467.

Green, G. M., and Lyman, R. L., 1972, Feedback regulation of pancreatic enzyme secretion as a mechanism for trypsin inhibitor-induced hypersecretion in rats, *Proc. Soc. Exp. Biol. Med.* **140**:6–12

Gumbmann, M. R., Spangler, W. L., Dugan, G. M., Rackis, J. J., and Liener, I. E., 1985, The USDA trypsin inhibitor study. IV. The chronic effects of soy flour and soy protein isolate on the pancreas in rats after two years, *Qual. Plant Foods Hum. Nutr.* **35**:275–314.

Howatson, A. G., and Carter, D. C., 1985, Pancreatic carcinogenesis-enhancement by cholecystokinin in the hamster-nitrosamine model, *Br. J. Cancer* **51**:107–114.

Johnson, F. E., LaRegina, M. C., Martin, S. A., and Bashiti, H. M., 1983, Cholecystokinin inhibits pancreatic carcinogenesis, *Cancer Detect. Prevent.* **6**:389–402.

Levison, D. A., Morgan, R. G. H., Brimacombe, J. S., Hopwood, D., Coghill, G., and Wormsley, K. G., 1979, Carcinogenic effects of di(2-hydroxypropyl)nitrosamine (DHPN) in male Wistar rats: Promotion of pancreatic cancer by raw soya flour diet, *Scand. J. Gastroenterol.* **14**:217–224.

Lhoste, E. F., and Longnecker, D. S., 1987, Effect of bombesin and caerulein on early stages of carcinogenesis induced by azaserine in the rat pancreas, *Cancer Res.* **47**:3273–3277.

Lhoste, E. F., Roebuck, B. D., and Longnecker, D. S., 1988, Stimulation of the growth of azaserine-induced nodules in the rat pancreas by dietary camostate (FOY-305), *Carcinogenesis* **9**:901–906.

Longnecker, D. S., 1987, The azaserine-induced model of pancreatic carcinogenesis in rats, in: *Experimental Pancreatic Carcinogenesis* (D. G. Scarpelli, J. K. Reddy, and D. S. Longnecker, eds.), CRC Press, Boca Raton, Fla., pp. 117–130.

McGuinness, E. E., Morgan, R. G. H., Levison, D. A., Frape, D. L., Hopwood, D., and Wormsley, K. G., 1980, The effects of long-term feeding of soya flour on the rat pancreas, *Scand. J. Gastroenterol.* **15**:497–502.

McGuinness, E. E., Morgan, R. G. H., Levison, D. A., Hopwood, D., and Wormsley, K. G., 1981, Interaction of azaserine and raw soya flour on the rat pancreas, *Scand. J. Gastroenterol.* **16**:49–56.

McGuinness, E. E., Morgan, R. G. H., and Wormsley, K. G., 1984, Effects of soybean flour on the pancreas of rats, *Environ. Health Perspect.* **56**:205–212.

Mack, T. M., 1982, Pancreas, in: *Cancer Epidemiology and Prevention* (D. Schottenfeld and J. Fraumeni, eds.), Saunders, Philadelphia, pp. 638–667.

Melmed, R. N., El-Aaser, A. A. A., and Holt, S. J., 1976, Hypertrophy and hyperplasia of the neonatal rat exocrine pancreas induced by orally administered soybean trypsin inhibitor, *Biochim. Biophys. Acta* **421**:280–288.

Mills, P. K., Beeson, W. L., Abbey, D. E., Fraser, G. E., and Phillips, R. L., 1988, Dietary habits and past medical history as related to fatal pancreas cancer risk among Adventists, *Cancer* **61**:2578–2585.

Miyasaka, K., Nakamura, R., Funakoshi, A., and Kitani, K., 1989, Stimulatory effect of monitor peptide and human pancreatic secretory trypsin inhibitor on pancreatic secretion and cholecystokinin release in conscious rats, *Pancreas* **4**:139–144.

Moore, M. A., Takahashi, M., Ito, N., and Bannasch, P., 1983a, Early lesions during pancreatic carcinogenesis induced in Syrian hamsters by DHPN or DOPN. I. Histologic, histochemical, and radioautographic findings, *Carcinogenesis* **4**:431–437.

Moore, M. A., Takahashi, M., Ito, N., and Bannasch, P., 1983b, Early lesions during pancreatic carcinogenesis induced in Syrian hamsters by DHPN or DOPN. II. Ultrastructural findings, *Carcinogenesis* **4**:439–448.

Morgan, R. G. H., 1987, Raw soy flour and pancreatic cancer in experimental animals, in: *Experimental Pancreatic Carcinogenesis* (D. G. Scarpelli, J. K. Reddy, and D. S. Longnecker, eds.), CRC Press, Boca Raton, Fla., pp. 159–174.

Morgan, R. G. H., Levison, D. A., Hopwood, D., Saunders, J. H. B., and Wormsley, K. G., 1977, Potentiation of the action of azaserine on the rat pancreas by raw soya bean flour, *Cancer Lett.* **3**:87–90.

Norell, S. E., Ahlbom, A., Erwald, R., Jacobson, G., Lindberg-Navier, I., Olin, R., Tornberg, B., and Wiechel, K. L., 1986, Diet and pancreatic cancer: A case–control study, *Am. J. Epidemiol.* **124**:894–902.

Ohkoshi, M., and Fujii, F., 1983, Effect of the synthetic protease inhibitor N,N-dimethylcarbamoylmethyl 4-(4-guanidinobenzoyloxy) phenylacetate methanesulfate on carcinogenesis by 3-methylcholantrene in mouse skin, *J. Natl. Cancer Inst.* **71**:1053-1057.

Pour, P. M., and Lawson, T., 1984, Pancreatic carcinogenic nitrosamines in Syrian hamsters, in: *N-Nitroso Compounds: Occurrence, Biological Effects and Relevance to Human Cancer* (I. K. O'Neil, R. C. von Borstel, C. T. Miller, J. Long, H. Bartsch, and C. York, eds.), International Agency for Cancer Research, Lyon, France, pp. 683-688.

Pour, P. M., and Wilson, R., 1980, Experimental tumors of the pancreas, in: *Tumors of the Pancreas* (A. R. Moossa, ed.), Williams & Wilkins, Baltimore, pp. 37-158.

Pour, P. M., Lawson, T., Helgeson, S., Donnelly, T., and Stepan, K., 1988, Effect of cholecystokinin on pancreatic carcinogenesis in the hamster model, *Carcinogenesis* **9**:597-601.

Roebuck, B. D., 1986a, Effects of high levels of dietary fats on the growth of azaserine-induced foci in the rat pancreas, *Lipids* **21**:281-284.

Roebuck, B. D., 1986b, Enhancement of pancreatic carcinogenesis by raw soy protein isolate: Quantitative rat model and nutritional considerations, in: *Nutritional and Toxicological Significance of Enzyme Inhibitors in Foods* (M. Friedman, ed.), Plenum Press, New York, pp. 91-107.

Roebuck, B. D., 1987, Enhancement of pancreatic carcinogenesis in the rat by dietary fats, in: *Experimental Pancreatic Carcinogenesis* (D. G. Scarpelli, J. K. Reddy, and D. S. Longnecker, eds.), CRC Press, Boca Raton, Fla., pp. 187-206.

Roebuck, B. D., Baumgartner, K. J., and Thron, C. D., 1984, Characterization of two populations of pancreatic atypical acinar cell foci induced by azaserine in the rat, *Lab. Invest.* **50**:141-146.

Roebuck, B. D., Baumgartner, K. J., and Longnecker, D. S., 1987a, Growth of pancreatic foci and development of pancreatic cancer with a single dose of azaserine in the rat, *Carcinogenesis* **8**:1831-1835.

Roebuck, B. D., Kaplita, P. V., Edwards, B. R., and Praissman, M., 1987b, Effects of dietary fats and soybean protein on azaserine-induced pancreatic carcinogenesis and plasma cholecystokinin in the rat, *Cancer Res.* **47**:1333-1338.

Satake, K., Mukai, R., Kato, Y., and Umeyama, K., 1986, Effects of cerulein on the normal pancreas and on experimental pancreatic carcinoma in the Syrian golden hamster, *Pancreas* **1**:246-253.

Silverberg, E., and Lubera, J. A., 1989, Cancer statistics, *Ca-A Cancer J. Clin.* **39**:3-20.

Struthers, B. J., MacDonald, J. R., Dahlgren, R. R., and Hopkins, D. T., 1983, Effects on the monkey, pig and rat pancreas of soy products with varying levels of trypsin inhibitor and comparison with the administration of cholecystokinin, *J. Nutr.* **113**:86-97.

Watanabe, S., Shiratori, K., Takeuchi, T., and Chey, W. Y., 1986, Intrajejunal administration of a synthetic trypsin inhibitor (camostate) stimulates the release of endogenous secretin, but not cholecystokinin in humans, *Gastroenterology* **90**:1685.

Wynder, E. L., 1975, An epidemiological evaluation of the causes of cancer of the pancreas, *Cancer Res.* **35**:2228-2233.

Yamamura, M., Nakamura, N., Fukui, Y., Takamura, C., Yamamoto, M., Minato, Y., Tamura, Y., and Fujii, S., 1978, Inhibition of 7,12-dimethylbenz[a]anthracene-induced mammary tumorigenesis in rats by a synthetic protease inhibitor, N,N-dimethylamino-[p-(p'-guanidinobenzoyloxy)] benzilcarbonyloxyglycolate, *Gann* **69**:749-752.

Yamauchi, Y., Kobayashi, M., and Watanabe, A., 1987, Anticarcinogenic effects of a serine protease inhibitor (FOY-305) through the suppression of neutral serine protease activity during chemical hepatocarcinogenesis in rats, *Hiroshima J. Med. Sci.* **36**:81-87.

Yokoyama, Y., Ohyama, K., and Takebe, T., 1985, Effect of a synthetic trypsin inhibitor FOY-305 on di-isopropanol nitrosamine-induced carcinoma of the pancreas in Syrian golden hamsters, *Gendai Iryo* **17**:2331-2335.

Index

The manufacturer's authorised representative in the EU is Springer
Nature Customer Service Centre GmbH, Europaplatz 3, 69115 Heidelberg,
Germany. If you have any concerns regarding our products, please
contact ProductSafety@springernature.com

Printed and bound by CPI Group (UK) Ltd, Croydon, CR0 4YY

23/04/2026

02095625-0006